OH SHE GLOWS
EVERY DAY

ALSO BY ANGELA LIDDON

The Oh She Glows Cookbook

QUICK AND SIMPLY SATISFYING PLANT-BASED RECIPES

OH SHE GLOWS
EVERY DAY

ANGELA LIDDON

MICHAEL JOSEPH

an imprint of

PENGUIN BOOKS

MICHAEL JOSEPH

UK | USA | Canada | Ireland | Australia
India | New Zealand | South Africa

Michael Joseph is part of the Penguin Random House group of companies whose addresses can be found at global.penguinrandomhouse.com.

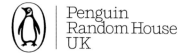

First published in Canada by Penguin Canada Books, Inc, 2016
First published in Great Britain by Michael Joseph 2017

001

Copyright © Glo Bakery Corporation, 2016
Photography, food and prop styling by Ashley McLaughlin
Lifestyle photography © Sandy Nicholson
Photographs on pages 4, 142, 156 and 193 by Angela Liddon
Interior design by Lisa Jager

The moral right of the author has been asserted

Printed in Italy by LEGO S.P.A.

A CIP catalogue record for this book is available from the British Library

ISBN: 978-0-718-18458-2

www.greenpenguin.co.uk

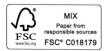

MIX
Paper from
responsible sources
FSC® C018179

Penguin Random House is committed to a
sustainable future for our business, our readers
and our planet. This book is made from Forest
Stewardship Council® certified paper.

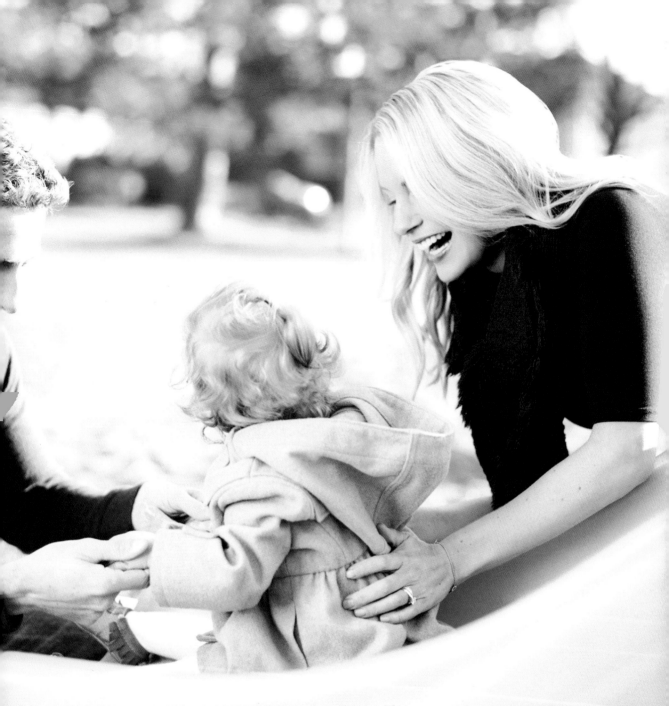

Adriana,

The love I have for you takes my breath away. The immense joy you've brought your dad and me is beyond anything we could have imagined. I also love that you get so excited about the food I make you (well, most of the time!). My dream for you is to never stop chasing the passions that make you feel alive.

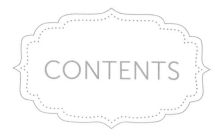

CONTENTS

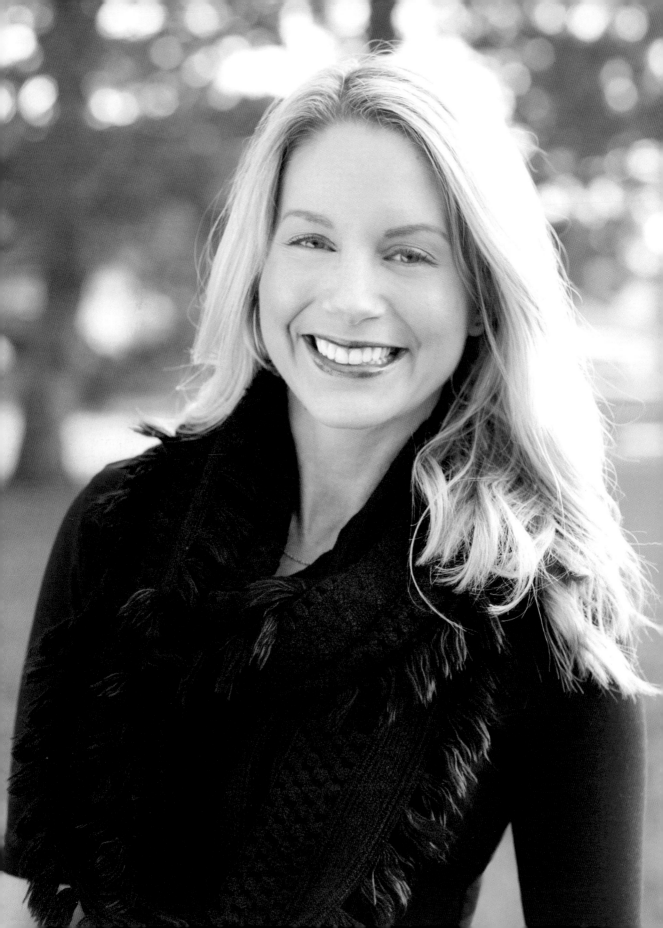

INTRODUCTION

I t's been almost two and a half years since the release of my first cookbook, but it feels like the blink of an eye. When *The Oh She Glows Cookbook* came out in March 2014, I was a few months pregnant with our first baby, and my husband, Eric, and I were going through a move and major house renovation all at once. Miraculously, our marriage survived, but not without the help of a freezer full of vegan cookie dough ice cream! Beyond that, 2014 was easily my most exciting year on record, as it brought the birth of our daughter, Adriana. With these major life experiences also came big changes in me and in our family dynamic. After 2014, I knew that life would never be the same again, and I soon found out that I wouldn't want it to be.

When our daughter was just a few months old, I signed on to write this second cookbook. Some friends and family thought I was overly ambitious (or sleep-deprived and not thinking clearly!) for taking on such a big project with a baby, but I was yearning to awaken my creative side again. During pregnancy, my love for food often dwindled, but the postpartum period was a totally different story. My creativity and passion for food returned quickly after I gave birth, which was a relief for this plant-based-food lover. I had such a ravenous appetite while breastfeeding that I found myself dreaming of recipes around the clock. In fact, some of my favourite recipes in this cookbook were created during middle-of-the-night nursing sessions (Ultimate Flourless Brownies [page 199], anyone?).

Once the creative juices were flowing, there was no stopping me! I discovered that as long as I fuelled myself with healthy food (including a steady supply of green smoothies), my energy levels remained quite high, in spite of the lack of sleep. My friends couldn't understand how I had so much energy, but I'm convinced that a balanced diet can do wonders for energy levels, mood and general well-being. Of course, there were weeks when I ate poorly and didn't feel my best (hello, leftover pie for breakfast!), but those times only reminded me to stay on a healthy path. I was also motivated by the immense encouragement of you, my amazing readers, who let me know loud and clear that you were eagerly awaiting another cookbook. I started to do cookbook work on the sly, adding recipe ideas to my Google document in the middle of the night and testing recipes whenever I had a spare moment. Soon enough this cookbook took shape. Eric and I (and eventually, Adriana) happily ate our way through the recipes, as did our dedicated group of recipe testers.

Many of us know that big life changes tend to decrease the time we have for food preparation. As a new parent, I found myself looking for ways to save time on the preparation and execution of my favourite recipes, without compromising taste and nutrition. I discovered rather quickly that I would go hungry if I didn't have a balanced breakfast waiting for me in the morning, so I relied on breakfasts that could be prepared in advance more than ever, as well as dinner recipes that could be thawed and reheated, or whipped up in about a half-hour and provide ample leftovers for the next day's lunch. Of course, things didn't always go as planned, and on many occasions we had to rely on a bowl of cereal or takeout for dinner. I won't try to tell you that we eat perfect, cooked-from-scratch meals all the time (does anyone?), but devoting a bit of time each day to food preparation and sitting down together to enjoy healthy food is definitely a goal we continually strive for.

Finding a solution that works for my family has taken some trial and error, but now that I have a collection of nutritious, easy-to-prepare meals by my side, it's time to share them, in hopes that you'll be inspired, too. I've perfected the recipes in this book to be sure that, if you have children, they'll love most of these dishes (for more info, see the 'kid-friendly' label, page xii), but really, the recipes in *Oh She Glows Every Day* are great for anyone with a busy, active lifestyle! And they are definitely all omnivore-approved, so have no fear if you are new to plant-based cuisine. I have no doubt that you are going to feel energized, happy and healthy as you cook your way through this book!

Oh She Glows Every Day includes a mix of 'weekday' recipes as well as special occasion, holiday, or 'Sunday dinner' recipes. A weekday menu might feature easy recipes such as 9-Spice Avocado Hummus Toast for breakfast, leftover Golden French Lentil Stew and Endurance Crackers for lunch, and Sun-Dried Tomato Pasta for dinner. An elaborate holiday menu could be a hearty spread featuring my Shepherd's Pie with Cosy Gravy, The Best Shredded Kale Salad, Roasted Brussels Sprouts and Coconut 'Bacon,' and High-Rise Pumpkin Cupcakes with Spiced Buttercream Frosting for dessert. Whether you need something fast or you want to take a bit of time to cook (while enjoying some good wine, perhaps?), I'm confident you'll find what you need within these tasty pages!

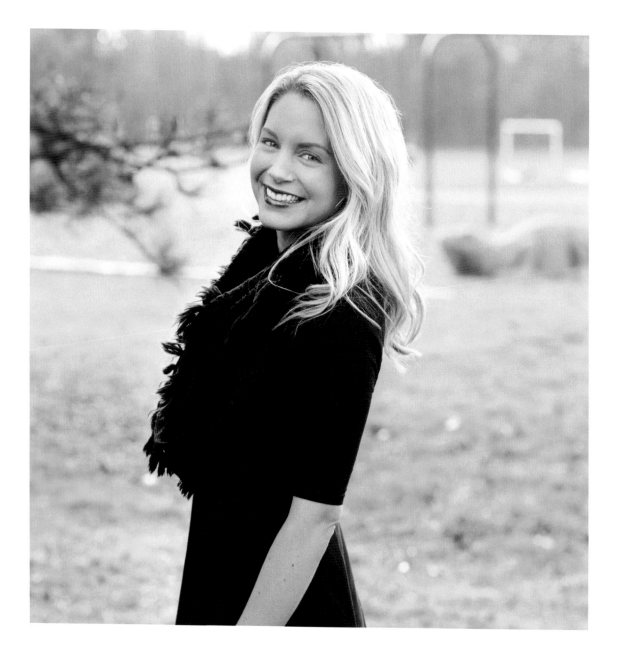

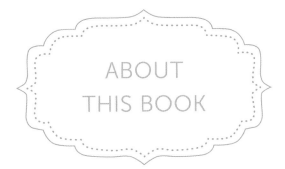

ABOUT THIS BOOK

O*h She Glows Every Day* features more than 100 plant-based, vegan recipes made from whole foods. I created these accessible, foolproof recipes for those of us with busy, active lifestyles. The better I fuel my body, the better I feel and the more energy I have to power through my days, and I want you to feel this way too! If your goal is to nourish yourself—and your family—with delicious meals that'll have you bursting with energy, this book is for you. Throughout the book, you'll find oodles of helpful tips and tricks for getting the most out of each recipe. Keep your eyes peeled for things like kid-friendly or allergy-friendly versions, as well as suggestions on how to freeze and reheat leftovers.

Oh She Glows Every Day is divided into nine different chapters to nourish you throughout the day:

Smoothies and Smoothie Bowls

Breakfast

Snacks

Salads

Sides and Soups

Entrées

Cookies and Bars

Desserts

Homemade Staples

Oh She Glows Every Day also includes my favourite kitchen tools, as well as a handy resource chapter (page 289), The Oh She Glows Pantry, which is packed with useful information detailing the ingredients I use in my every day recipes. Even though the majority of my recipes call for familiar ingredients, this section is great for providing background information, and my favorite tips and preparation methods for each ingredient.

Allergy and Preparation Labels

Near the top of each recipe, you'll find various allergy and preparation labels. The allergy labels help you quickly identify which recipes will fit into your diet. Always be proactive, however, and check the labels of your ingredients to ensure the food is safe for you to consume.

vegan: The recipe does not contain any animal products, such as meat/fish, dairy, honey, etc. All recipes in this book are vegan.

gluten-free: The recipe does not contain any gluten. Be sure to check the ingredient lists of the products you use to ensure that they are certified gluten-free. I've labelled all recipes including oats as gluten-free, but oats processed in facilities that also process other foods can be cross-contaminated, so if you cannot tolerate gluten at all, please be sure to buy certified gluten-free oats.

nut-free: The recipe does not contain any tree nuts, excluding coconut. Health Canada classifies coconut as 'a seed of a fruit' and they do not classify coconut as a tree nut. Health Canada states that '[coconuts] are not usually restricted from the diet of someone allergic to tree nuts,' but of course, some reactions can occur. On the other hand, the US Food and Drug Administration classifies coconut as a tree nut, while the American College of Allergy, Asthma & Immunology classifies it as a fruit, and states that most people who are allergic to tree nuts can safely consume coconut. As you can see, there is some discrepancy over its classification. If you think you might be allergic to coconut, be sure to talk to your allergist before consuming coconut products.

soy-free: The recipe does not contain any soy products. Soy products include things like dark chocolate made with soy lecithin or tamari made from soybeans. Whenever possible I provide soy-free alternatives, such as swapping coconut aminos for tamari.

grain-free: The recipe does not contain any grains or grain flours, such as rice, oats, sorghum, millet, wheat, spelt, quinoa (even though it's technically a seed), etc.

oil-free: The recipe does not contain any added oil.

advance prep required: The recipe requires some advance preparation, such as soaking nuts, chilling a can of coconut milk, freezing a banana, etc. It will also be listed in recipes for which you need to prepare another recipe (like a sauce or a topping) in advance.

kid-friendly: The recipe is wildly popular with children! All the recipes in *Oh She Glows Every Day* were tested by many kids, from one-year-olds to teenagers. Along with the feedback from my testers, and personal experience of feeding my own daughter and young relatives, I narrowed my recipe list to identify more than fifty recipes that were popular with kids. You can be confident that the recipes marked 'kid-friendly' are big hits (such as Mac and Peas, page 177)! Keep in mind that many recipes that do not have the kid-friendly label are still popular with kids. Also, I sometimes include a 'make it kid-friendly' tip at the bottom of a recipe for advice on how to transform a recipe so kids will enjoy it, too. For example, my Golden French Lentil Stew (page 145) is easier for little ones to enjoy if you purée their servings in a blender and serve the soup with my Easiest Garlic Croutons (page 257) cut into strips for dipping.

freezer-friendly: This recipe freezes beautifully! When you see this label you can be confident that you can make extra portions and freeze them for later. Whenever possible, I provide tips on the best method for freezing and how to reheat the recipe.

Before You Begin

I know you might be rolling your eyes here, but it's worth reminding you to read the entire headnote, recipe and tips before beginning a recipe. Some recipes require advance preparation (such as soaking nuts or chilling a can of coconut milk), so it helps to plan ahead whenever possible. I also pride myself on providing as many helpful tips as I can, so be sure to read those, too. Often I'll provide a tip detailing how to modify the recipe to create something new, or how to make a recipe allergy-friendly. You wouldn't want to miss out on that, would you?

Following Recipes and Experimentation

I'm a big advocate for having fun and experimenting with recipes, but I always recommend that the first time you make a recipe, you follow it exactly as it's written, so you know how it's supposed to turn out. If you'd like to experiment after that, you have a 'baseline' to compare it to. Keep in mind that I can't guarantee the recipe will turn out if you deviate from the recipe; I've tested these recipes hundreds of times, as have my testers, and even small changes can drastically change the outcome of a recipe. That said, as an experienced cook, I now find that experimenting with recipes is one of my greatest joys in cooking! Don't be afraid to get creative once you're comfortable.

A Note on Salt

I provide a suggested salt amount (or range) in my recipes rather than simply saying 'Add salt to taste.' My husband likes to remind me that as a beginner cook, he has no idea what a recipe is 'supposed to taste like,' so he's not a fan of recipes that don't provide a little salt guidance! In this cookbook, I'll almost always tell you the amount of salt that I use as a guide, but keep in mind that you can tailor this amount to suit your own tastes. Over time, knowing how much salt to add will become intuitive, if it's not already. When I provide a range, I recommend you add the lesser amount first, taste, and add more salt from there, if you desire. When sautéing vegetables, I always add a generous pinch of salt early on in the cooking process (such as when sautéing garlic and onion as a first step). Salting early on (as opposed to only at the end) has been found to reduce the overall amount of salt you will need in a recipe.

Oven Cooking

As a rule of thumb, I *never* use the oven's convection setting when developing recipes. Convection settings tend to cook foods much faster. For the best outcome, I don't recommend using your oven's convection setting when following recipes in this book. Additionally, it might be helpful to test your oven's true temperature with an oven thermometer.

Measuring Flour

I use the 'scoop and shake' method for measuring flour; in other words, I place the measuring cup into the bag/container of flour, scoop the flour so the flour is slightly heaping over the cup, and then I shake the cup back and forth until the flour is level with the rim of the cup. This isn't the 'traditional' way of measuring flour (spooning the flour into the cup and then leveling it off with a knife), but my method seems faster and feels more natural to me. My 'scoop and shake' method can result in a slightly heavier cup compared to the traditional method, which is why this distinction is worth noting. When I feel a recipe calls for a *very precise* flour measurement, I'll provide you with the various flour weights and recommend that you weigh the flours with kitchen scales.

The Oh She Glows Pantry

The Oh She Glows Pantry (page 289) gives a detailed overview of the ingredients I use most often in my cooking and, consequently, in this cookbook. I recommend reading through this chapter before you start cooking to get some great information and tips about these key ingredients.

Nutritional Information

While I don't focus a great deal on the nutritional information of my recipes (aside from striving for a nice balance of protein, carbs, fat, flavour, etc.), I do realize that many of you appreciate nutritional information, whether it's for a health condition, a weight loss or weight gain goal, or simply because it helps you enjoy a balanced plant-based diet. For this reason, I've provided nutritional information for this cookbook on my website at www.ohsheglows.com/OSG2nutrition. Keep in mind that the nutritional information provided is only an estimate, as nutrition can vary greatly based on the specific brand of food, and there's some variation depending on the nutritional software program used.

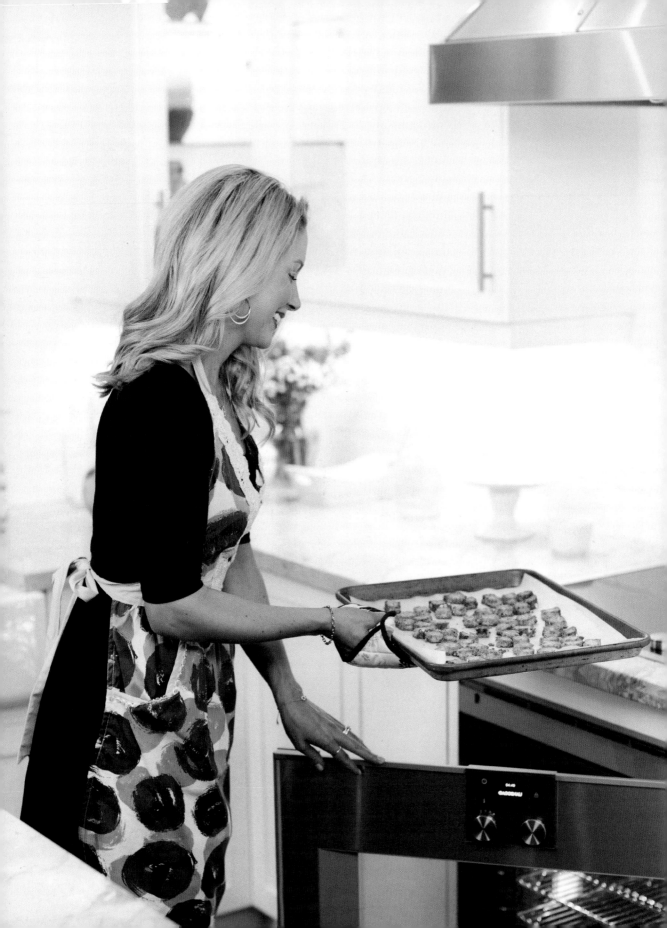

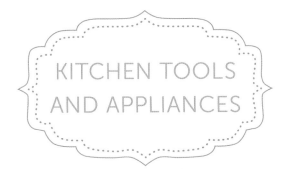

KITCHEN TOOLS AND APPLIANCES

Here is a list of the tools and appliances I use most frequently. As you'll see, some of these are big investments (like a high-speed blender), but many are humble tools that most home cooks have hiding in a kitchen drawer already.

FOOD PROCESSOR

I have a beloved 3.5l Cuisinart food processor, which gets used on average once a day. Sometimes it seems as though I use it for everything: desserts, snack bars, vegetable chopping, nut butters, sauces, hummus, pesto, and more. A model this big isn't necessary—anything that has a 1.75l capacity or higher will serve you well—but a capacity of at least 2.5l may be helpful for many of my recipes. I also own a Cuisinart mini food processor. I don't recommend using mini food processors for anything other than mincing garlic or making salad dressings; most don't have the motor power to grind and mix ingredients efficiently.

HIGH-SPEED BLENDER

If you're just starting out with plant-based recipes, then a regular blender will probably cover your needs. If you get hooked on green smoothies, though, or if you want to blend soaked nuts into silky smooth sauces, then it's really worth investing in a Vitamix 5200. It's pricey, but it creates perfect textures with even the toughest ingredients, and it has a fantastic warranty, so it's built to last. We use our Vitamix a minimum of twice a day (for green smoothies), but often more, especially when I'm recipe testing!

GLASS CANNING JARS

Plastic containers—especially cheap ones—may contain chemical residues that can leach into your food. I use glass for storage whenever possible, and Mason jars are my favourite! I use them for storing nut milks, smoothies, leftovers (such as soups or grain salads) and dry ingredients. I recommend investing in a variety of sizes, from 125ml to 2l.

CHEF'S KNIFE AND PARING KNIFE

A good chef's knife and paring knife are essential for any kitchen—especially kitchens where lots of vegetables get sliced, diced and chopped. Be sure to invest in a knife sharpener, so that you can keep your chef's knife (and your hands) safe. I won't name the family member who I scold each time I visit because his (or her) chef's knife is duller than a butter knife!

MICROPLANE RASP GRATER

Microplane graters are wonderful for zesting citrus, grating ginger or spices (such as whole nutmeg), or grating chocolate directly onto a dessert (my favourite use!). They're inexpensive and versatile, and they handle fine jobs more easily than box graters.

LARGE RIMMED BAKING SHEETS

Rimmed baking sheets are perfect for roasting things like vegetables and chickpeas. They prevent spills as you move the baking sheet into and out of the oven, and they also help keep ingredients from falling to the oven floor and burning. I recommend getting the largest size that will fit in your oven so that you can maximize space. I have an extra-large 38 by 53cm rimmed baking sheet that gets tons of use!

ENAMELLED DUTCH OVEN

Enamelled Dutch ovens are not cheap, but they are invaluable for creating soups and stews, and for roasting and braising. The cast iron distributes heat evenly, while the lid keeps heat trapped within the oven as you cook. They last for ever, so you may be able to find one at a local garage sale. If not, the Le Creuset and Staub brands can't be beaten. I also have a large enamelled Dutch oven from Costco (Kirkland brand) that (over the years) has proven to be durable and high quality.

ELECTRIC HAND MIXER OR STAND MIXER

If you do a lot of baking or home-made bread making, then a stand mixer is a worthwhile investment. It will allow you to create perfect cookies and cakes, knead bread, whip up some of my Coconut Whipped Cream (page 275), and more. That said, I use an inexpensive, handheld electric mixer most of the time for convenience and easy cleaning, and all the recipes in this book will work just fine with either type of mixer.

CAST-IRON SKILLET

I think that a 10- or 12-inch (25 or 30cm) cast-iron skillet is essential for perfectly charred tofu cubes, as well as for grilling on the hob and occasional baking. It's sturdier than a regular frying pan, and it distributes heat more evenly. As an added bonus, trace amounts of the iron in the pan will be released into food as you cook, which will help you meet your iron requirements! Be sure to check the manufacturer's instructions for seasoning and re-seasoning the pan.

MINI FOOD PROCESSOR

While I don't use mini food processors for heavy-duty jobs like hummus or nut butter, I think they're very useful for quickly mincing garlic or making quick sauces. The Cuisinart brand is always reliable.

JULIENNE PEELER OR VEGETABLE SPIRAL SLICER

Julienne peelers and vegetable spiral slicers (or 'spiralizers') will allow you to create fun, ribbon- and spaghetti-shaped strands of fresh vegetables, including courgettes, carrots, beets, sweet potatoes and more. I use a Kuhn Rikon julienne peeler and a World Cuisine vegetable spiralizer for quick-and-easy veggie 'pasta' dishes.

PASTRY ROLLER

A pastry roller is a small rolling pin with a short handle. I use it to make snack bars (such as my Mocha Empower Glo Bars, page 69) or to roll out small amounts of dough for some desserts.

SPRING-RELEASE COOKIE SCOOP

A spring-release cookie scoop is my go-to for scooping even portions of batter into muffin tins and creating consistently sized cookies. I typically use a 2-tablespoon (30ml) stainless-steel scoop, but many sizes are available.

STAINLESS-STEEL WHISK

My trusty OXO 23cm stainless-steel whisk is one of my most frequently used kitchen tools. I'm a bit obsessed with it! I love using it to create super-smooth gravies, matcha teas, sauces and dressings, and also to whisk together dry ingredients when I bake.

NUT MILK BAG

I love creating creamy, homemade nut milks from scratch. A nut milk bag makes it easy to strain home-made nut milk, creating a perfectly silky texture, and it'll leave you with almond (or other nut) pulp that you can repurpose in other ways.

FINE-MESH STAINLESS-STEEL SIEVE

I recommend rinsing grains like quinoa and millet before cooking, and a fine-mesh sieve will do the job easily. I also use it to sift cocoa powder or confectioner's sugar, when necessary.

CITRUS JUICER

I'm pretty obsessed with my OXO double-sided citrus juicer. It's a small, non-electric device that collects all the juice in a container while keeping out most of the pulp and seeds. I've had it for years, it's dishwasher-friendly, and I find it also extracts much more juice compared to simply squeezing citrus by hand. It always helps to get every last drop!

KITCHEN SCALES

Kitchen scales will only set you back a few pounds, but they're worth their weight in gold. I use mine frequently for measuring ingredients whenever a recipe requires precision.

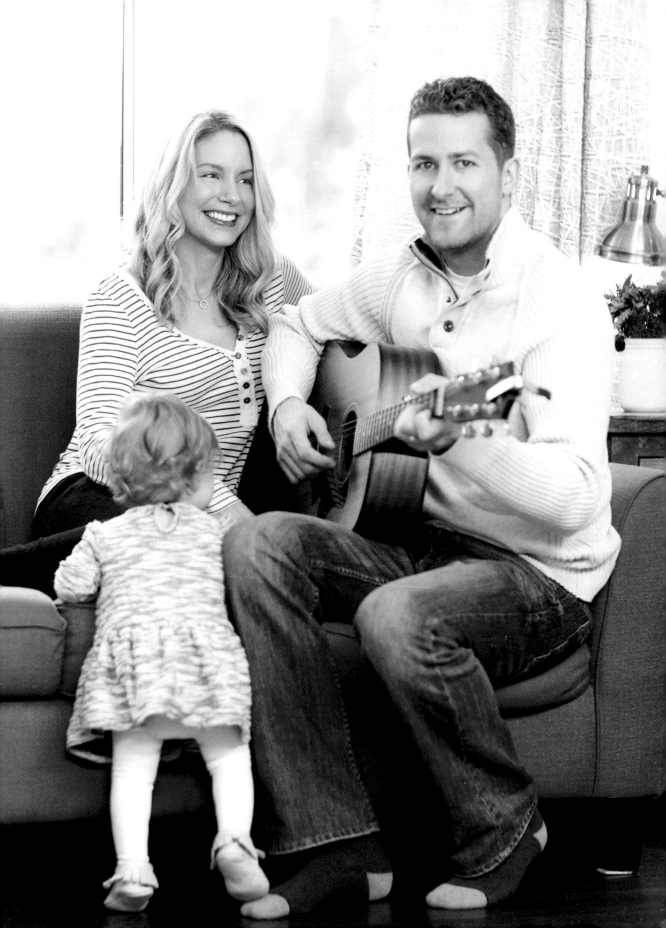

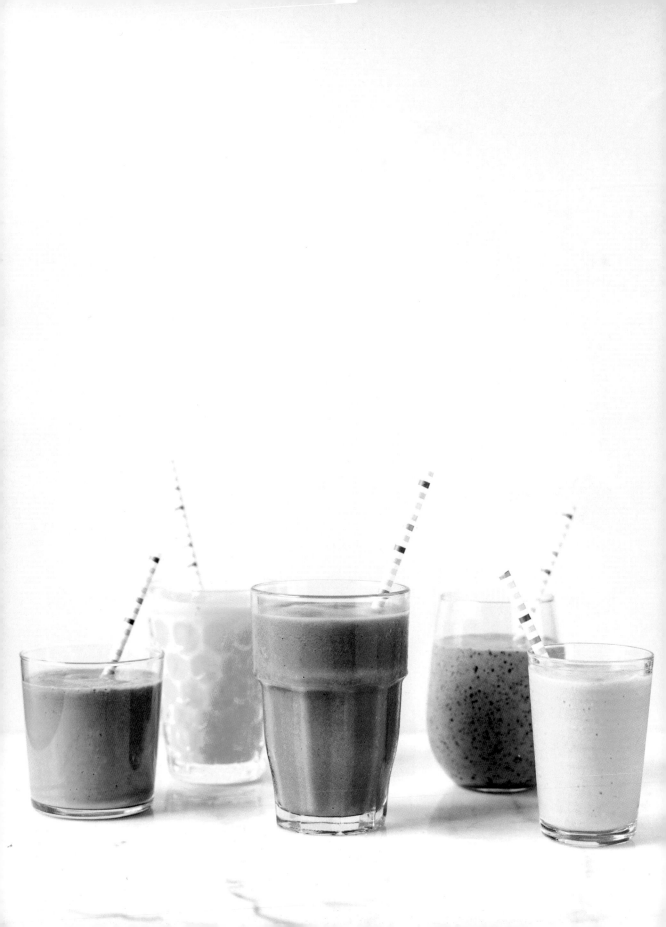

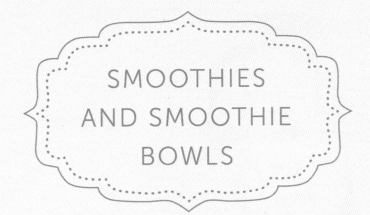

SMOOTHIES AND SMOOTHIE BOWLS

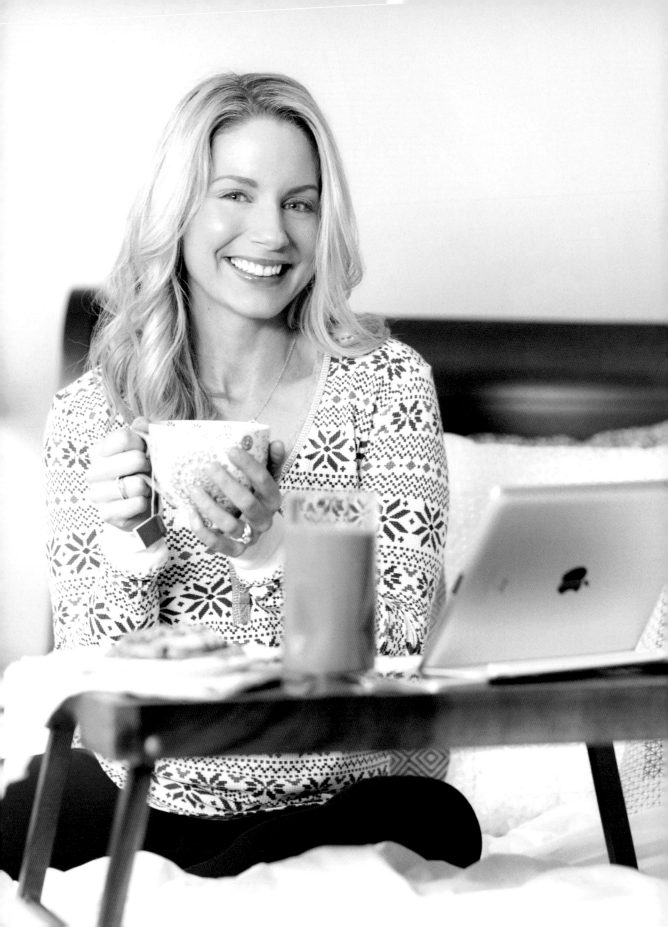

I WASN'T ALWAYS a smoothie aficionado. I know it's probably hard for you to believe, but there was once a time when my smoothie-making game was so bad, I had to choke down each concoction. Lumpy, gritty, swamp water-hued smoothies. Yummy? Would you also believe that I still drank each one because I couldn't justify pouring once beautiful vegetables down the drain? It's true. But as they say, practice makes perfect. After endless testing over the years, my smoothie game is stronger than ever. Even my husband jumped on board the green smoothie train, and it wasn't long before Adriana was asking for her own blends.

I love to throw together a family-size Reset Button Green Smoothie and share it among the three of us. Large-batch smoothies are always a great time saver, and if I'm thinking in advance, I will sometimes gather the ingredients the night before so it's even faster in the morning. When I have just a few minutes, The Satiety Smoothie comes together in a flash, with ingredients I almost always have on hand, and it's packed with more than 20 grams of protein. I created it when I was nursing because I needed something that would tame my intense hunger; I'd often devour a big bowl of overnight oats when I woke up and then I'd make this smoothie shortly after.

Smoothie bowls are a fun change if you want to enjoy the cool creaminess of a smoothie while also treating yourself to a sit-down meal (which, if you are anything like me, feels like a total luxury in the morning!). As an added bonus, you can pack in even more protein and nutrients by loading on different toppings. You must try my Magical 'Ice Cream' Smoothie Bowl; it's one of my most popular smoothie recipes (smoothie ice cream, anyone?), loved by kids and adults alike! I make it at least once a week in the summer, along with my Green Tea Lime Pie Smoothie Bowl. If you are in the mood for something decadent-tasting but still nutritious, try my Chocolate Dreams Protein Smoothie Bowl as a fun morning breakfast, or the Salted Chocolate Hemp Shake for Two is a splurge-worthy afternoon pick-me-up and hot summer evening treat.

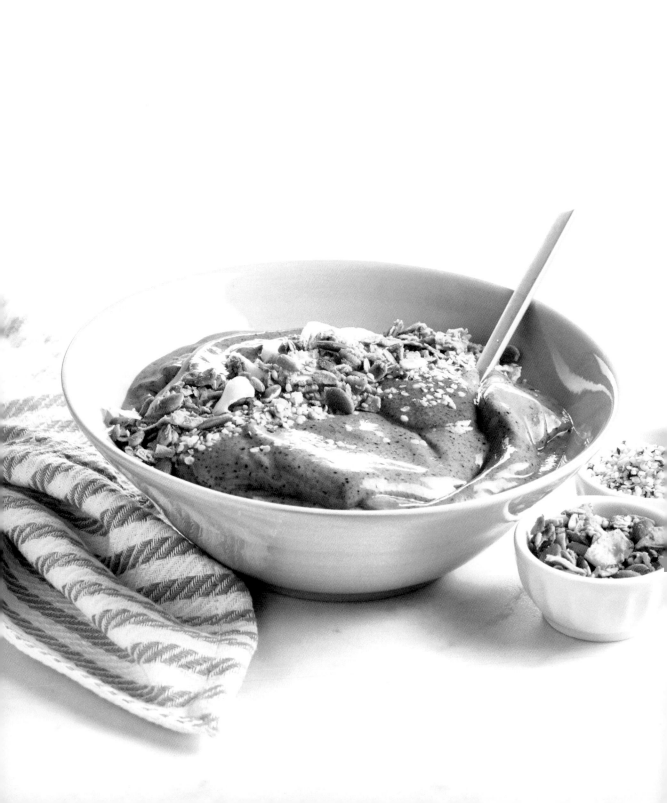

Magical 'Ice Cream' Smoothie Bowl

VEGAN, GLUTEN-FREE, SOYA-FREE, GRAIN-FREE, OIL-FREE,
KID-FRIENDLY OPTION

MAKES 2 BOWLS

PREP TIME: **10 MINUTES**

I originally created this smoothie bowl as a single-serving recipe, but my friends and family went so crazy for it that I expanded the portion to serve two people. When a smoothie bowl is this good, it needs to be shared! Frozen banana, blueberries and avocado create a super-thick texture, which makes the smoothie feel rich and decadent in spite of how healthy it is. Roasted almond butter adds additional creaminess, nuttiness and depth of flavour. My friend's three-year-old calls this 'breakfast ice cream', and I'd have to agree! I think it's essential to serve smoothie bowls with a generous amount of toppings, and I always recommend adding a crunchy topping, such as my Vanilla Super-Seed Granola with Coconut Chips (page 33), for textural contrast. Of course, you can also serve this smoothie in a glass if you are short of time (thin it with additional almond milk as needed). I like the mild sweetness of this bowl, but you can add a touch of liquid sweetener or a pitted date, if desired.

1. In a high-speed blender, combine all the smoothie ingredients and blend on high until smooth. If your blender is having trouble blending, add more almond milk, a tablespoon at a time, and blend again until the desired consistency is reached. Keep in mind that the smoothie should be very thick so the toppings can 'float' on top. If you have a Vitamix, use the tamper to get things moving while blending.

2. Pour the smoothie into a bowl. Add your desired toppings and serve immediately.

Make it kid-friendly Serve a kid-size portion in a parfait glass with sliced bananas. It makes a fun and healthy snack!

FOR THE SMOOTHIE

280ml unsweetened almond milk

80g frozen blueberries

2 large frozen bananas, roughly chopped

55g avocado

2 tablespoons roasted almond butter

1 teaspoon pure vanilla extract

Pinch of fine sea salt (omit if using salted almond butter)

$1/8$ to $1/4$ teaspoon ground cinnamon, to taste (optional)

2 ice cubes, or as needed

TOPPING SUGGESTIONS

Sliced banana

Hemp hearts

Roasted almond butter

Shredded or large-flake coconut, or Maple Cinnamon Coconut Chips (page 283)

Vanilla Super-Seed Granola with Coconut Chips (page 33)

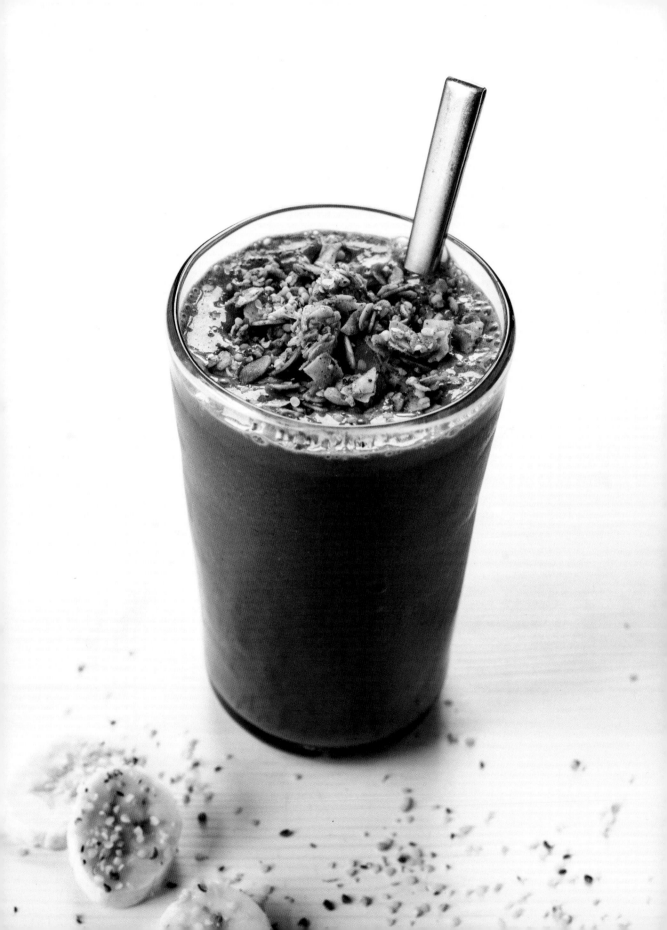

Salted Chocolate Hemp Shake for Two

VEGAN, GLUTEN-FREE, NUT-FREE OPTION, SOYA-FREE, GRAIN-FREE,
OIL-FREE, KID-FRIENDLY OPTION

MAKES 1L

PREP TIME: **5 MINUTES**

Cool down and bliss out with this creamy chocolate hemp smoothie. You'll be amazed at how a pinch of sea salt brings out the rich, complex chocolate flavour. In spite of the fact that it tastes like a milk shake, the smoothie is actually incredibly nutritious! Hemp hearts provide both protein and omega-3 fatty acids, while cocoa powder adds a concentrated dose of antioxidants. I love the addition of coconut butter, which has a rich, buttery taste and luxurious texture. If your blender has a hard time blending dates, I recommend using the maple syrup option instead, or you can soak the pitted dates in boiling water for twenty to thirty minutes before you begin.

1. In a high-speed blender, combine all the ingredients and blend on high until super-smooth.

Tip Coconut butter can be difficult to locate, so feel free to substitute peanut or almond butter in this recipe (or simply make coconut butter at home—see page 281).

Make it nut-free Swap the almond milk for 1 400ml can light coconut milk (chilled) and use coconut butter in lieu of the nut butter.

Make it kid-friendly Reduce or omit the salt.

425ml unsweetened almond milk

1 large frozen banana, roughly chopped

3 or 4 large pitted Medjool dates, to taste, or 2 tablespoons pure maple syrup

3 tablespoons unsweetened cocoa powder

3 tablespoons hemp hearts

1 tablespoon coconut butter or nut butter

$1/4$ teaspoon ground cinnamon (optional)

$1/8$ to $1/4$ teaspoon fine sea salt, to taste

4 ice cubes

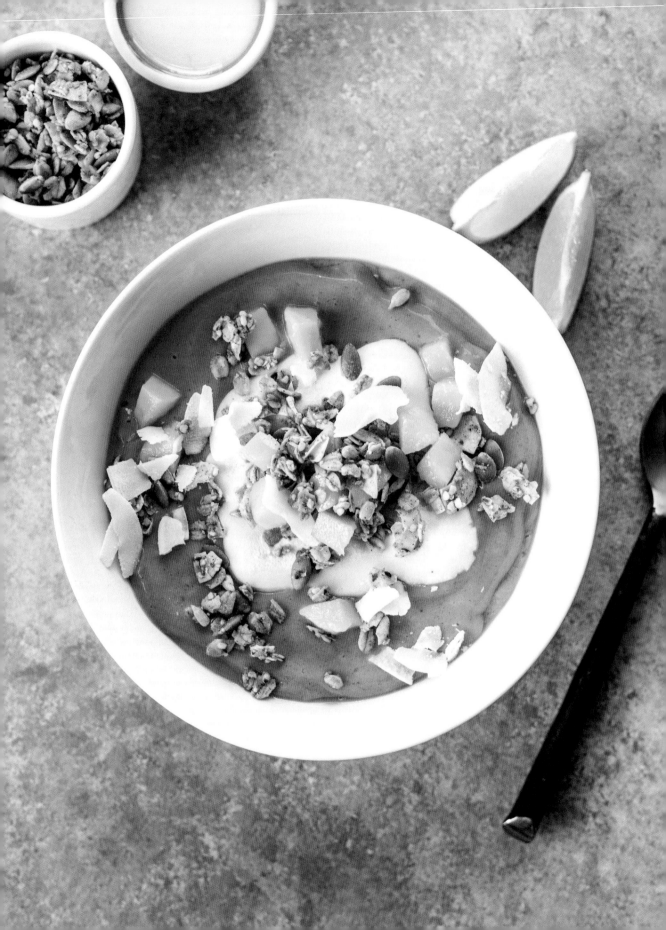

Green Tea Lime Pie Smoothie Bowl

VEGAN, GLUTEN-FREE, NUT-FREE, SOYA-FREE, GRAIN-FREE, OIL-FREE, KID-FRIENDLY OPTION

MAKES 1 BOWL (500ML)

PREP TIME: **10 MINUTES**

This smoothie offers the tropical flavours of lime, coconut, banana and avocado in a rich, exotic blend that's enhanced with the nutritional benefits of fresh greens and matcha green tea powder. If you've never tried matcha in a smoothie before, prepare yourself for an energizing kick! Matcha is a natural source of caffeine, and it's rich in disease-fighting antioxidants. On its own, it has a slightly bitter, toasted flavour, but you won't detect so much as a hint of bitterness when you blend the powder into a sweet, refreshing smoothie bowl. I happen to think that this smoothie tastes like key lime pie: creamy, tart, tropical and sweet all at once. Ahh, now this is living!

1. In a high-speed blender, combine all the smoothie ingredients and blend on high until smooth. Taste and adjust the sweetness, if desired.

2. Pour into a bowl and add the toppings of your choice. Enjoy with a spoon!

Make it kid-friendly Omit the matcha powder and reduce the quantity of lime juice.

FOR THE SMOOTHIE

125ml coconut water

225g fresh baby spinach

1 large frozen banana, chopped

55g avocado

2 teaspoons lime zest (from 1 large lime)

1 tablespoon plus 1 teaspoon fresh lime juice (from 1 large lime)

2 or 3 ice cubes, as needed

2 teaspoons pure maple syrup, or to taste

1/2 teaspoon matcha green tea powder, or to taste

TOPPING SUGGESTIONS

Vanilla Super-Seed Granola with Coconut Chips (page 33)

Fresh sliced mango, pineapple, and/or banana

Melted coconut butter

Large-flake coconut or Maple Cinnamon Coconut Chips (page 283)

Hemp hearts

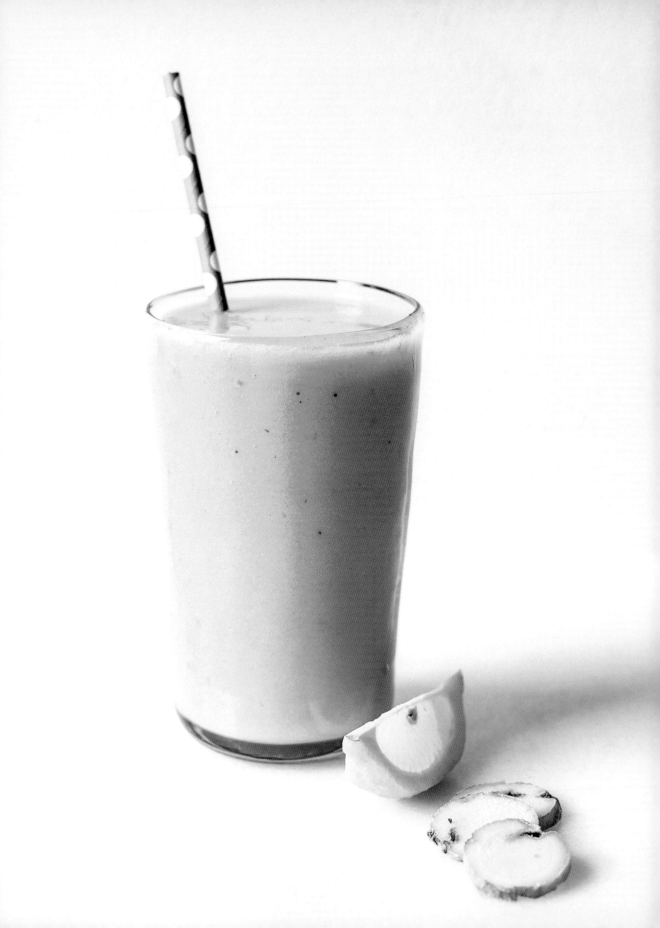

Morning Detox Smoothie

VEGAN, GLUTEN-FREE, NUT-FREE, SOYA-FREE, GRAIN-FREE, OIL-FREE,
ADVANCE PREP REQUIRED, KID-FRIENDLY OPTION

MAKES 500ML

CHILL TIME: **A FEW HOURS (FOR THE TEA)**

PREP TIME: **10 MINUTES**

We usually associate bright green smoothies with detoxing and cleansing. This sunny yellow blend looks nothing like your typical green detox smoothie, but I promise you that it packs a healthful punch! It's invigorating and sweet, and the addition of white tea means that it also provides some natural energy in the form of caffeine without any unpleasant jitters. Preparing the tea in advance does take a bit of forethought, but the wonderful sweet and zesty flavors in this drink make chilling a cup of white tea in the fridge overnight well worth the effort. In some cultures, lemon is thought to help aid the liver in its natural detoxification processes, while ginger can help to soothe and assist digestion. Cayenne pepper is rich in capsaicin, which has anti-inflammatory and pain-fighting properties, and it adds a pleasant heat to the smoothie. That said, if you prefer something milder, feel free to leave out the cayenne.

1. Put the tea bag in a mug and pour the boiling water over the top. Place the mug in the fridge (with the tea bag left in) and chill for several hours, or overnight. Remove and discard the tea bag and pour the chilled tea into a high-speed blender.

2. Add the remaining ingredients and blend until smooth.

Tip 1. If you swap the fresh mango for 250ml frozen mango chunks, I recommend using a non-frozen banana to avoid an icy consistency.
2. If you are a fan of ginger and lemon, feel free to add more to taste (or conversely, reduce the amount if you're not a fan).

Make it kid-friendly Swap the tea for coconut water or water. Omit the ginger and cayenne pepper for a less spicy flavor.

1 white tea bag

250ml boiling water

1 large fresh mango, pitted and flesh scooped out, or 250ml frozen mango chunks

1 large frozen banana, roughly chopped

1 tablespoon fresh lemon juice

1 teaspoon grated fresh ginger

Tiny dash of cayenne pepper (optional)

Ice cubes (optional)

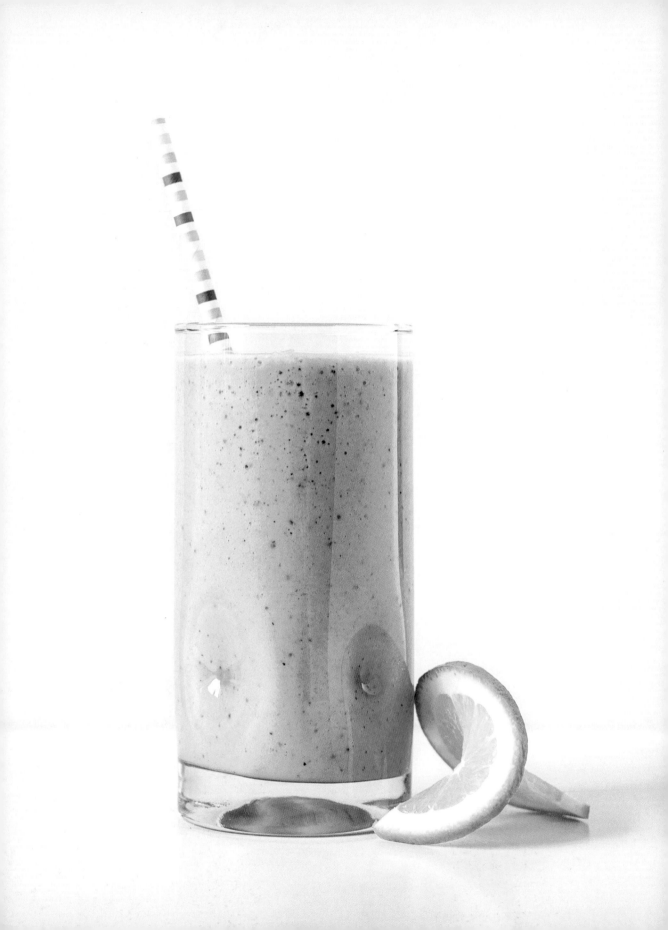

Green-Orange Smoothie

VEGAN, GLUTEN-FREE, NUT-FREE, SOYA-FREE, GRAIN-FREE, OIL-FREE, KID-FRIENDLY

MAKES 1L (2 SERVINGS)

PREP TIME: 5 MINUTES

I used to be obsessed with orange Creamsicles as a child. Those creamy vanilla centers and icy orange shells just stole my heart. After looking at the ingredient list on a box of Creamsicles and seeing that it was full of additives, I decided to combine the delicious flavours of vanilla and orange in this creamy, ice-cold smoothie. Coconut milk creates plenty of creamy texture and taste without a hint of dairy, while spinach and avocado add nutrient power. This drink is great for hot summer days or any time you need a little sunshine in your life. It's also a perfect 'starter' green smoothie for kids, who will fall in love with its sweet flavour!

1. In a high-speed blender, combine all the ingredients and blend on high until smooth. Taste and adjust the sweetness, if desired.

Tip If your dates are on the dry side, I recommend soaking them in boiling water for 20 to 30 minutes before making this smoothie.

1 400ml can light coconut milk, chilled

300ml fresh or prepared orange juice

225g baby spinach

2 tablespoons avocado

½ teaspoon pure vanilla extract

4 or 5 large pitted Medjool dates, to taste

6 ice cubes, or as needed

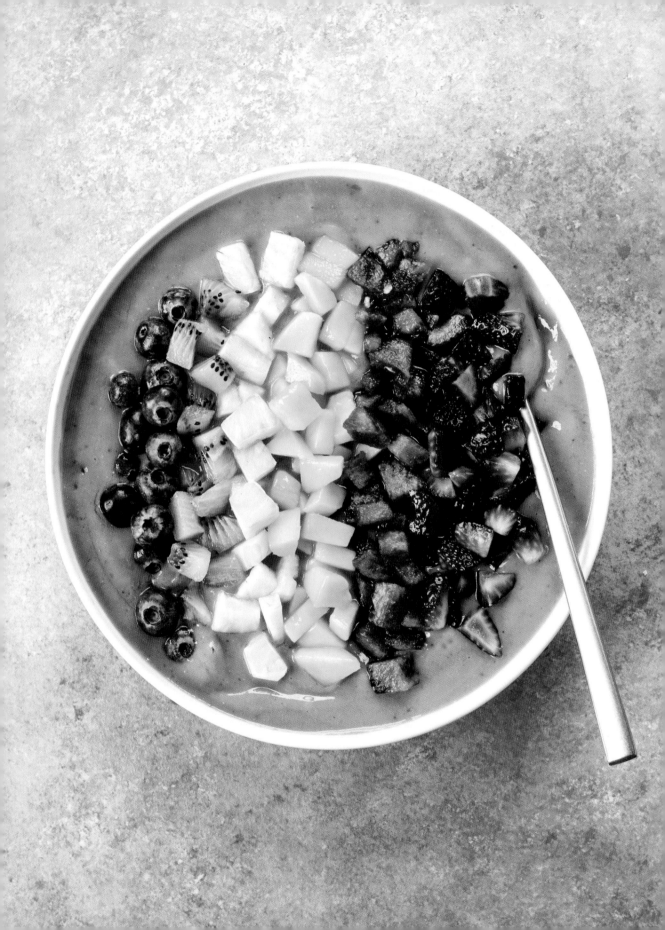

Glowing Rainbow Smoothie Bowl

VEGAN, GLUTEN-FREE, NUT-FREE, SOYA-FREE, GRAIN-FREE, OIL-FREE, ADVANCE PREP REQUIRED, KID-FRIENDLY

MAKES 1 BOWL (500ML)

PREP TIME: 5 TO 10 MINUTES

This is a lovely, refreshing summer snack for a really hot day, when all you can face eating is fruit. Kids love this smoothie bowl, and you can get them involved in its preparation by asking them to help choose and add toppings! This recipe makes one bowl, but you can easily double it if you want to make a larger portion. Be sure to freeze the watermelon and strawberries (or simply use frozen strawberries) overnight or for several hours before using them. This will give the smoothie bowl a very cold and creamy texture.

1. Freeze 150g of the watermelon (and the hulled strawberries, if using fresh) overnight, or for several hours.

2. In a high-speed blender, blend the remaining 190g fresh watermelon on low-medium speed until watery.

3. Add the frozen watermelon, frozen strawberries and avocado. Blend until smooth. If you have a Vitamix, I recommend using the tamper to help it blend.

4. Taste and add the maple syrup, if desired. Blend again until smooth.

5. Pour the smoothie into a shallow bowl. If desired, add the toppings in the pattern of a rainbow, as shown in the picture. If you have kids, I've discovered they love helping with this step. Enjoy immediately before it melts!

FOR THE SMOOTHIE

340g diced watermelon

200g hulled fresh or frozen strawberries

56g avocado

1 to 2 teaspoons pure maple syrup, or 1 or 2 pitted Medjool dates, to taste (optional)

TOPPING SUGGESTIONS

Blueberries

Diced kiwi or grapes

Diced pineapple

Diced mango

Diced watermelon

Diced strawberries

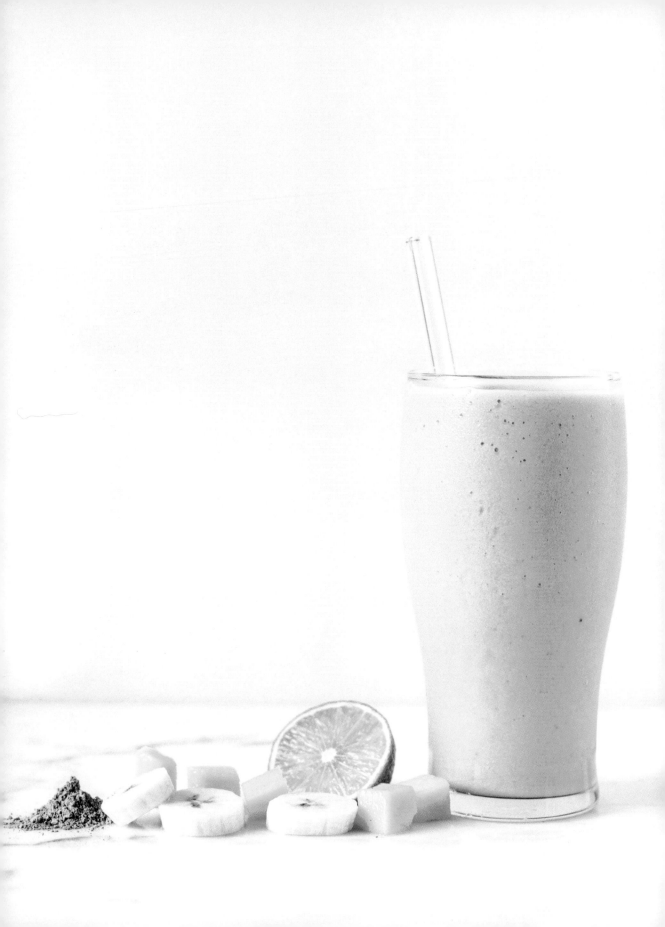

Green Matcha Mango Ginger Smoothie

VEGAN, GLUTEN-FREE, NUT-FREE OPTION, SOYA-FREE, GRAIN-FREE, OIL-FREE

PREP TIME: **10 MINUTES**

MAKES 750ML (2 SERVINGS)

Matcha powder is the perfect pick-me-up for busy mornings. It provides natural caffeine along with polyphenols, plant compounds that have been shown to help prevent numerous diseases. One of the compounds in matcha might even help boost metabolism. Well, sign me up! I highly recommend using in-season Ataulfo mangoes in this smoothie, if you can get your hands on some. They're smaller and more tender than the large, oval-shaped mangoes. They are also exceptionally sweet and have a buttery texture, which is so perfect in this smoothie. If you can't find them or they aren't in season, Tommy Atkins mangoes (which are more common in North America) can be very sweet and soft when they're ripe, too. Otherwise, feel free to use 400g of any chopped fresh or frozen mango. If your mango isn't very sweet, you might wish to add a teaspoon or two of liquid sweetener to the blend.

1. In a high-speed blender, combine all the ingredients and blend on high until smooth. Serve and enjoy!

Tip 1. Some grocery stores carry single-serving packets of matcha. This smoothie uses one single-serving packet (about ¾ teaspoon), but it's best to measure just to be sure. 2. For extra green power, feel free to add a handful of baby spinach to the mix.

Make it nut-free Use coconut milk instead of almond milk.

250ml unsweetened almond milk or coconut milk

2 ripe medium Ataulfo mangoes, pitted and flesh scooped out (400g chopped)

1 medium frozen banana, roughly chopped

¾ teaspoon matcha powder, or to taste (see Tip)

1 teaspoon grated fresh ginger

1 to 2 teaspoons fresh lime juice, to taste

2 or 3 ice cubes

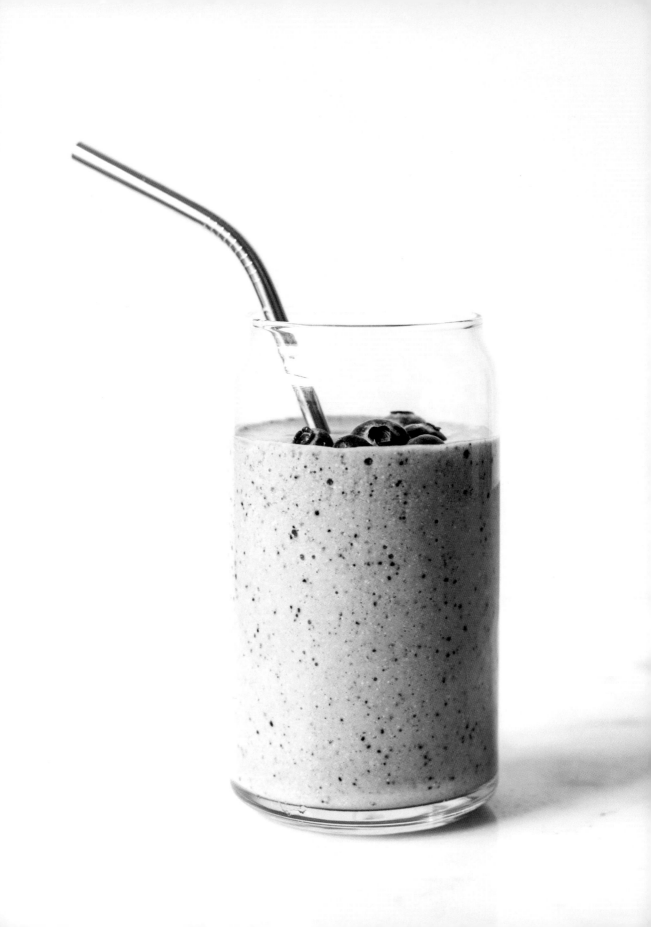

The Satiety Smoothie

VEGAN, GLUTEN-FREE, NUT-FREE OPTION, SOYA-FREE, GRAIN-FREE, OIL-FREE, KID-FRIENDLY OPTION

MAKES 625ML (1 SERVING)

PREP TIME: 5 MINUTES

This stick-to-your-ribs smoothie is packed with more than 20 grams of protein (depending on the type of protein powder you use) as well as all kinds of healthy fats thanks to the hemp hearts, coconut butter and avocado. You'd be hard pressed to find a healthier or more nutrient-dense smoothie without superfood powders. I recommend using a high-speed blender for this smoothie, as some blenders have a difficult time blending the hemp hearts. Be sure to use a neutral-tasting protein powder so it doesn't overwhelm the natural (and delightful) tastes of banana, blueberries and cinnamon. I use Omega Nutrition Pumpkin Seed Protein Powder or Sunwarrior Warrior Blend protein powder in natural/unflavoured.

1. In a high-speed blender, combine all the ingredients and blend until smooth. Add more water or ice cubes as needed to achieve the desired consistency.

Make it nut-free Use coconut milk instead of almond milk.

Make it kid-friendly Omit the protein powder for the child's serving. You can simply pour his/her smoothie and then add the protein powder to the blender, blend again, and pour into your own glass.

250ml unsweetened almond milk

60ml water or coconut water, plus more as needed

2 tablespoons avocado

3 to 4 tablespoons unflavoured or vanilla protein powder

2 tablespoons plus 1½ teaspoons hemp hearts

½ teaspoon ground cinnamon

1 large frozen banana, roughly chopped

40g frozen blueberries

1 tablespoon Homemade Coconut Butter (page 281; optional)

1 teaspoon pure maple syrup (optional)

1 or 2 ice cubes (optional)

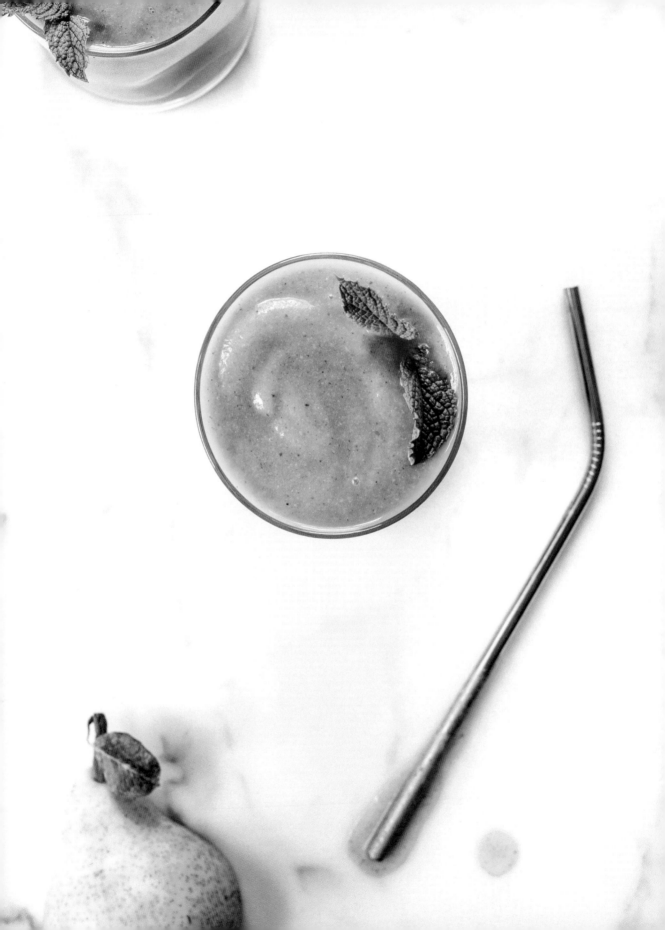

Pear Vanilla Mint Green Smoothie

VEGAN, GLUTEN-FREE, NUT-FREE, SOYA-FREE, GRAIN-FREE, OIL-FREE, KID-FRIENDLY

MAKES 1L (2 SERVINGS)

PREP TIME: **10 MINUTES**

A blend of sweet pear, fragrant vanilla and refreshing mint, this smoothie is energizing and restorative at the same time. It's an ideal choice as a pre- or post-workout snack because the electrolytes in the coconut water and the vitamin E in the fresh avocado are great for rehydration. Vitamin E also has anti-inflammatory and immunity-boosting effects—both of which can help the body recover and repair after exercise. Fresh mint is beneficial for the digestion, while baby spinach offers iron, folate, and a slew of antioxidants. These nutrition benefits, coupled with the smoothie's mildly sweet taste, make it one of my very favourites. I love juicy and sweet Bartlett pears, but you can use any variety of pear you like.

1. In a high-speed blender, combine all the ingredients and blend on high until smooth. Taste and adjust the sweetness, if desired. Serve and enjoy!

Tip You can skip the ice and use frozen chopped pears instead. You might need to increase the amount of coconut water a bit since it'll be quite thick.

300ml coconut water

2 ripe pears, cored and chopped (about 450g)

2 tablespoons avocado

225g baby spinach

10g fresh mint leaves

½ to 1 teaspoon pure vanilla extract, to taste

1 to 2 teaspoons pure maple syrup, to taste (optional)

5 to 7 ice cubes, as needed

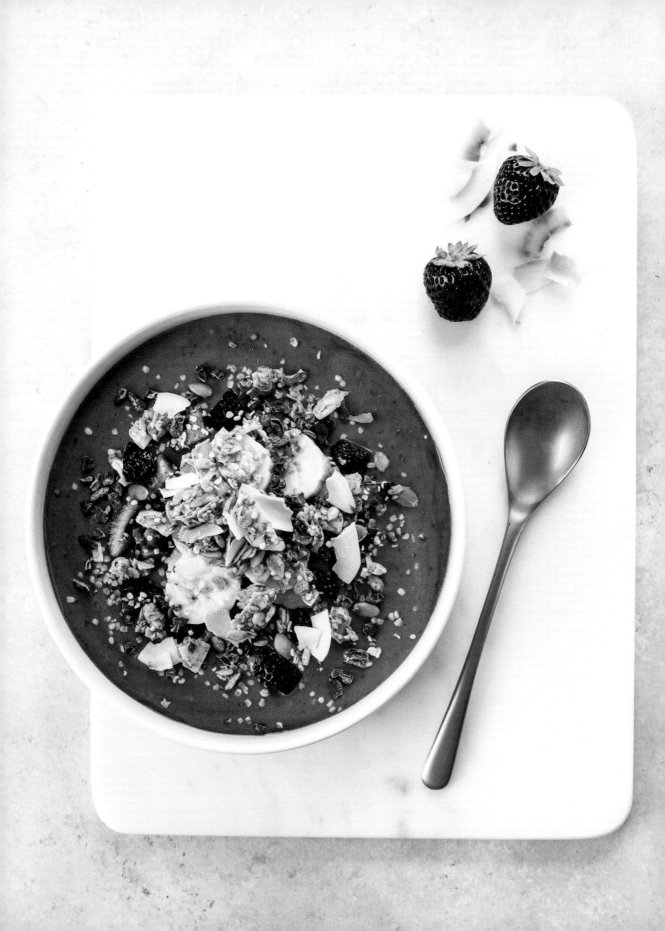

Chocolate Dreams Protein Smoothie Bowl

VEGAN, GLUTEN-FREE, NUT-FREE OPTION, SOYA-FREE, GRAIN-FREE,
OIL-FREE

MAKES 375ML (1 SERVING)

PREP TIME: **5 TO 10 MINUTES**

This smoothie bowl is the perfect fix for those mornings when you wake up dreaming of chocolate! (Or am I the only one who does that?) The light, almost fluffy texture will remind you of chocolate soft-serve ice cream, and it's garnished with an array of fun toppings like strawberries, coconut chips and granola. It's a great option for summer mornings because it's cold and sweet—think of it as dessert for breakfast! Better still, it packs in at least 15 grams of protein, depending on which type of protein powder you use. I recommend choosing a neutral-tasting protein powder, as the smoothie will take on the flavor of the protein powder you use, and some of them can be bland and chalky, or overly sweet. I use Sunwarrior Warrior Blend in unflavoured/natural and Omega Nutrition Pumpkin Seed Protein Powder with great success, but feel free to use your preferred protein powder. Chocolate or vanilla will be nice, as long as they're not overpowering. Note that you can also turn this smoothie bowl into a portable smoothie by adding more almond milk to thin it out.

1. Put the almond milk in a high-speed blender, then add the remaining ingredients and blend until smooth. The smoothie should have a thick, soft texture. If using a Vitamix, use the tamper to move things along. You can add a bit more milk if your blender is having a hard time blending it.

2. Spoon the smoothie into a bowl and add your desired toppings. Enjoy immediately!

Tip 1. Be sure to use very soft Medjool dates. If yours are firm, try soaking them in boiling water for 20 to 30 minutes. 2. If your blender has a hard time blending dates completely smooth (which many do), feel free to use liquid sweetener instead. 3. Be sure to use a very ripe banana in this smoothie for the sweetest flavour.

Make it nut-free Swap the almond milk for a nut-free milk, such as coconut milk.

FOR THE SMOOTHIE BOWL

125ml unsweetened almond milk, plus more if needed

1 very large frozen banana, chopped (about 120g chopped)

2 tablespoons avocado

1 scoop (60ml) neutral-flavoured protein powder

2 tablespoons unsweetened cocoa powder

1 to 3 pitted Medjool dates or liquid sweetener, to taste

1 or 2 ice cubes (optional)

TOPPING SUGGESTIONS

Chopped strawberries

Shredded or large-flake unsweetened coconut, or Maple Cinnamon Coconut Chips (page 283)

Sliced banana

Vanilla Super-Seed Granola (page 33) or Roasted Hazelnut-Almond Granola Clusters (page 71)

Hemp hearts

Cacao nibs

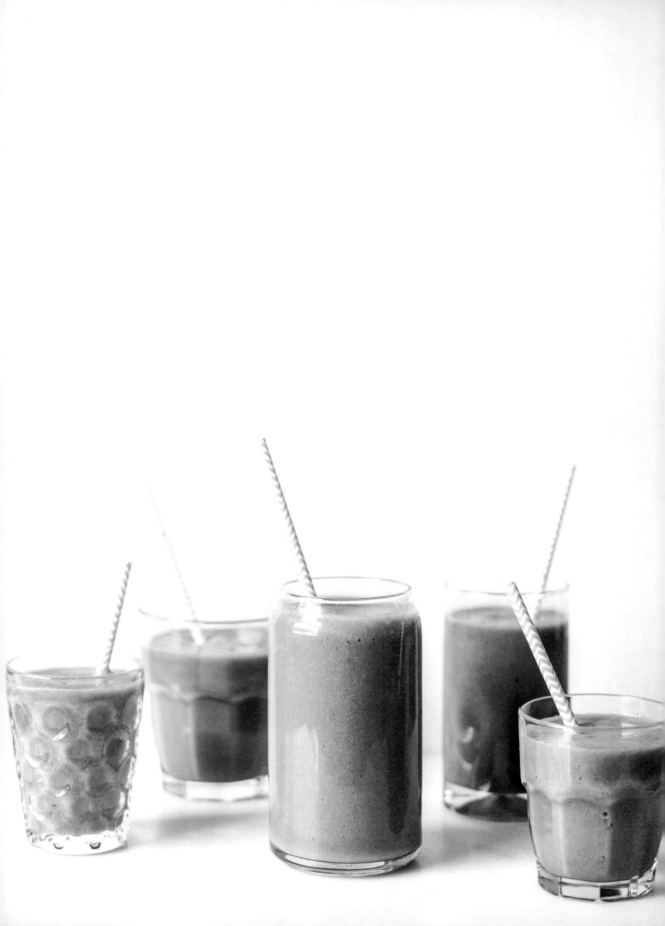

Reset Button Green Smoothie (Family-Size)

VEGAN, GLUTEN-FREE, NUT-FREE, SOYA-FREE, GRAIN-FREE, OIL-FREE,
KID-FRIENDLY OPTION

MAKES 1.25L (3 SERVINGS)

PREP TIME: **15 MINUTES**

This is what I like to call a 'family-size' smoothie. It packs in an incredible 8 servings of vegetables, and includes 1.25l of leafy greens. Mellow, hydrating cucumber, along with pears, bananas, and pineapple, help to balance out all that leafy green goodness with just the right amount of natural sweetness, while still tasting healthy and fresh. Just a word of warning: All the ingredients *just* fit into a (2l) Vitamix blender, so if your blender is smaller, I recommend making the half-batch version (page 27).

1. In a high-speed blender (2l capacity), combine all the ingredients and blend until smooth. If using a Vitamix, use the tamper to press the ingredients down into the blade. You can add a bit more water if necessary to get the blender going.

Make it kid-friendly Omit the mint (the flavour can be a bit strong for some kiddos) and use all spinach instead of a mix of spinach and kale or romaine.

60ml water or coconut water, plus more if desired

150g chopped cucumber (unpeeled is fine)

450g de-stemmed kale leaves, chopped romaine lettuce or baby spinach

675g baby spinach

15g fresh mint leaves

1 very large or 2 small ripe pears, cored and chopped (280g)

1½ large frozen bananas, roughly chopped

245g frozen pineapple chunks

1 tablespoon fresh lime juice

2 or 3 ice cubes (optional)

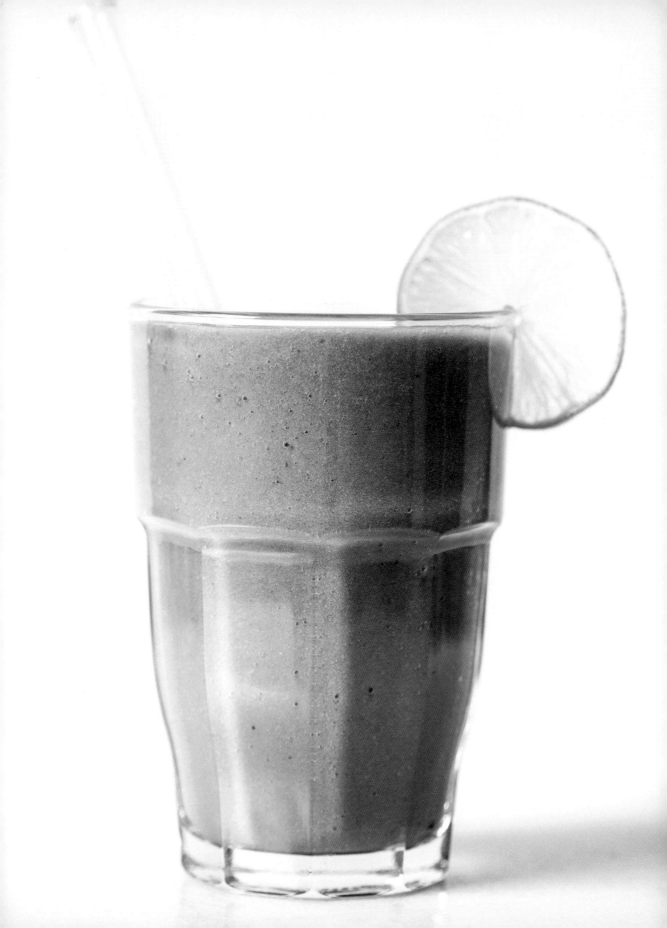

Reset Button Green Smoothie (Half Batch)

VEGAN, GLUTEN-FREE, NUT-FREE, SOYA-FREE, GRAIN-FREE, OIL-FREE,
KID-FRIENDLY OPTION

MAKES 750ML (2 SERVINGS)

This smoothie has all the same goodness of the 'family-size' Reset Button Green Smoothie, but this is a half batch for when you just want one large serving or two smaller servings. If you aren't a big mint fan, feel free to start with half the amount and add from there.

1. Put the water and cucumber in a high-speed blender and blend until the cucumber is liquid. (This step helps the rest of the smoothie ingredients blend more easily.)

2. Add the remaining ingredients and blend until smooth. If using a Vitamix, use the tamper to press the ingredients down into the blade. You can add a bit more water if necessary to get the blender going.

Make it kid-friendly Omit the mint (the flavour can be a bit strong for some kiddos) and use all spinach instead of a mix of spinach and kale or romaine.

60ml water, more if desired

75g chopped cucumber (peeled or unpeeled)

225g stemmed kale leaves chopped romaine lettuce, or baby spinach

340g fresh baby spinach

5g fresh mint leaves

1 ripe medium pear, cored and chopped 170g

1 medium frozen banana, roughly chopped

125g frozen pineapple chunks

1½ teaspoons fresh lime juice

1 or 2 ice cubes (optional)

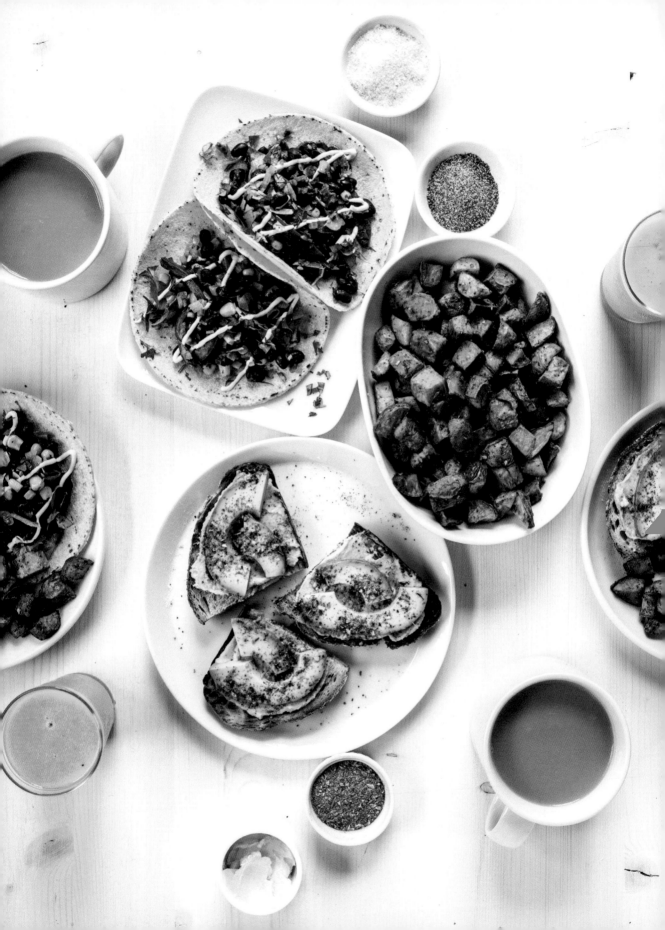

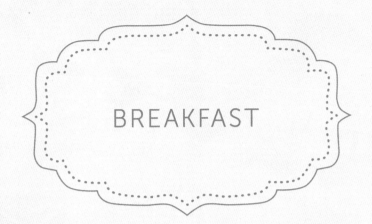

BREAKFAST

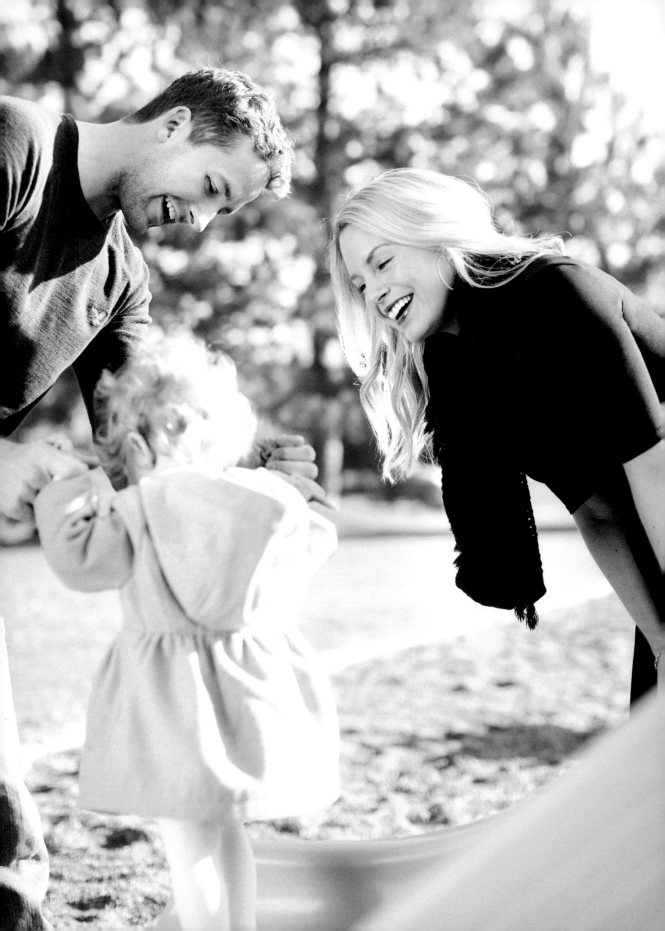

BEFORE ADRIANA CAME into our lives, mornings were a bit slower (not to mention quieter!), and I'd often spend time dreaming up new breakfast creations at least once a week. These days, we're busy feeding a growing toddler—quickly—and then we're often out the door! I like to rely on a handful of easy, go-to breakfast recipes that I know will be both nourishing and a hit with my whole family.

I love breakfasts that can be prepared (at least in part) the night before, such as my Overnight Hot Oatmeal Power Bowl or the Fastest Sprouted Steel-Cut Oatmeal; both are warming, cold-weather recipes (however, I discovered we love them chilled, too). I also love breakfast foods that can be frozen and thawed overnight like my PB&J Thumbprint Breakfast Cookies, Vanilla Super-Seed Granola with Coconut Chips and Strawberry Oat Crumble Bars. It's rare that I don't have a batch of granola or breakfast bars in the freezer! Of course, smoothies are a staple in my morning routine, as you saw in the previous chapter. We drink smoothies every day (yes, even in the winter!), often for pre- or post-workout fuel (see Smoothies and Smoothie Bowls, page 1).

Weekends tend to be a bit slower-paced for us, and I love to take a bit more time to make a Sunday brunch filled with savoury dishes like my 9-Spice Avocado Hummus Toast, Black Bean Rancheros or Roasted Breakfast Hash. All these dishes make a satisfying breakfast-for-dinner option, too!

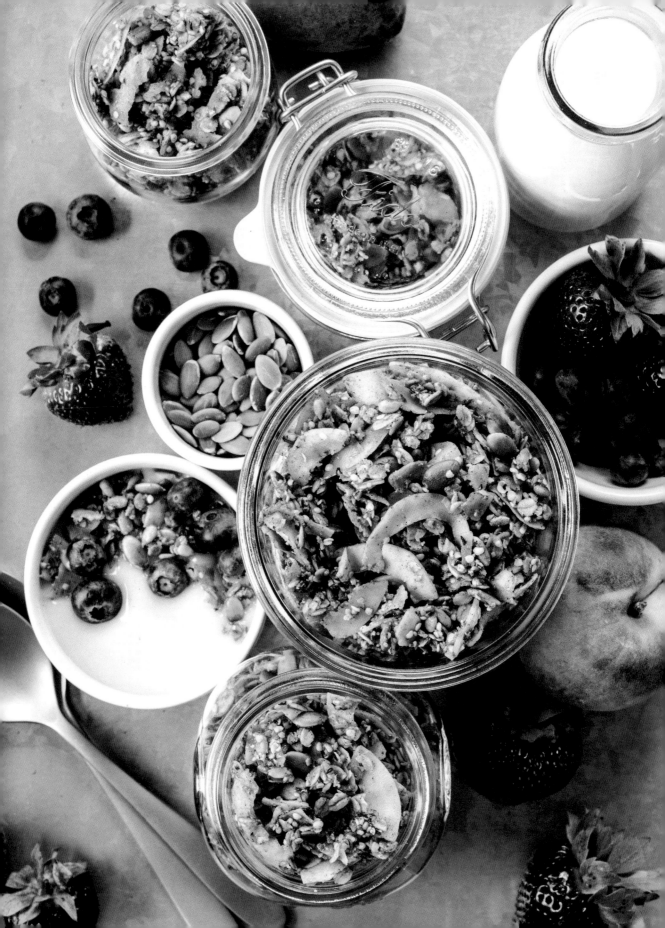

Vanilla Super-Seed Granola with Coconut Chips

VEGAN, GLUTEN-FREE, NUT-FREE, SOYA-FREE, KID-FRIENDLY, FREEZER-FRIENDLY

MAKES 1.65L (ABOUT TWENTY 75ML SERVINGS)

PREP TIME: **20 MINUTES**

BAKE TIME: **23 TO 28 MINUTES**

I've made a lot of granola recipes in my day, but they all contain nuts. That's why I'm so excited about this nut-free granola. It still has an incredibly crunchy texture and nutty flavour, but it's great for those with tree-nut allergies, and is kid-approved to boot! Best of all, its amazing toasted aroma of coconut, vanilla, cinnamon and maple will make your home smell absolutely delectable as it bakes. I've been known to throw in a batch just before company comes over and delight in everyone's curiosity about what is about to emerge from the oven! Be sure to use large-flake coconut (also known as raw coconut chips) in this recipe, rather than shredded coconut—the coconut chips give this granola its amazing, crunchy texture. Try it on top of my Overnight Hot Oatmeal Power Bowl (page 49), any smoothie bowl (see Smoothies and Smoothie Bowls, page 1), or Tropical Overnight Oats (page 57), or simply enjoy it by the handful as a snack on the go!

1. Preheat the oven to 300°F (150°C). Line an extra-large rimmed baking sheet (38 x 53cm) with parchment paper.

2. In a large bowl, combine the flaked coconut, oats, pumpkin seeds, hemp hearts, sunflower seeds, sugar, cinnamon and salt.

3. In a small saucepan, melt the coconut oil, then remove from the heat. Whisk in the maple syrup, sunflower seed butter and vanilla until combined. Stir in the vanilla pod seeds (or vanilla powder) and set aside the vanilla bean pods, if using.

4. Pour the wet mixture on top of the dry mixture and stir until the dry mixture is fully coated.

5. Spoon the granola mixture onto the prepared baking sheet (along with the reserved vanilla pods). Spread the granola into an even layer.

6. Bake for 15 minutes. Remove the baking sheet from the oven and stir. Bake for 8 to 13 minutes more, until the granola is *just* starting to turn a bit golden along the edges. The granola will be soft when it comes out of the oven, but it will harden as it cools. Let cool completely on the baking sheet, about 1 hour or so, then transfer to glass jars for storing. If you used vanilla beans, feel free to place the pods in the glass jar too for even more vanilla aroma.

7. The granola will keep in an airtight container in the fridge for 3 to 4 weeks, or you can freeze it for a couple of months. My preferred storage method is freezing cooled granola in zip-top freezer bags for easy grab-and-go portions. Be sure to press out all the air before sealing.

190g unsweetened large-flake coconut

170g gluten-free rolled oats

35g raw (pumpkin seeds)

80g hemp hearts

35g raw sunflower seeds or more pumpkin seeds

2 tablespoons coconut sugar or granulated sweetener of choice

1½ teaspoons ground cinnamon

½ teaspoon fine sea salt

90ml virgin coconut oil, melted

105ml pure maple syrup

2 tablespoons Homemade Sunflower Seed Butter (page 79), or store-bought

1 teaspoon pure vanilla extract

2 vanilla pods, halved lengthwise and seeds scraped, or ½ teaspoon vanilla powder

Tip 1. Feel free to change up the seeds and incorporate nuts (such as walnuts or sliced almonds) if your diet allows them. 2. You can also swap the sunflower seed butter for a nut butter, if you prefer.

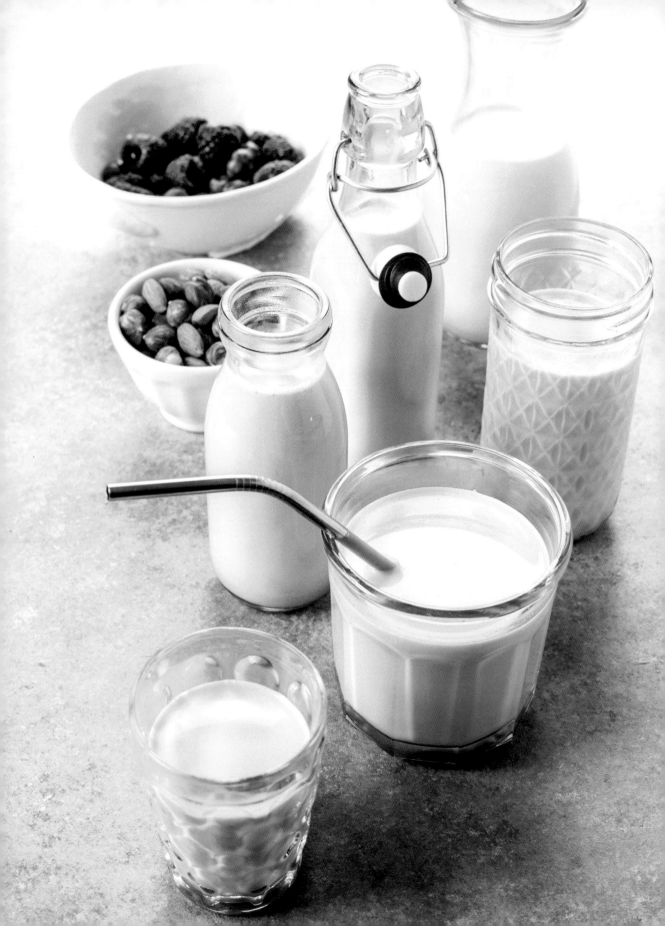

Coffee Shop-Worthy Hazelnut Milk

VEGAN, GLUTEN-FREE, SOYA-FREE, GRAIN-FREE, OIL-FREE,
ADVANCE PREP REQUIRED

MAKES 875ML

SOAK TIME: **1 TO 12 HOURS**

PREP TIME: **10 MINUTES**

Decadent, luxurious, and totally splurge-worthy, this homemade hazelnut milk is fit for a high-end coffee shop! It's perfect for a cup of coffee or black tea, as well as for whipping up dairy-free lattes at home. For a truly decadent treat, try mixing it with unsweetened cocoa powder and a touch of maple syrup for a creamy hot chocolate flavour, or pairing it with chai spices for a warming chai latte. I use a mix of soaked hazelnuts and almonds in this recipe, but feel free to use all hazelnuts if you prefer their unique flavour. Drink the milk alone, add it to cereal or smoothies, or use it to make hot oatmeal or overnight oats that are particularly creamy. No matter how you use it, you'll fall in love with its light notes of caramel (thanks to the Medjool dates), cinnamon and vanilla pod. If you don't have a nut milk bag (see page xvi), you can use a fine-mesh sieve lined with cheesecloth. The milk won't get quite as smooth, but if you strain it a few times, it turns out pretty well.

1. Place the hazelnuts and almonds in a bowl and cover with 5 to 8cm of water. Soak overnight for 8 to 12 hours. Drain and rinse.

2. Place the nuts in a blender along with the remaining ingredients. Blend on high for about 1 minute.

3. Place a nut milk bag over a large bowl and slowly pour the milk into the bag. Gently squeeze the bottom of the bag to release the milk. This process can take 3 to 5 minutes. You should left with 175 to 250ml of pulp in the bag. (See Tip for uses for the leftover pulp.)

4. Using a funnel, carefully transfer the milk into a large Mason jar and secure with lid. Chill in the fridge. The milk will stay fresh for 2 to 3 days. Give the jar a good shake each time before enjoying.

90g raw hazelnuts

25g raw almonds

875ml water

3 large pitted Medjool dates, or 1 to 2 tablespoons pure maple syrup, to taste

1 vanilla pod, roughly chopped, or ½ to 1 teaspoon pure vanilla extract, to taste

½ teaspoon ground cinnamon

Dash of fine sea salt

Tip 1. If your dates or vanilla pod are dry or stiff, soak in boiling water to soften before use for 20 to 30 minutes. 2. For a quick-soak method, cover the hazelnuts and almonds with boiling water and soak for 1 hour. 3. Ideas for using leftover pulp: Spread it onto a baking sheet and dry it out in a preheated 300°F (150°C) oven for 25 to 30 minutes until lightly golden in some spots. Let cool completely before storing. You can use the toasted pulp in granola recipes or any other baked goods you like.

For Cashew-Almond Milk Use 65g raw cashews in place of the hazelnuts and increase the almonds to 50g. Proceed as directed.

For Almond Milk Omit the hazelnuts and use 100g raw almonds. Proceed as directed.

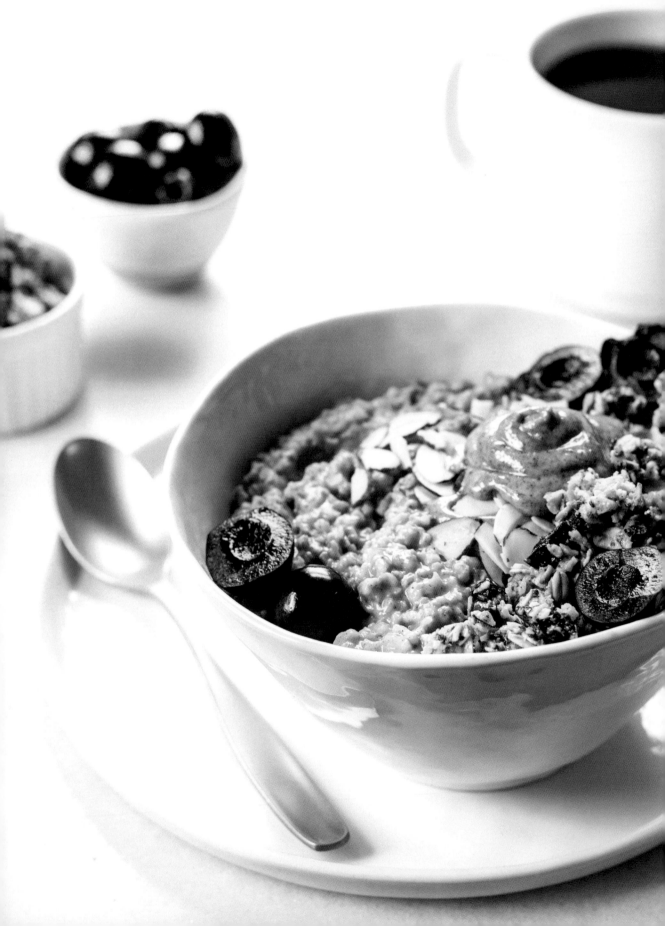

The Fastest Sprouted Steel-Cut Oatmeal

VEGAN, GLUTEN-FREE, NUT-FREE OPTION, SOYA-FREE,
ADVANCE PREP REQUIRED, KID-FRIENDLY

SERVES 3

SOAK TIME: **OVERNIGHT**

PREP TIME: **5 MINUTES**

COOK TIME: **9 TO 11 MINUTES**

I absolutely love steel-cut oatmeal, but rarely make it because it requires at least a half hour on the hop. So I came up with a way to cut the cooking time by almost 75 per cent simply by soaking or 'sprouting' the steel-cut oats in water overnight. Now I enjoy this breakfast regularly because it's so quick and easy! Soaking softens and expands the grain so you only need to cook the oats for a mere ten minutes. If you're concerned that this will detract from the characteristic texture of the oats, don't be! The oats retain all their lovely creaminess and chew. This recipe includes mashed banana and cinnamon, which turns it into a lovely tasting bowl of 'banana bread'-flavoured oats. It makes enough for a few breakfasts too; I've been known to enjoy the leftovers cold, straight from the fridge, with a drizzle of maple syrup. Pure heaven.

1. Place the oats in a medium bowl and cover with a couple of inches of water. Soak the oats overnight on the counter, uncovered. In the morning, drain and rinse the oats.

2. In a medium pot, melt the coconut oil over low heat. Stir in the oats. Increase the heat to medium and toast the oats in the oil for a few minutes, stirring frequently.

3. Stir in the milk, banana, sugar (if using), cinnamon and salt. Simmer the mixture, stirring frequently, for 9 to 11 minutes, until thickened. Remove from the heat and stir in the vanilla.

4. Portion into bowls and add your desired toppings. Any leftovers will keep in an airtight container in the fridge for 3 to 5 days.

Tip 1. Try stirring the seeds from 1 vanilla pod into this oatmeal for intense vanilla flavour! It's also lovely topped with some fresh lemon zest. 2. Bob's Red Mill Quick Cooking Steel Cut Oats will work in this recipe, too (just note that they are not certified gluten-free). Soak the oats overnight and rinse before using, but use only 175 to 250ml almond milk when preparing the oatmeal. Or you can skip soaking the quick-cooking steel-cut oats, and simply rinse the oats before cooking; cook for 5 to 7 minutes using 375 to 425ml almond milk.

Make it nut-free Swap the almond milk for a nut-free milk, such as coconut milk. Top the oatmeal with toasted seeds (rather than nuts) and my nut-free Vanilla Super-Seed Granola with Coconut Chips (page 33).

FOR THE OATMEAL

130g gluten-free steel-cut oats

1 tablespoon virgin coconut oil

425ml almond milk, homemade (page 35) or store-bought

1 large ripe banana, mashed

2 teaspoons coconut sugar (optional)

1½ teaspoons ground cinnamon

Good pinch of fine sea salt

1 to 1½ teaspoons pure vanilla extract, to taste

TOPPING SUGGESTIONS

Roasted Hazelnut-Almond Granola Clusters (page 71)

Fresh pitted cherries, other berries or sliced banana

Chopped toasted walnuts

Toasted unsweetened shredded or large-flake coconut

Nut or seed butter

Pure maple syrup

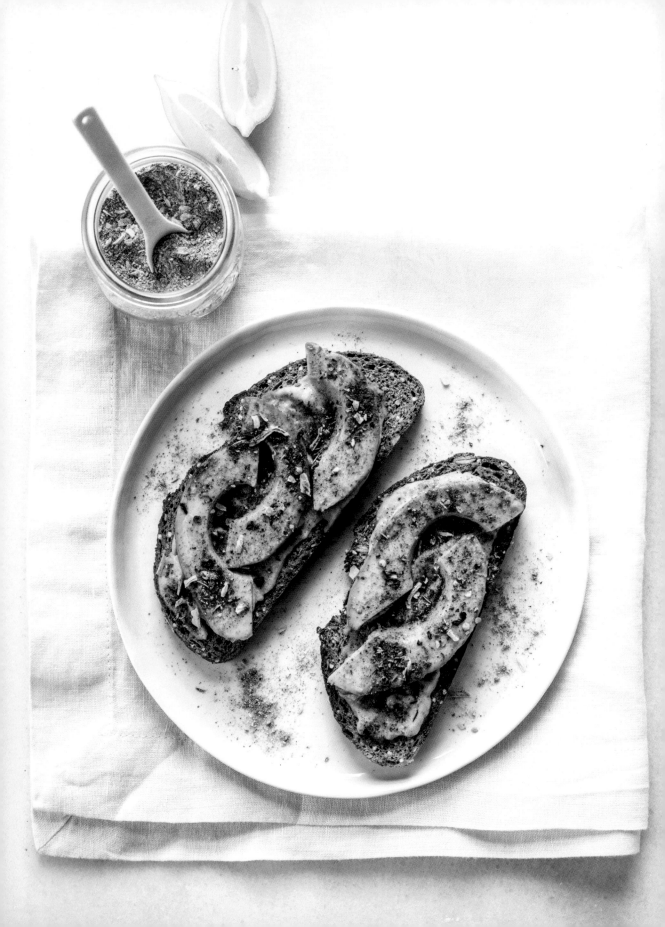

9-Spice Avocado Hummus Toast

VEGAN, GLUTEN-FREE OPTION, NUT-FREE, SOYA-FREE,
ADVANCE PREP REQUIRED, KID-FRIENDLY

MAKES 4 SLICES (2 SERVINGS)

PREP TIME: **10 MINUTES**

COOK TIME: **5 MINUTES**

You know that age-old question, 'What meal could you live off of for the rest of your life?' Well, I'm pretty sure this one ranks high for me. Avocado toast isn't anything new for most of us, but I can promise you've never had it this flavourful before. The secret is in my favourite homemade 9-Spice Mix, which is incredibly flavourful, a little smoky, and also lightly sweet. I like to keep the spice mix on hand so it's ready whenever a craving strikes (which is often). This recipe starts with infusing the toast with fresh garlic. Once you try it prepared this way, you'll never make avocado toast without it. Then it's topped with hummus, sliced avocado, a generous amount of spice mix, red pepper flakes, sea salt and a drizzle of olive oil. I recommend having all your ingredients ready to go before you put the toast in the toaster; that way, once the toast pops, it's go time! This recipe serves two, because anyone else in your house is likely to become insanely jealous if you eat this alone; I speak from experience. However, feel free to halve the recipe if it's just for you.

4 slices of your favourite bread

1 large clove garlic, halved lengthwise

60ml Every Day Lemon-Garlic Hummus (page 91) or hummus of choice

1 Hass avocado, pitted and sliced

1 to 2 teaspoons 9-Spice Mix (page 258), to taste

Fine sea salt

Red pepper flakes (optional)

2 teaspoons extra-virgin olive oil or avocado oil

Squeeze of fresh lemon or lime juice, for garnish (optional)

1. Toast the bread until golden and fairly crisp, so that it stands up well to the toppings without getting soggy.

2. Rub the sliced garlic, cut-side down, all over each piece of toast. This will infuse the bread with garlic flavor without it being overpowering.

3. Spread 1 tablespoon of the hummus over each piece of toast and top with avocado slices.

4. Shake the spice mix to combine, if necessary, and sprinkle ¼ to ½ teaspoon onto each piece of toast.

5. Add salt and red pepper flakes (if using) to taste and drizzle with olive oil and lemon juice, if desired. Serve immediately.

Tip Short of time? This toast still tastes great even without the spice mix.

Make it gluten-free Use gluten-free bread. (I like to state the obvious, apparently.)

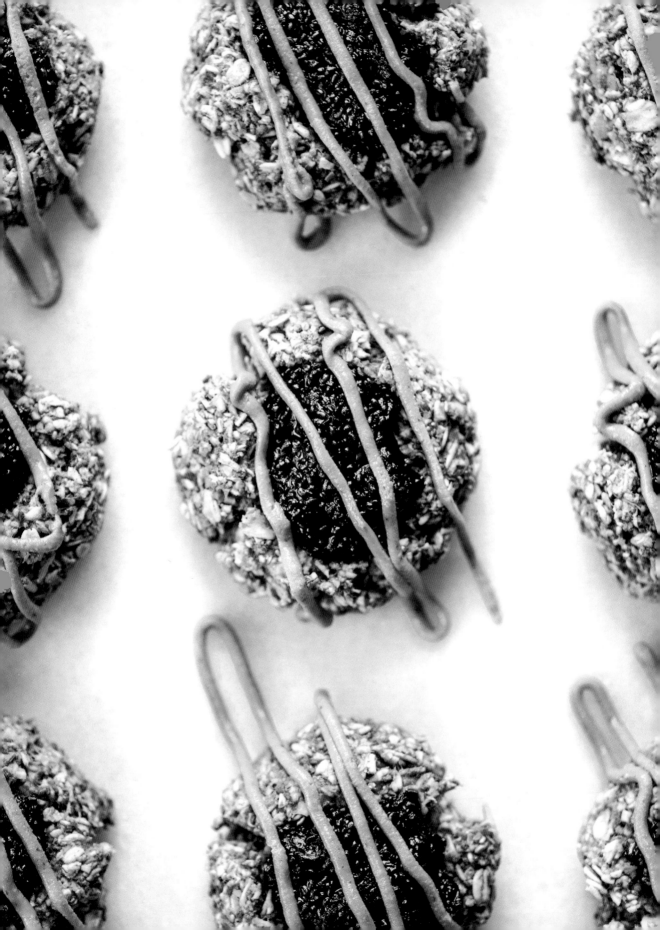

Peanut Butter & Jam Breakfast Cookies

VEGAN, GLUTEN-FREE, NUT-FREE OPTION, SOYA-FREE, OIL-FREE, ADVANCE
PREP OPTION, KID-FRIENDLY, FREEZER-FRIENDLY

MAKES 8 LARGE COOKIES

PREP TIME: **10 MINUTES**

COOK TIME: **12 MINUTES**

These wholesome cookies are soft, very dense, and mildly sweet, thanks to the addition of fresh, ripe banana. Rolled oats give them a pleasantly chewy texture. I like to think of them as portable baked oatmeal. They're also a perfect option for breakfast on the go . . . that's if you can keep yourself from eating them that long (I never can). Prepare them at the start of the week and grab a few as you leave the house on busy mornings, or simply have them on hand for a healthy snack. Have fun adding different mix-ins to the recipe, like chopped nuts or seeds, or using different flavours of jam. I always pop some in the freezer for later, as they freeze and thaw beautifully.

1. Preheat the oven to 350°F (180°C). Line a baking sheet with parchment paper.

2. In a food processor, add the oats and pulse until the oats are coarsely chopped. Avoid processing them into a powder—you still want some texture.

3. Transfer the oats to a large bowl. Add the banana, chia seeds, cinnamon, and salt and stir to combine. The mixture should be very wet and dense.

4. With a retractable ice cream scoop or a spoon, scoop the dough into 8 mounds, placing them at least 2.5cm apart on the baking sheet. Press your thumb into the center of each cookie to create a well. Fill each well with 1 heaped teaspoon of jam.

5. Bake the cookies for 11 to 13 minutes, until they are slightly firm, but still soft and doughy in the middle. Transfer the cookies to a cooling rack and let cool for 10 minutes or so.

6. Spoon the nut butter into a plastic bag and snip off one corner. Pipe the nut butter over the cookies. Alternatively, you can skip this step and simply enjoy the cookies as they are, or serve them with a pat of coconut oil or coconut butter. The cookies will keep in an airtight container in the fridge for a few days, or you can wrap them in clingfilm and place into an airtight container or zip-top bag in the freezer for 2 to 3 weeks.

Make it nut-free Omit the peanut or almond butter topping and use sunflower seed butter instead.

170g gluten-free rolled oats

250ml mashed very ripe banana (about 2 extra-large)

3 tablespoons chia seeds or milled linseed

1 teaspoon ground cinnamon

1/8 teaspoon fine sea salt

8 heaped teaspoons Berry Chia Seed Jam (page 43) or your favourite jam

65g smooth peanut, almond, or sunflower seed butter, for serving (optional)

Coconut oil or coconut butter, for serving (optional)

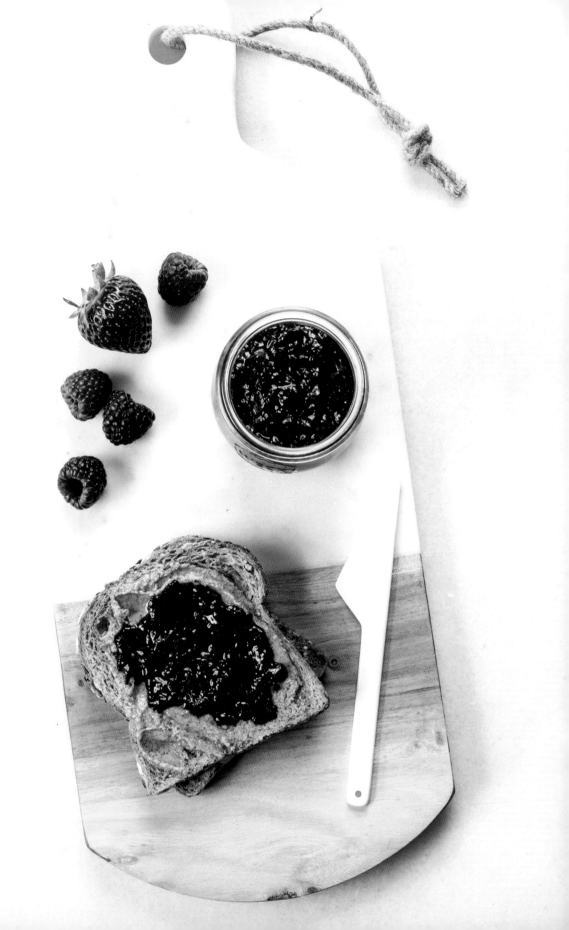

Berry Chia Seed Jam

VEGAN, GLUTEN-FREE, NUT-FREE, SOYA-FREE, GRAIN-FREE, OIL-FREE,
KID-FRIENDLY, FREEZER-FRIENDLY

MAKES 325 TO 375ML

PREP TIME: **5 MINUTES**

COOK TIME: **13 TO 22 MINUTES**

Chia seed jam has been my go-to quick-and-easy jam recipe for years. While not a traditional jam by any means, I certainly don't miss all the refined sugar of traditional versions when I enjoy this fresh, vibrant spread. You can use any kind of berry you prefer, and have fun changing it up with different mix-ins like lemon juice or zest, orange juice or zest, vanilla pod seeds or extract, cinnamon, cardamom, and any other spices or extracts you enjoy. Since berries vary in terms of sweetness, feel free to adjust the sweetener to suit your own taste with each batch. You'll be happy to know that chia seed jam also freezes well. I like to portion individual servings into a silicone mini-muffin tray, freeze them until they're solid, and then pop them out and store them in a freezer bag. This way you can have chia seed jam ready anytime! Simply thaw it in the fridge or at room temperature. If I'm making overnight oats, I will often thaw a cube of chia seed jam in the fridge overnight while the oats thicken. Then it's all ready for me to enjoy in the morning without any fuss. How's that for easy?

475g frozen strawberries, raspberries, pitted sweet cherries or blueberries, or a mix

60ml pure maple syrup, or to taste

Dash of fine sea salt

2 tablespoons chia seeds

½ teaspoon pure vanilla extract

½ teaspoon pure vanilla powder, or 1 large vanilla pod, split lengthwise and seeds scraped out

Squeeze of fresh lemon juice (optional)

1. In a medium pot, stir together the berries, maple syrup and salt until combined. Bring to a simmer over medium-high heat and cook for 5 to 7 minutes, until the berries have softened (they will release a lot of liquid during this time).

2. Reduce the heat to medium and carefully mash the berries with a potato masher until mostly smooth. The jam will still look very watery at this point, but this is normal!

3. Add the chia seeds and stir until combined. Simmer over low-medium heat, stirring frequently (reducing heat if necessary to avoid sticking) for 8 to 15 minutes more, until a lot of the liquid has cooked off and the mixture has thickened slightly.

(recipe continues)

4. Remove from the heat and stir in the vanilla extract, vanilla powder and lemon juice (if using). Transfer the mixture to a bowl and refrigerate, uncovered, until cool, at least a couple of hours. For quicker cooling, pop the jam into the freezer, uncovered, for 45 minutes, stirring every 15 minutes. The chia seed jam will keep in an airtight container in the fridge for up to 2 weeks. It also freezes well for 1 to 2 months.

For the Strawberry-Vanilla Chia Seed Jam Use 475g frozen strawberries, 60ml pure maple syrup, a dash of salt, 2 tablespoons chia seeds, 1 teaspoon fresh lemon juice and 2 seeded vanilla pods or ½ teaspoon pure vanilla bean powder.

For the Raspberry-Almond Chia Seed Jam Use 300g frozen or fresh raspberries, 60ml pure maple syrup, 2 tablespoons chia seeds, ¼ teaspoon pure almond extract, and a pinch of fine sea salt.

Strawberry Oat Crumble Bars

VEGAN, GLUTEN-FREE, NUT-FREE, SOYA-FREE, ADVANCE PREP REQUIRED,
KID-FRIENDLY, FREEZER-FRIENDLY

SERVES 12 TO 16

PREP TIME: **20 TO 25 MINUTES**

BAKE TIME: **33 TO 40 MINUTES**

These delicious 'anytime' bars are vegan, lunchbox-friendly, gluten-free, and made with a refined sugar-free strawberry-vanilla chia seed jam. (With the chia jam, the bars will be lightly sweet; if you use store-bought jam, they'll be much sweeter.) It's hard to resist gobbling them up once you slice them, but I actually find that they taste better the following day, after the flavours have had a chance to meld in the fridge overnight. I also recommend making the chia jam in advance, so it has time to cool in the fridge before you begin making the recipe. Once chilled, the bars firm up (thanks to the coconut oil), but at room temperature they soften and will virtually melt in your mouth while you eat them! Hubba, hubba. Either way, you are going to go crazy over the roasted sunflower seed 'cookie' crust. Enjoy these as a quick breakfast with tea or coffee, as an afternoon snack when you need a boost, or warmed up for dessert with a scoop of ice cream (it'll remind you of a berry crisp!).

1. If desired, roast the sunflower seeds: Preheat the oven to 325°F (160°C). Spread the seeds over a large rimmed baking sheet in an even layer. Roast for 9 to 12 minutes, until lightly golden in some spots. Remove from the oven and set aside.

2. Increase the oven temperature to 350°F (180°C). Line a 23cm square pan (or a 20cm pan for a slightly thicker bar) with parchment paper, leaving some overhang, which will make it easy to lift out the bars later.

3. In a food processor, combine the sunflower seeds, oats, and salt and process until you have a coarse flour.

4. In a small pot, melt the oil over low heat. Remove from the heat and whisk in the maple syrup, brown rice syrup and sunflower seed butter until combined. Pour the wet mixture on top of the oat mixture in the food processor and process until the mixture comes together, 10 to 15 seconds. The dough should feel quite heavy and oily, and there shouldn't be any dry patches. If there are, process for 5 seconds more. If for some reason it's still too dry, try adding water, a teaspoon at a time, and processing until it comes together.

300ml Strawberry-Vanilla Chia Seed Jam (see page 44) or store-bought jam

140g hulled sunflower seeds

255g gluten-free rolled oats

¼ teaspoon plus ⅛ teaspoon fine sea salt

125ml virgin coconut oil

60ml pure maple syrup

3 tablespoons brown rice syrup

1 tablespoon Homemade Sunflower Seed Butter (page 79), or store-bought

(recipe continues)

5. Set aside some of the oat mixture for the topping. Crumble the remaining oat mixture over the base of the prepared pan in an even layer. Starting at the center, push down with your fingers (you can lightly wet them if they stick) to spread out and pack down the crust. Press the dough down tightly. Even out the edges with your fingertips. Prick the crust with the tines of a fork about 9 times to allow steam to escape.

6. Parbake the crust for 10 minutes. Remove from the oven and let cool for 5 minutes. (If the crust puffed up while baking, gently press down on it to release the air.) Spread the jam in an even layer over the crust. Crumble the reserved oat mixture evenly over the jam.

7. Bake, uncovered, for 14 to 18 minutes more, until the topping is lightly firm to the touch. The topping will not turn golden in colour; it will remain the same shade as it was before baking. Let cool in the pan on a cooling rack for 45 to 60 minutes, then transfer the pan to the freezer for 30 minutes until completely cool. Lift out the slab and slice it into squares or bars. Leftovers can be stored in an airtight container in the fridge for several days, or wrapped up and stored in the freezer for 4 to 5 weeks.

Tip If you have a food processor with less than a 2.6l capacity, you might need to process the crust in two batches and then stir it all together in a large bowl before measuring.

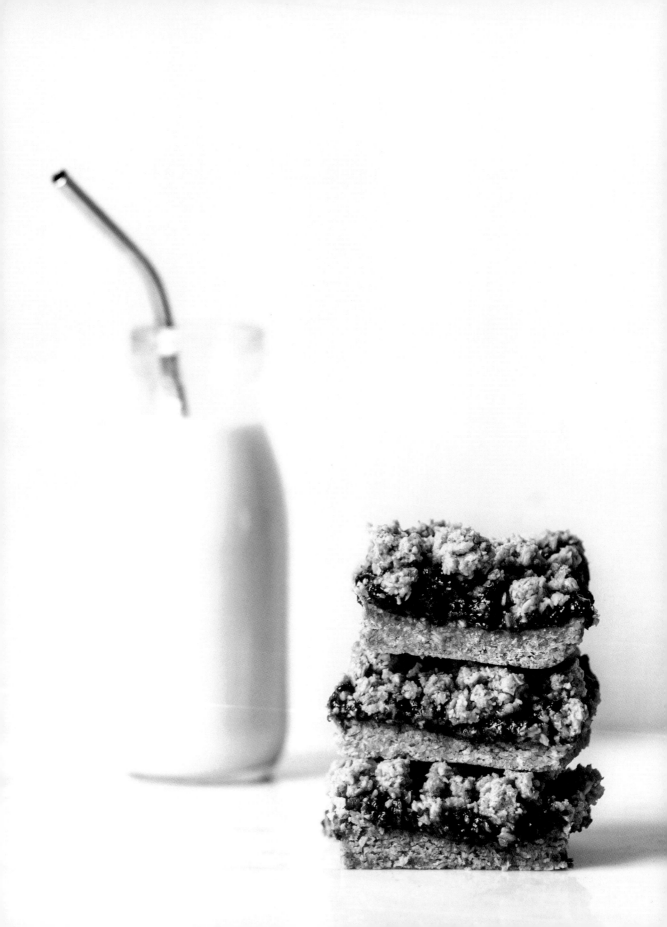

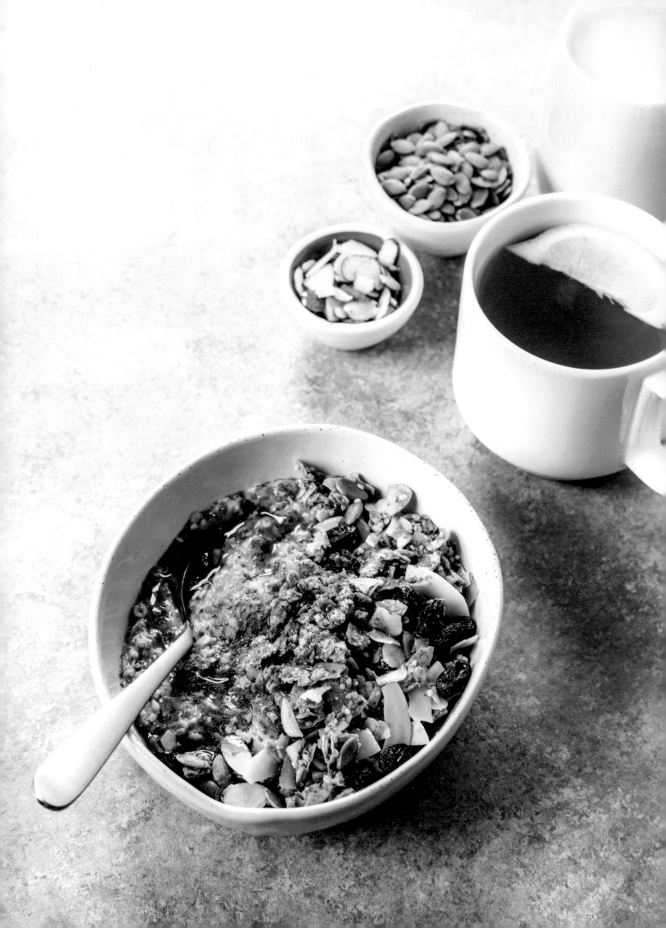

Overnight Hot Oatmeal Power Bowl

VEGAN, GLUTEN-FREE, SOYA-FREE, OIL-FREE, ADVANCE PREP REQUIRED

MAKES 1 LARGE BOWL (ABOUT 375ML)

SOAK TIME: **OVERNIGHT OR 8 HOURS**

PREP TIME: **5 MINUTES**

COOK TIME: **3 MINUTES**

This is an easy bowl of hot oatmeal, as it comes together in just a few minutes in the morning! Soaking the oatmeal mixture overnight significantly cuts down the cooking time; all you have to do is heat it on the stove for a minute or two in the morning, and it's ready to be enjoyed. This is my go-to breakfast during the cooler fall and winter months, and it's a staple for any busy period of time. When Adriana was a newborn, I practically lived off this oatmeal for the first several weeks because it's just so easy and nutritious. In the summer, you can simply soak the ingredients and enjoy a chilled bowl of overnight oats in the morning—no heat required.

1. The night before: In a medium bowl, stir together the banana, chia seeds, oats, cinnamon, milk, water, vanilla (if using) and salt until combined. Cover and refrigerate overnight.

2. In the morning, scoop the oat mixture into a medium pot and bring to a simmer over medium-high heat, stirring frequently. Reduce the heat to medium-low and cook, stirring frequently, until heated through and thickened, 2 to 3 minutes.

3. Pour the oats into a bowl. Garnish with toppings as desired and enjoy immediately.

Tip I love soaking the almonds, pumpkin seeds, and raisins in a mug of water overnight. This 'sprouts' the nuts and seeds, removing some of their natural anti-nutrients and allowing the body to digest them better, and it also plumps the raisins. In the morning, simply drain and rinse before adding them on top of the oatmeal. Alternatively, you can use toasted almonds or pumpkin seeds.

FOR THE OATMEAL

1 ripe, spotty medium banana, mashed

2 tablespoons chia seeds

30g gluten-free rolled oats

¼ teaspoon ground cinnamon

150ml unsweetened almond milk

75ml water

½ teaspoon pure vanilla extract (optional)

Small pinch of fine sea salt

TOPPING SUGGESTIONS

30g Vanilla Super-Seed Granola with Coconut Chips (page 33) or Roasted Hazelnut-Almond Granola Clusters (page 71)

1 tablespoon sliced almonds, soaked or toasted (see Tip)

1 tablespoon pumpkin seeds, soaked or toasted (see Tip)

1 teaspoon raisins (optional)

1 teaspoon unsweetened shredded or large-flake coconut, toasted, if preferred

Pinch each of ground cinnamon, ginger and allspice (or customize the spices to your liking)

1 to 2 teaspoons pure maple syrup or coconut sugar, to taste (optional)

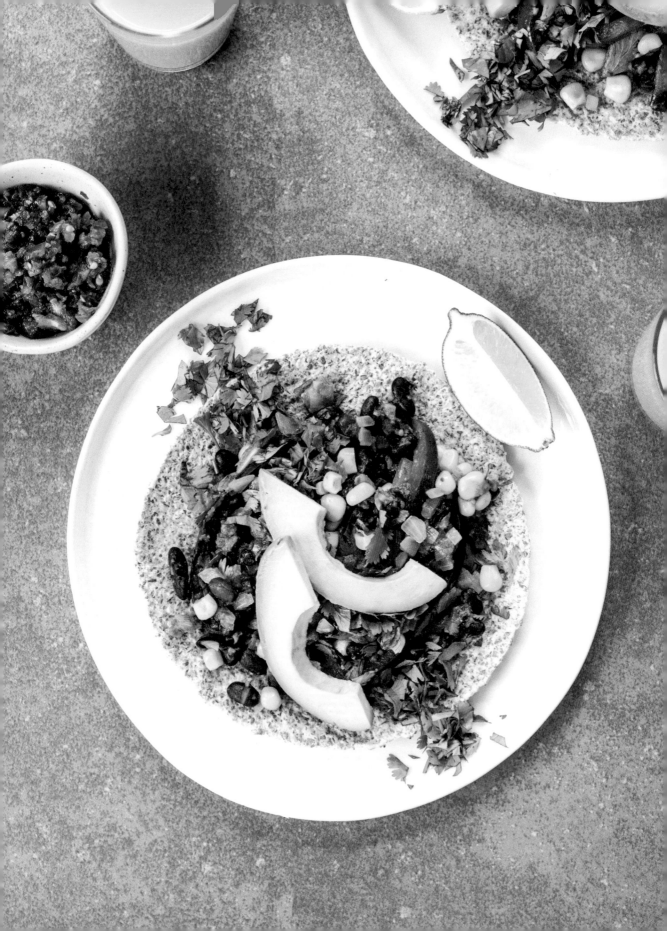

Black Bean Rancheros

VEGAN, GLUTEN-FREE, NUT-FREE, SOYA-FREE, GRAIN-FREE OPTION, KID-FRIENDLY, FREEZER-FRIENDLY

SERVES 3 OR 4

PREP TIME: **10 MINUTES**

COOK TIME: **15 MINUTES**

This recipe is a great savoury breakfast option, and it comes together in less than 30 minutes. Try making it at the peak of summer, when you can enjoy the fresh, sweet flavours of corn, bell pepper and juicy cherry tomatoes. To incorporate it into a complete brunch spread, serve it with my 9-Spice Avocado Hummus Toast (page 39) and Roasted Breakfast Hash (page 53). You can also try serving it with brown rice, Crispy Smashed Potatoes (page 123), or even grilled corn. A dollop of Cashew Sour Cream (page 261) brings the recipe to life and adds cool, tart flavor to an otherwise spicy, savory dish. I love to make these rancheros with my Fresh Cherry Tomato Salsa (page 63), but any store-bought salsa will work in a pinch.

1. In a large skillet or wok, heat the oil over medium heat. Add the onion and sauté for 5 minutes, or until the onion is translucent.

2. Add the bell pepper, jalapeño (if using), and corn and cook for 5 minutes more, or until the peppers soften.

3. Stir in the beans, salsa, cumin, garlic powder and salt. With a fork, lightly mash some of the beans, if desired, leaving most of the beans intact. (This gives it a bit of a refried bean texture, but it's optional.) Cook for 3 to 5 minutes more, until the mixture is heated through and the vegetables are tender. Stir in the coriander just before serving.

4. Warm the tortillas just before serving, if desired (see Tip).

5. Divide the bean mixture among the tortillas, and serve with sliced avocado, salsa, and coriander. Squeeze some fresh lime juice on top of each tortilla.

6. Store any leftover bean mixture in an airtight container in the fridge for up to 3 days, or you can freeze the rancheros for up to 1 month. Simply assemble each ranchero in a wrap, wrap it in a layer of parchment paper and foil, and place in a freezer bag. To thaw, remove the foil-wrapped rancheros from the bag and place in a 400°F (200°C) oven for 20 to 25 minutes, flipping halfway through, until warmed throughout.

Make it grain-free Omit the sweetcorn kernels and corn or flour tortillas, and use a lettuce wrap instead.

1 tablespoon extra-virgin olive oil

1 small onion, diced (about 225g)

1 red bell pepper, sliced into thin strips

1 medium jalapeño, seeded and minced (optional)

175g frozen or fresh sweetcorn

1 400g can black beans, drained and rinsed, or 255g cooked black beans

125ml Fresh Cherry Tomato Salsa (page 63), plus more for serving

1 teaspoon ground cumin

1 teaspoon garlic powder, or to taste

1/2 to 3/4 teaspoon fine sea salt, to taste

50g fresh coriander, roughly chopped, plus more for garnish

6 medium or 8 small corn or flour tortillas

1 large avocado, pitted and sliced

Fresh lime juice, for serving

Tip To warm tortillas in the oven, preheat the oven to 350°F (180°C) and wrap up to 6 tortillas in aluminum foil. Place them directly on the oven rack and heat for 15 to 20 minutes, until warmed through. To warm the tortillas in the microwave, place up to 6 tortillas on a large plate and cover with a damp paper towel. Microwave in 20-second intervals until the tortillas are warmed to your liking. Last, you can reheat the tortillas on the hob by placing a single tortilla in a dry frying pan and heating it over medium heat for about 30 seconds on each side.

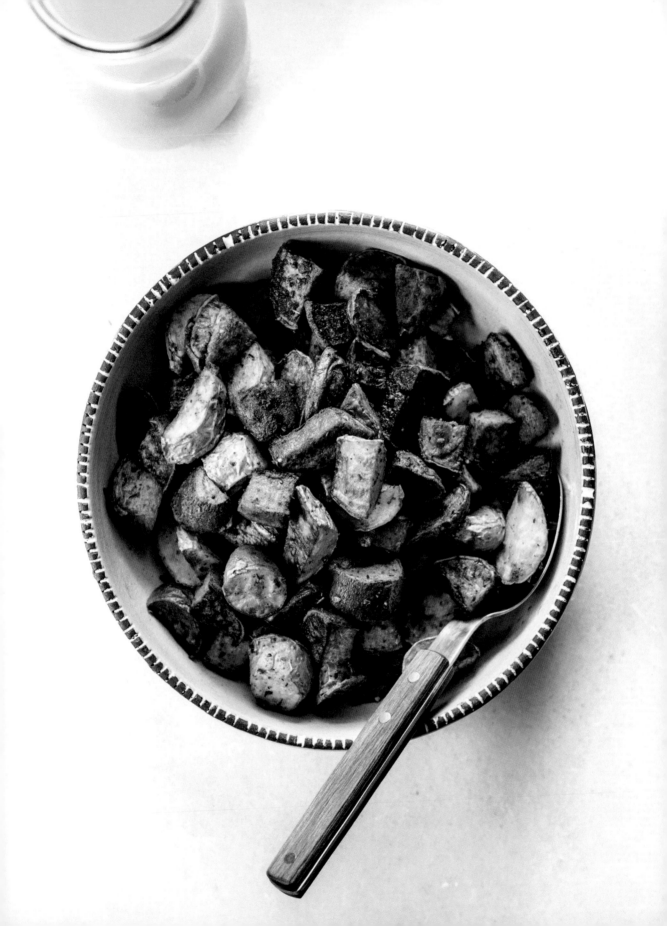

Roasted Breakfast Hash

VEGAN, GLUTEN-FREE, NUT-FREE, SOYA-FREE, GRAIN-FREE, KID-FRIENDLY

SERVES 6 AS A SIDE DISH

PREP TIME: **10 MINUTES**

COOK TIME: **25 TO 35 MINUTES**

I created this easy, roasted potato hash as a side dish option for my Black Bean Rancheros (page 51) and 9-Spice Avocado Hummus Toast (page 39). If you're looking to serve a fabulous brunch, serve all three recipes together along with my Green Matcha Mango Ginger Smoothie (page 17) or Morning Detox Smoothie (page 11). My 9-Spice Mix gives this hash a sweet and smoky flavour, and the textures of the creamy sweet potatoes and the crispy, buttery new potatoes work together beautifully. For a decadent topping, try serving this with my Avocado Coriander Crema (see page 165). If you can't find fingerling potatoes, feel free to use Yukon Gold or red potatoes instead.

450g sweet potatoes, unpeeled, cut into 1cm chunks or cubes

450g small new potatoes, unpeeled, cut into 1cm chunks or cubes

40ml extra-virgin olive oil or avocado oil

1 tablespoon 9-Spice Mix (page 258)

½ teaspoon garlic powder

½ to ¾ teaspoon fine sea salt, to taste

1. Preheat the oven to 425°F (220°C). Line a large rimmed baking sheet with parchment paper.

2. Place the potatoes in a large bowl and toss with the oil. Sprinkle on the 9-Spice Mix, garlic powder and salt and stir to combine.

3. Spoon the potatoes onto the baking sheet and spread them into an even layer, making sure they don't overlap.

4. Roast the potatoes for 15 minutes, flip, and roast for 10 to 20 minutes more, until fork-tender and lightly charred on the bottoms. Serve immediately.

Smoky Sweet Potato Breakfast Hash Use 900g chopped unpeeled sweet potatoes (omit the fingerling potatoes) and replace the 9-Spice Mix with the following spices: 1½ teaspoons smoked paprika, 1 teaspoon ground coriander, ½ teaspoon ground cumin, ½ teaspoon garlic powder, ½ to ¾ teaspoon salt, to taste, and ¼ teaspoon cayenne pepper. Top with chopped fresh coriander and fresh lime juice.

Curried Roasted Potatoes Use 900g chopped unpeeled Yukon Gold, fingerling or red potatoes and replace the 9-Spice Mix with 1 tablespoon good-quality curry powder (I love Simply Organic brand).

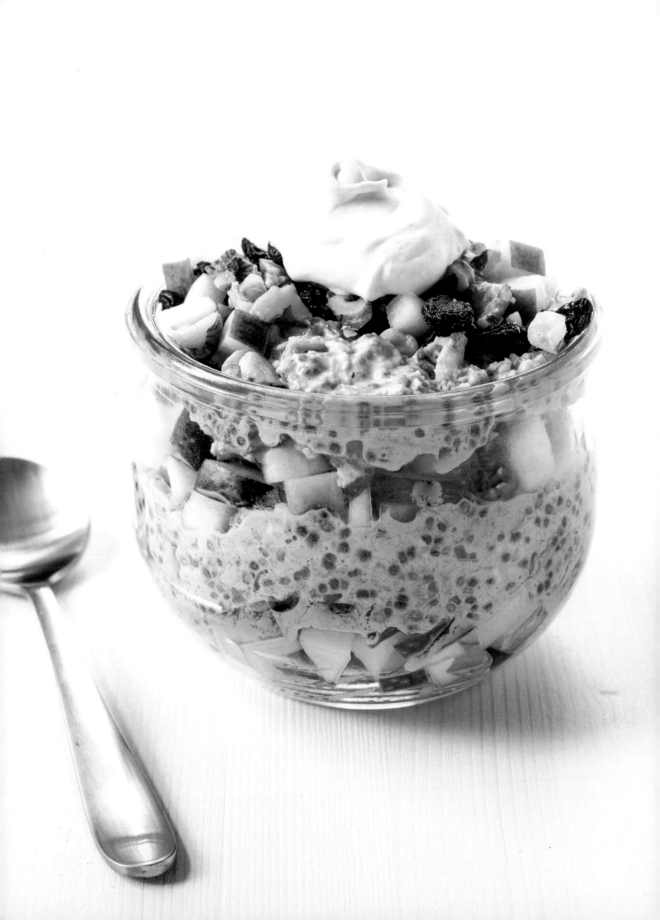

Apple Pie Overnight Oats

VEGAN, GLUTEN-FREE, NUT-FREE OPTION, SOYA-FREE, OIL-FREE, ADVANCE
PREP REQUIRED, KID-FRIENDLY

SERVES 2 OR 3

SOAK TIME: **OVERNIGHT, OR FOR A
MINIMUM OF 1 HOUR**

PREP TIME: **10 MINUTES**

This recipe tastes like a freshly baked apple pie, while still being incredibly nutritious and light. I soak the oat mixture overnight and serve it
chilled. If you've never tried oats this way before, expect to fall in love
with their soft, creamy texture and incredible convenience. I love that
overnight oats let me enjoy all the heartiness and texture of oatmeal
while also keeping cool; they're a perfect breakfast option for summer
months. This recipe is great for August and September, when apples are
just coming into season but the temperature is still too warm for a
piping-hot breakfast. I especially love Honeycrisp apples in this recipe—
their sweet and tangy flavour complements the cool oats and hints of
cinnamon and maple syrup perfectly. If you're truly not a fan of cool
oats, don't worry: You can heat this up and enjoy it warm, too. If you
have some on hand, my Coffee Shop-Worthy Hazelnut Milk (page 35) is
superb as a substitute for regular almond milk!

1. In a medium bowl, stir together the oats, milk, maple syrup, cinnamon,
vanilla, salt, grated apple and chia seeds until thoroughly combined.
Taste and season with allspice and ginger. Cover and refrigerate for a
minimum of 1 to 2 hours, or up to overnight. The mixture will thicken
and the oats will soften. If the mixture is too thick for your liking, you can
add a splash or two of almond milk and stir until combined.

2. Portion into bowls and add your desired toppings. Serve chilled, or
reheat it in a saucepan on the hop and serve warm, if you prefer.
Leftovers will keep in an airtight container in the fridge for a few days.

Make it nut-free Swap the almond milk for nut-free milk and the pecans
or walnuts for toasted pumpkin seeds.

For Banana Bread Overnight Oats Mash 1 large or 2 small spotty banana(s)
and use them in place of the apple. Omit the ground allspice and ginger
and add a dash of ground nutmeg instead.

FOR THE OVERNIGHT OATS

85g gluten-free rolled oats

375ml unsweetened almond milk,
plus more as needed

1 tablespoon pure maple syrup

½ to 1 teaspoon ground cinnamon,
to taste

½ teaspoon pure vanilla extract

Small pinch of fine sea salt

1 large Honeycrisp or Gala apple,
unpeeled, grated

3 tablespoons chia seeds

Ground allspice

Ground ginger

TOPPING SUGGESTIONS

Raisins or chopped dates

Ground cinnamon

Chopped walnuts or pecans

Diced apple

Drizzle of pure maple syrup

Coconut Whipped Cream (page 275)

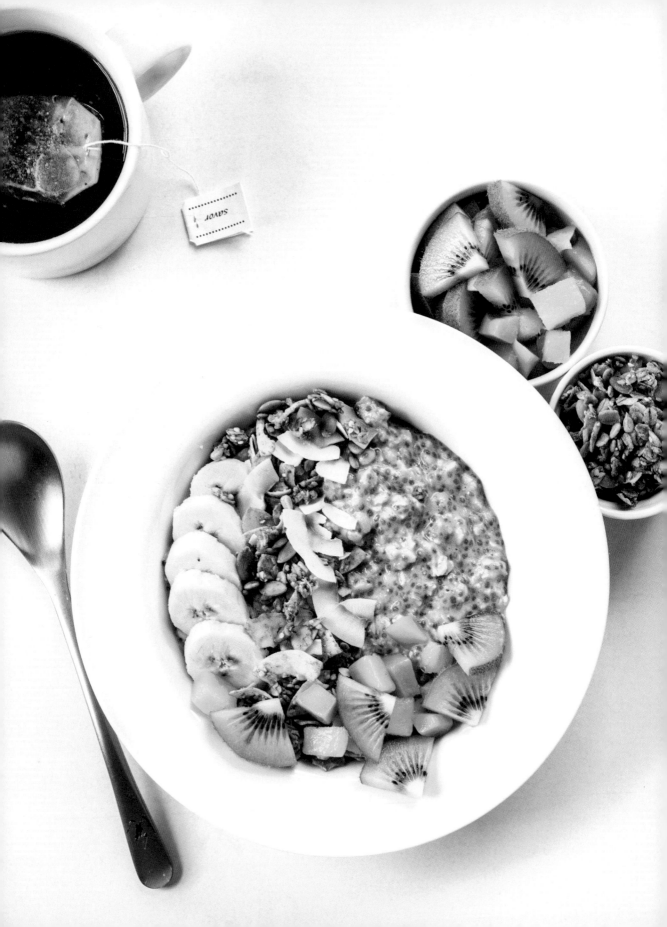

Tropical Overnight Oats

VEGAN, GLUTEN-FREE, NUT-FREE, SOYA-FREE, OIL-FREE,
ADVANCE PREP REQUIRED

SERVES 3

SOAK TIME: **OVERNIGHT, OR FOR A
MINIMUM OF 1 HOUR**

PREP TIME: **10 MINUTES**

This is an ultra-creamy, tropical twist on overnight oats. Rather than adding almond milk to the oat and chia base, here I blend together light coconut milk, banana, and dates. The result is a decadent 'milk' bursting with tropical, summery flavours. I love the way a combination of oats and chia seeds creates texture in this creamy bowl, and I especially love that the chia seeds give the recipe a boost of protein and calcium. Throw this breakfast together before bed and wake up to a playful, sweet and energizing morning meal. If you love the coconut-banana-date milk as much as I do, you may find yourself sipping it on its own for a sweet treat!

1. In a high-speed blender, combine the coconut milk, banana, pitted dates and salt. Blend on high until smooth.

2. Pour the coconut milk mixture into a medium bowl or a medium-size food storage container with a lid.

3. Stir the oats and chia seeds into the coconut milk mixture until thoroughly combined. Cover and refrigerate overnight, or for at least 1 hour. The oat mixture will thicken and soften.

4. Stir the oats after chilling. If the oat mixture is too thick for your liking, thin it out with a bit of coconut milk or almond milk and stir again.

5. Portion the oats into bowls and add your desired toppings, or layer the oats and toppings in glass jars. Serve immediately. Leftovers will keep in an airtight container in the fridge for up to a few days.

Tip If you plan on eating this recipe after only 1 hour of chilling, be sure to refrigerate your can of coconut milk before making this recipe. This will help the oats chill faster.

FOR THE OVERNIGHT OATS

1 400ml can light coconut milk, plus more if needed

1 large ripe banana, peeled

3 large Medjool dates, pitted

Small pinch of fine sea salt

85g gluten-free rolled oats

3 tablespoons chia seeds

Almond or coconut milk (optional)

TOPPING SUGGESTIONS

Sliced banana, kiwi and mango

Unsweetened large-flake or shredded coconut, toasted, if preferred

Vanilla Super-Seed Granola with Coconut Chips (page 33)

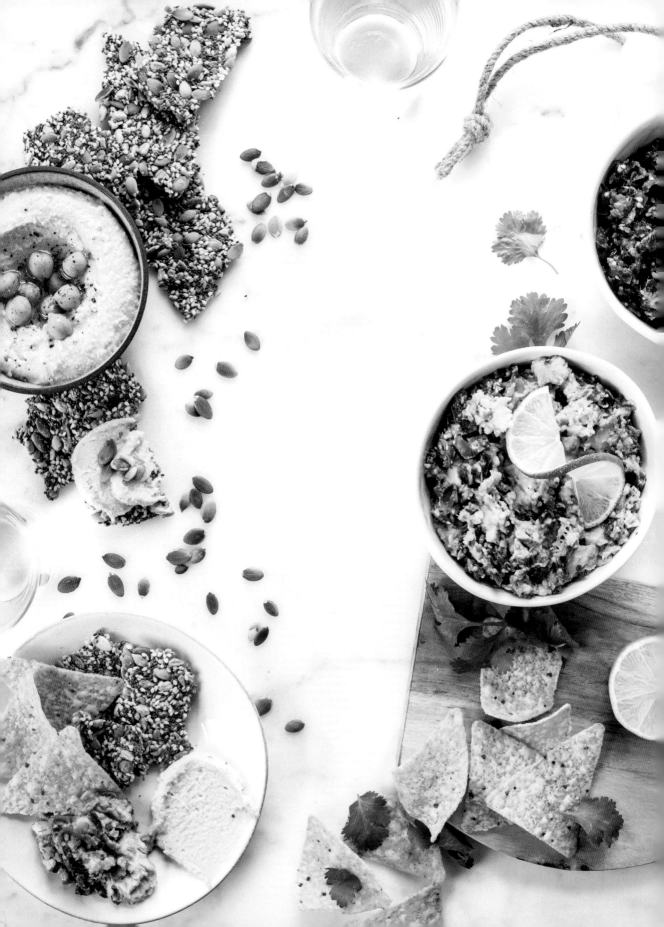

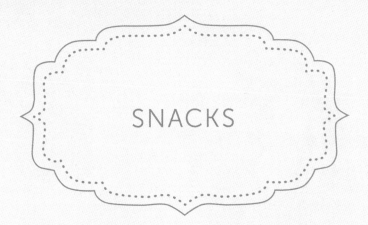

SNACKS

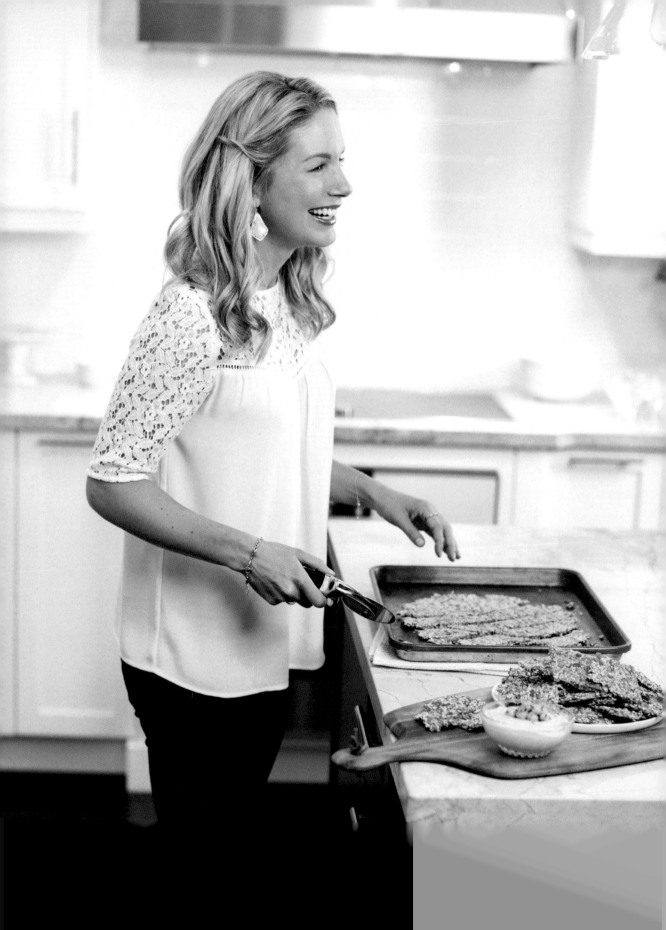

I TRIED A JUICE CLEANSE once. After chugging my first green juice of the day, it seemed easy enough. *I so got this*, I thought. But the hours passed ever so slowly, and after what felt like years I looked at the clock and it read eleven a.m. *How do people do this!?* I thought. *I can't even think straight.* After four torturous hours, my juice cleanse came to an abrupt end. What can I say? I love to eat!

Now that I'm a parent, I appreciate snacks even more, and I find myself trying to come up with wholesome snacks my daughter will love, too. Plus, snacks are a great way to power yourself through a busy day when four to six hours between meals just won't cut it. I've included a mix of savoury and lightly sweetened treats to suit any occasion or craving. On the sweeter side of things, my Coconut Chia Seed Pudding, Roasted Hazelnut-Almond Granola Clusters, and Cookie Dough Balls V are delicious, and portable, too. My Mocha Empower Glo Bars, which were a best-selling Glo Bar in Glo Bakery, are easy to wrap up individually and toss into your bag when you're running out the door in the morning; they also store well in the freezer, so feel free to make a double or triple batch!

For savoury options, try my Sun-Dried Tomato and Garlic Super-Seed Crackers or Endurance Crackers with Fresh Cherry Tomato Salsa and The Freshest Guacamole, Roasted Garlic and Sun-Dried Tomato Hummus or Every Day Lemon-Garlic Hummus. Wholegrain toast topped with my Berry Chia Seed Jam (page 43), sliced banana and Homemade Sunflower Seed Butter is always an easy option (for a quick breakfast, too), and both condiments keep well in the fridge.

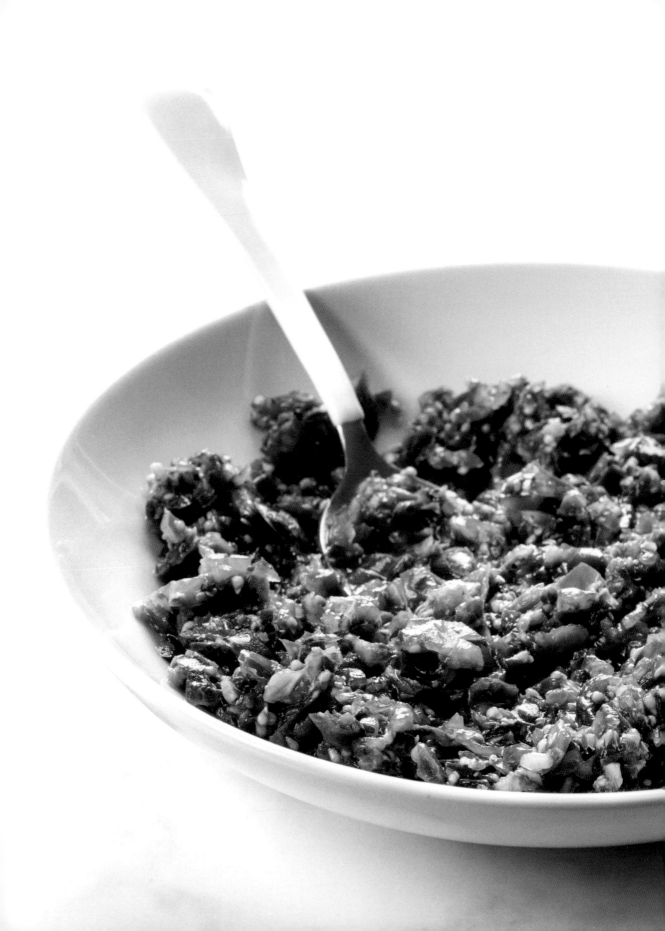

Fresh Cherry Tomato Salsa

VEGAN, GLUTEN-FREE, NUT-FREE, SOYA-FREE, GRAIN-FREE, KID-FRIENDLY

MAKES 625ML

PREP TIME: **15 MINUTES**

REST TIME: **30 MINUTES**

This fresh, no-cook salsa is a cinch to whip up! After testing countless batches of fresh salsa that were just too watery, I came up with an easy trick to create the perfect texture. All you have to do is put the processed tomato mixture in a colander in the sink, salt it well and let it sit for half an hour. A lot of the water will drain off into the sink, resulting in a much less watery fresh salsa. It's life-changing! Be sure to see The Freshest Guacamole (page 65) for instructions on how to easily turn this salsa into mouth-watering guacamole. Both recipes are great to serve at gatherings along with corn chips or even my 9-Spice Super-Seed Crackers (page 82). This salsa is also delicious with Black Bean Rancheros (page 51), Ultimate Green Taco Wraps (page 191) and Stuffed Avocado Salad (page 109). Feel free to substitute grape or hothouse tomatoes instead of cherry tomatoes at a pinch. If you aren't a big coriander fan, you can either adjust the amount to your taste or try swapping it for fresh parsley.

1. Mince the garlic in a food processor. Add the spring onions, jalapeño and coriander. Process until finely chopped.

2. Add the tomatoes and pulse until the mixture is chunky, or pulse longer if you prefer a smoother salsa.

3. Spoon the salsa into a fine-mesh colander placed in the sink. Add ½ teaspoon (2ml) of the salt on top of the salsa and gently stir to combine. Let the salsa drain in the colander for 30 minutes. Stir it every now and then to help it drain.

4. Transfer the salsa to a medium bowl and stir in lime juice, oil, pepper, and red pepper flakes to taste. I also like to give it a generous dusting of Herbamare to enhance the flavor even more. This fresh salsa is best enjoyed the same day, but it'll stay fresh in an airtight container in the fridge for 24 to 48 hours.

1 large clove garlic, or more to taste

2 spring onions, roughly chopped

1 jalapeño, seeded, if desired (leave the seeds in for more heat)

15g fresh coriander leaves

675g cherry tomatoes

½ to ¾ teaspoon fine sea salt, to taste

3 to 4 teaspoons fresh lime juice, to taste

1½ teaspoons to 1 tablespoon extra-virgin olive oil, to taste

Freshly ground black pepper

Red pepper flakes

Herbamare (see page 307) or fine sea salt, for seasoning (optional)

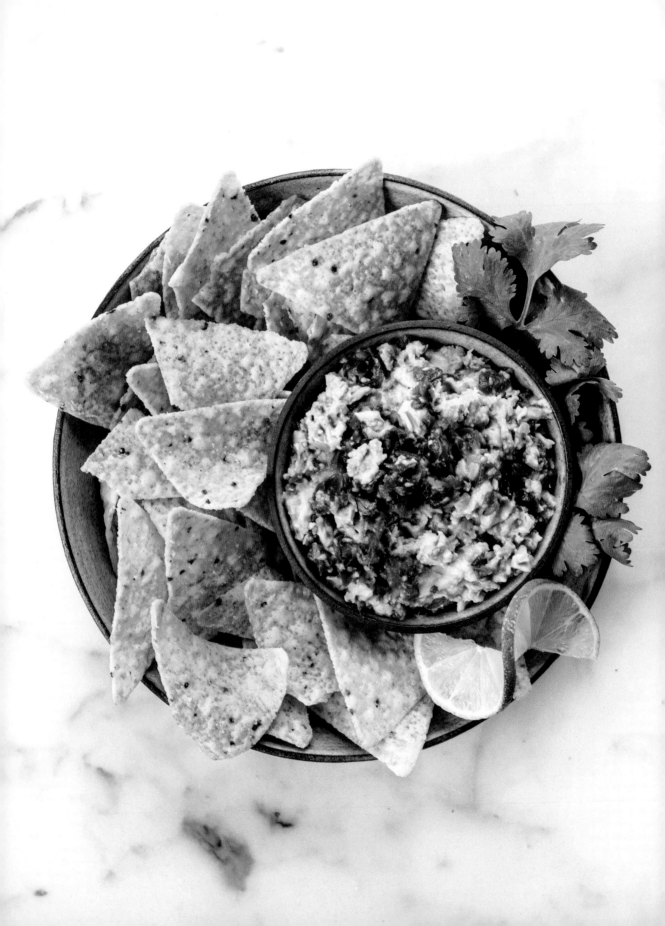

The Freshest Guacamole

VEGAN, GLUTEN-FREE, NUT-FREE, SOYA-FREE, GRAIN-FREE, ADVANCE PREP REQUIRED

MAKES 375ML

PREP TIME: **5 MINUTES**

This is my go-to guacamole. I whip it up whenever I have a batch of my Fresh Cherry Tomato Salsa (page 63) on hand. Just fold the salsa into the creamy avocados and season to taste—that's it! The resulting guacamole is incredibly flavourful and fresh, and cherry tomatoes make it a little sweeter and more summery than traditional guacamole mixes. I usually enjoy it with corn chips, but it's also great to spread on a wrap, rice crackers or toast, or to scoop on top of a salad or baked potatoes for a fun twist. There are just so many exciting ways to enjoy homemade guacamole!

1. In a medium bowl, mash the avocado until it reaches your desired consistency.

2. Fold in the salsa and season with Herbamare and lime juice, to taste. Guacamole is best when you eat it immediately, or within a few hours, since the avocado oxidizes quickly. You can get a bit more life out of it if you store the guacamole with the pit in an airtight container in the fridge.

2 large ripe avocados, pitted

125 to 175ml Fresh Cherry Tomato Salsa (page 63), to taste

Herbamare (see page 307) or fine sea salt

Fresh lime juice

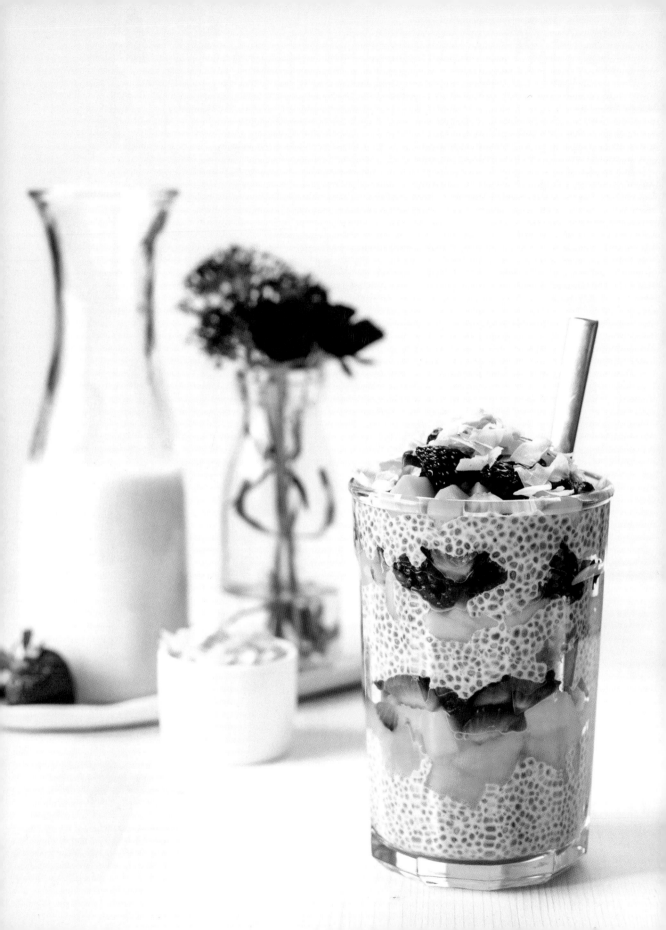

Coconut Chia Seed Pudding

VEGAN, GLUTEN-FREE, NUT-FREE, SOYA-FREE, GRAIN-FREE, OIL-FREE,
ADVANCE PREP REQUIRED, KID-FRIENDLY OPTION, FREEZER-FRIENDLY
MAKES 4 PARFAITS

PREP TIME: **15 MINUTES**

CHILL TIME: **MINIMUM 3 HOURS OR OVERNIGHT**

Chia seed pudding is so easy to prepare, and it's bursting with nutrients like calcium, iron, protein, and omega-3 fatty acids. When chia seeds are soaked in liquid, they expand and develop a gel-like texture. This results in a thick, tapioca-like pudding in just a few hours and without any heat. I love making parfaits with my chia pudding creations, and this is one of my favourite flavour combinations: coconut, strawberry and mango with a bit of lime or lemon zest for a refreshing kick! It keeps in the fridge for a couple of days, so you can have it handy for snacking on the go; just throw some into a small Mason jar before you leave the house. I recently discovered that you can freeze chia pudding, too. So if you don't plan to eat it within a few days, simply follow the instructions for freezing.

1. Make the chia seed pudding In a large Mason jar or bowl, whisk together the coconut milk, chia seeds, maple syrup, vanilla and salt until thoroughly combined. Screw on the lid or cover with plastic wrap and refrigerate for at least 3 hours or overnight, until thickened. Whisk the mixture two or three times during the chill time so the chia seeds don't clump together.

2. Preheat the oven to 300°F (150°C). Spread the coconut flakes over a small baking sheet. Toast in the oven for 3 to 6 minutes, until lightly golden and fragrant. Be careful not to burn them. Let cool.

3. Make the parfaits Grab four 250ml Mason jars or parfait glasses. Fill the jars or glasses with alternating layers of the chia pudding, mango and strawberries. (You will use about 80g of chia pudding per parfait.) Repeat until each jar or glass is filled to about 1cm from the top. Sprinkle 1 tablespoon of the toasted coconut on top of each, then drizzle on some maple syrup and sprinkle with fresh lime zest, if desired. Enjoy immediately or cover and store in the fridge for up to 2 days. You can also throw it into a freezer bag, push out as much air as possible, and seal. Freeze on a flat surface in the freezer for up to 1 month. Thaw in the fridge and enjoy as usual.

Tip If your chia pudding is still too runny after sitting overnight, stir in another tablespoon or two of chia seeds and let it chill for another hour or so.

FOR THE CHIA SEED PUDDING (MAKES 500ML

1 400ml can light coconut milk

45g chia seeds

2 tablespoons pure maple syrup, or to taste

½ teaspoon pure vanilla extract, or 1 vanilla pod, seeds scraped, or ½ teaspoon vanilla powder

Dash of fine sea salt

FOR THE PARFAITS

20g large-flake coconut or Vanilla Super-Seed Granola with Coconut Chips (page 33)

2 Ataulfo mangoes, pitted, peeled, and chopped (about 530g chopped mango)

300g chopped fresh strawberries

Drizzle of pure maple syrup (optional)

Fresh lime or lemon zest, for garnish (optional)

Make it kid-friendly Serve sliced fruit alongside the chia pudding so kids can scoop up the pudding with the fruit.

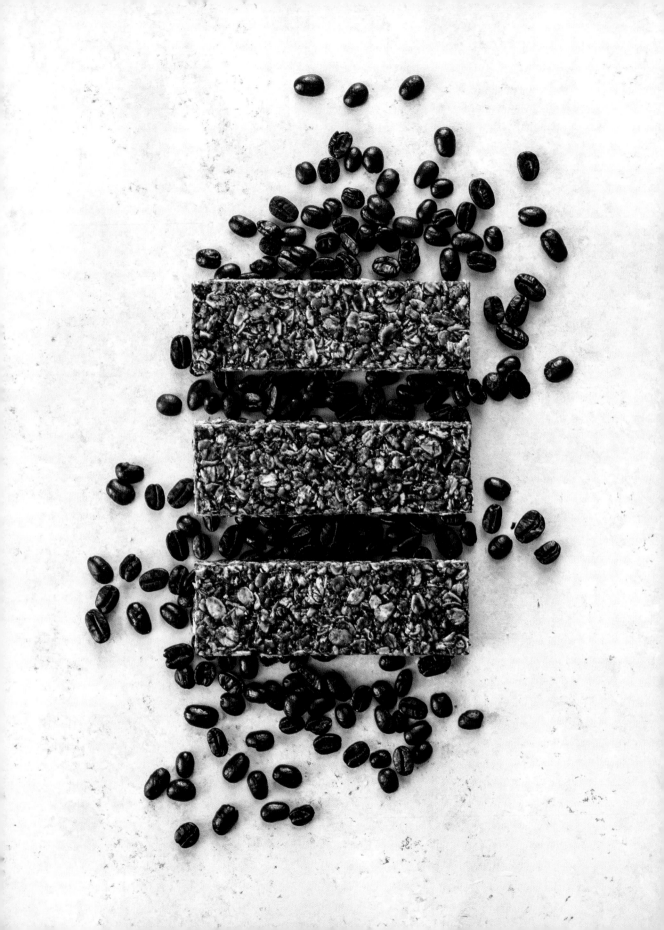

Mocha Empower Glo Bars

VEGAN, GLUTEN-FREE, SOYA-FREE OPTION, KID-FRIENDLY OPTION,
FREEZER-FRIENDLY

MAKES 12 BARS

PREP TIME: **15 MINUTES**

BAKE TIME: **6 TO 9 MINUTES**

CHILL TIME: **10 TO 15 MINUTES**

These bars have the perfect balance of sweet and salty flavour and crunchy, chewy texture. The real secret, though, is their mild coffee flavour and aroma, which pair perfectly with roasted almond butter and chocolate. They make for a perfect grab-and-go snack to enjoy with a coffee. When I ran Glo Bakery, this was a best-selling Glo Bar—it often sold out within an hour! I prefer to use freshly ground coffee beans for the best flavour. Caffeinated or decaf, it's your choice.

1. Preheat the oven to 325°F (160°C). Line a 23cm square pan with two pieces of parchment paper, one going each way.

2. Spread the almonds over a small baking sheet and toast in the oven for 6 to 9 minutes, until lightly golden in some spots. Transfer to a plate and let cool.

3. Grind the coffee beans in a coffee grinder until a fine powder forms. If you don't have a coffee grinder, you may be able to do this in a blender. Just make sure the beans are ground very fine.

4. In a large bowl, stir together the ground coffee, oats, cereal, chocolate chips, shredded coconut and salt.

5. In a small pot, stir together the brown rice syrup, almond butter, and coconut oil until combined. Bring the mixture to a low simmer over low heat, stirring carefully and being careful not to burn it, then remove from the heat. Stir in the vanilla.

6. Add the toasted almonds to the dry ingredients and stir. Immediately pour the brown rice syrup mixture over the dry ingredients and stir until the oats are fully coated in the syrup mixture. This can take some elbow grease, but it's worth it so you don't have dry patches. The chocolate chips will melt during this process to create a uniform chocolate flavour in the bars.

7. Scoop the mixture into the prepared pan and spread it out evenly with lightly wet hands or a spoon. Grab a rolling pin, if you have one, and roll out the mixture until even and smooth. Or simply press down firmly with your hands—the more you pack down the mixture, the better the bars hold together. Using your fingertips, press the mixture in along the edges to create straight edges.

35g chopped raw almonds

2 heaped tablespoons dark roast coffee beans (you can use decaf beans, if preferred)

115g gluten-free rolled oats

25g crispy rice cereal (not puffed rice)

40g non-dairy chocolate chips

20g unsweetened shredded coconut

¼ teaspoon fine sea salt

125ml brown rice syrup

60ml smooth Roasted Almond Butter (see page 75)

2 teaspoons virgin coconut oil

1 teaspoon pure vanilla extract

Make it soya-free Use soya-free non-dairy chocolate chips, such as Enjoy Life brand.

Make it kid-friendly Use decaf coffee beans, or simply omit the coffee altogether.

(recipe continues)

8. Place the pan in the freezer, uncovered, for 10 to 15 minutes, until the bars firm up enough to slice. With a pizza slice, slice the block into 12 bars. Wrap the leftover bars in plastic wrap and store in an airtight container in the fridge for up to 1 week or in the freezer for up to 4 weeks. The bars will firm up when chilled. You can let them sit at room temperature for 5 to 10 minutes before enjoying, if a softer texture is desired.

Roasted Hazelnut-Almond Granola Clusters

VEGAN, GLUTEN-FREE, SOYA-FREE OPTION, KID-FRIENDLY, FREEZER-FRIENDLY

MAKES 1.5 TO 1.75L

PREP TIME: **20 MINUTES**

BAKE TIME: **30 TO 36 MINUTES**

Oh, this granola. It has become an obsession for me and for Eric, who loves it as much as I do. The first time I made it, I knew it had to go into this book. It's stolen the hearts of everyone who has tried it, from my recipe testers to family and friends. The granola is brimming with fragrant toasted hazelnuts and almonds, and it's studded with chocolate chips and dried cherries. Binding it all together is a decadent mixture of maple syrup, coconut oil and my homemade Roasted Hazelnut-Almond Butter (page 77), which brings out the naturally nutty flavour of the granola. If you don't want to make the Roasted Hazelnut-Almond Butter, you can substitute raw or roasted almond butter (page 75) in at a pinch. Hard as it is not to keep this granola all to yourself, it makes a lovely homemade gift, too. Just allow it to cool completely and then fill up a Mason jar and add a ribbon and tag. It's easy and festive, and your friends and family will be just dying for the recipe!

1. Preheat the oven to 300°F (150°C). Spread the hazelnuts over a small baking sheet and the almonds over another small baking sheet. Put both in the oven and roast for 12 to 14 minutes, until the hazelnut skins have darkened, cracked, and are almost falling off. Let the nuts cool on the sheet for 5 minutes or so. Transfer the hazelnuts to a damp tea towel and rub vigorously until most of the skins fall off. The goal is to remove most of them, but a few stragglers are okay! Chop the hazelnuts and almonds and set aside.

2. Line a large baking sheet with parchment paper and keep the oven set to 300°F (150°C).

3. In a large bowl, stir together the chopped hazelnuts and almonds, oats, shredded coconut, chocolate chips, cherries, chia seeds and salt.

4. In a small pot, melt the coconut oil over low heat. Transfer it to a small bowl and whisk in the brown rice syrup, hazelnut-almond butter, maple syrup and vanilla until smooth. (Normally I would just whisk everything into the pot to save a dish, but for this recipe we don't want the wet mixture to become warm and melt the chocolate chips while mixing.)

5. With a spatula, scoop the wet mixture on top of the dry mixture, being sure to get every last drop. Stir well until thoroughly combined.

90g raw hazelnuts

50g raw almonds

115g gluten-free rolled oats

40g unsweetened shredded coconut

70g non-dairy mini chocolate chips

20g dried cherries, finely chopped

2 tablespoons chia seeds

$\frac{1}{4}$ teaspoon plus $\frac{1}{8}$ teaspoon fine sea salt

1 tablespoon virgin coconut oil

$4\frac{1}{2}$ teaspoons brown rice syrup

60ml Roasted Hazelnut-Almond Butter (page 77)

75ml pure maple syrup

2 teaspoons pure vanilla extract

(recipe continues)

6. Scoop the granola mixture onto the prepared baking sheet and spread it out into a thin layer, no more than 5mm to 1cm thickness. Try to space out the granola as much as possible so it has room to 'breathe' while cooking.

7. Bake for 10 minutes, then rotate the pan and bake for 8 to 12 minutes more, until the bottom and edges of the granola are just starting to turn golden (the granola itself will still look a bit pale in colour). The granola will get crispy as it cools.

8. Let the granola cool completely on the baking sheet, then break it apart into clusters. It will keep in an airtight container in the fridge for 3 to 4 weeks or in a large zip-top freezer bag in the freezer for a couple of months. Be sure to press all the air out before freezing (or use a straw to suck out all the air from the bag).

Make it soya-free Use soya-free non-dairy chocolate chips, such as Enjoy Life brand.

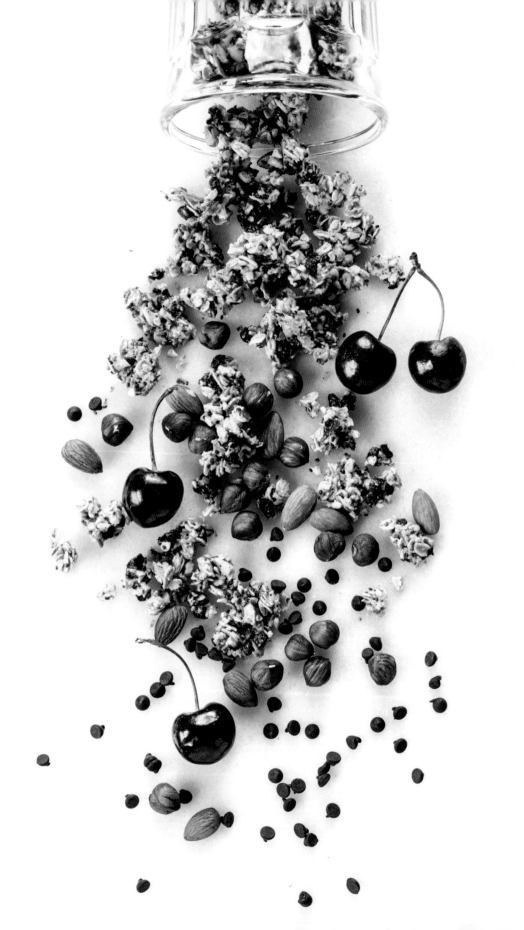

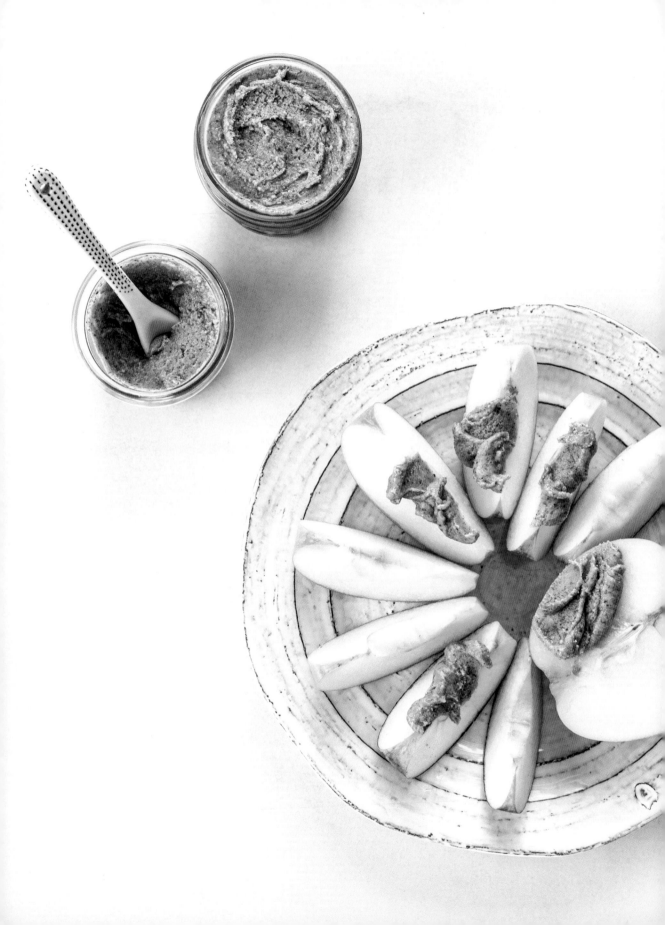

Homemade Almond Butter

VEGAN, GLUTEN-FREE, SOYA-FREE, GRAIN-FREE, OIL-FREE

MAKES 250ML

PREP TIME: **10 MINUTES**

200g raw almonds

Sure, picking up a jar of store-bought almond butter is easy enough (and I do it often!), but I never regret it when I make a fresh batch at home. I recommend using a heavy-duty food processor (see my recommendation on page xv) so that it can handle the hefty processing job. Smaller food processors might overheat or might not be able to get the almonds smooth enough. Use this in The Ultimate Flourless Brownies (page 199), on toast with Berry Chia Seed Jam (page 43), or in a Magical 'Ice Cream' Smoothie Bowl (page 5). The butter has a mild and simple flavour, so it can be added to a huge variety of recipes. See my other nut butter variations below.

1. In a heavy-duty food processor, process the almonds for 8 to 12 minutes, stopping to scrape down the bowl every 30 to 60 seconds as needed. Store the nut butter in an airtight container in the fridge for up to 1 month.

Tip You might be tempted to stop as soon as a butter forms, but if you keep going that extra minute or two you'll be rewarded with silky smooth, 'drippy' almond butter.

For Roasted Almond Butter Preheat the oven to 300°F (150°C). Spread the almonds over a baking sheet and roast for 10 to 14 minutes, until fragrant. Let cool for 5 minutes before proceeding with the recipe. Makes 250ml.

For Raw Cashew Butter Use 200g raw cashews and process for 7 to 10 minutes until a smooth butter forms, stopping to scrape down the bowl as necessary. Makes 250ml.

For Roasted Peanut Butter Use 290g roasted peanuts and process for 5 to 10 minutes until a smooth butter forms, stopping to scrape down the bowl as necessary. Makes 250ml.

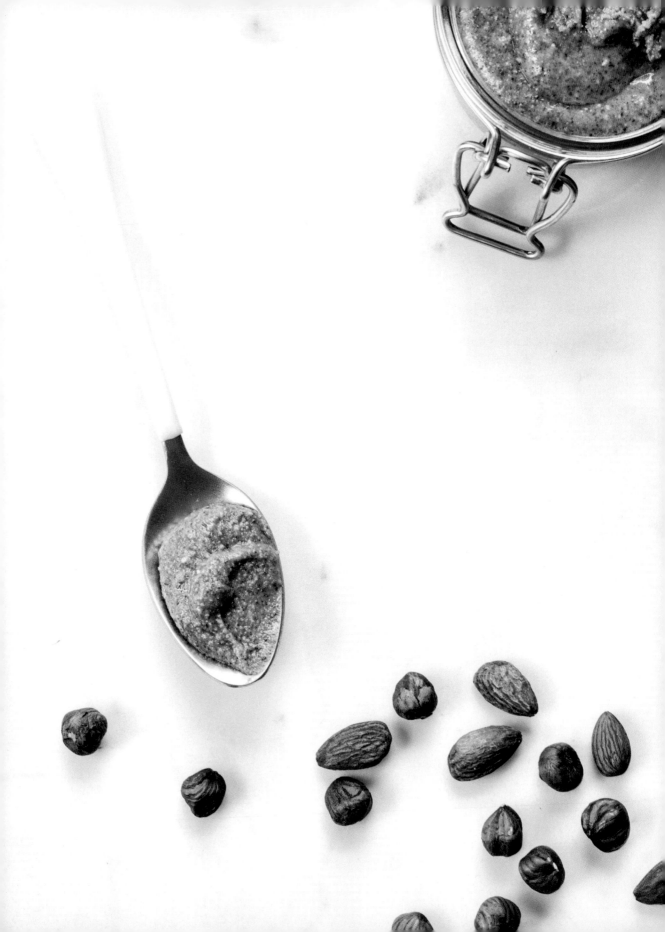

Roasted Hazelnut-Almond Butter

VEGAN, GLUTEN-FREE, SOYA-FREE, GRAIN-FREE, OIL-FREE, KID-FRIENDLY

MAKES 250ML

PREP TIME: **10 MINUTES**

BAKE TIME: **12 TO 14 MINUTES**

This is a delicious take on traditional roasted almond butter. The hazelnuts add a sweet and buttery flavour that goes well with the nutty, mild flavour of the almonds. Use it in my Roasted Hazelnut-Almond Granola Clusters (page 71), or simply spread some on toast with my Berry Chia Seed Jam (page 43).

1. Preheat the oven to 300°F (150°C). Spread the hazelnuts over a small baking sheet and the almonds over another small baking sheet. Put both in the oven and roast for 12 to 14 minutes, until the hazelnut skins have darkened, cracked, and are almost falling off. Let the nuts cool on the sheet for 5 minutes or so. Transfer the hazelnuts to a damp dishcloth and rub vigorously until most of the skins fall off. The goal is to remove most of them, but a few stragglers are okay!

2. Transfer the almonds and skinned hazelnuts to a heavy-duty food processor and process until a smooth butter forms, 5 to 10 minutes, stopping to scrape down the bowl as necessary.

3. With the processor running, slowly add the sugar, vanilla, cinnamon and salt to taste through the feed tube.

4. Store the nut butter in an airtight container in the fridge for up to 1 month.

120g raw hazelnuts

100g raw almonds

3 tablespoons coconut sugar or natural cane sugar, or to taste

½ teaspoon pure vanilla extract

Dash of ground cinnamon

Fine sea salt

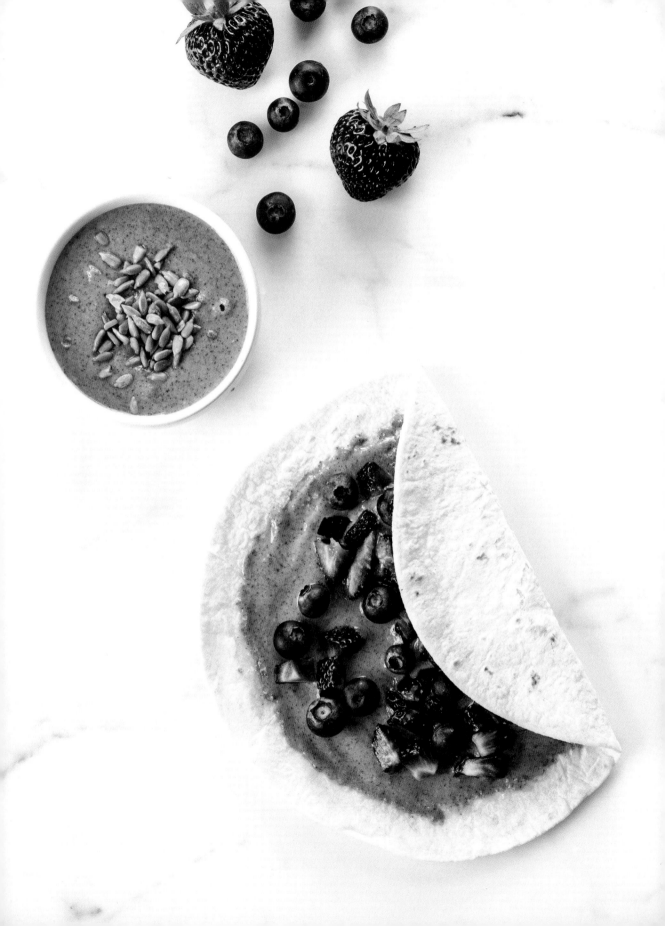

Homemade Sunflower Seed Butter

VEGAN, GLUTEN-FREE, NUT-FREE, SOYA-FREE, GRAIN-FREE, KID-FRIENDLY

MAKES 425ML

PREP TIME: **15 MINUTES**

BAKE TIME: **9 TO 12 MINUTES**

Peanut and almond butter get all the attention, but what about making a superb-tasting sunflower seed butter at home, too? This coconut oil, vanilla bean and sea salt sunflower seed butter is a great alternative to almond or peanut butter, especially if you or your kids suffer from tree nut allergies. I love the sweet, toasted flavour of this seed butter, and you'll see that I use it in a lot of my recipes, such as my Vanilla Super-Seed Granola with Coconut Chips (page 33) and my Nut-Free Dream Bars (page 211). Be sure to roast the sunflower seeds beforehand, which helps break down and release their oils—essential for the butter-making process. As always, when making nut or seed butter, I recommend using a heavy-duty food processor that can withstand the long motor-running time.

400g raw hulled sunflower seeds

50g coconut sugar

2 tablespoons virgin coconut oil, softened, plus more if needed

Pinch of fine sea salt

½ teaspoon ground cinnamon, or to taste (optional)

1 teaspoon pure vanilla extract

1 vanilla pod, seeds scraped, or ¼ teaspoon pure vanilla powder (optional)

1. Preheat the oven to 325°F (160°C). Line a large baking sheet with parchment paper and spread the seeds over the pan in an even layer. Roast for 9 to 12 minutes, until some of the seeds are lightly golden. Let cool for a few minutes before using.

2. In a high-speed blender, grind the sugar into a powder. Leave the lid on and set aside so the 'dust' can settle.

3. Spoon the toasted seeds into a heavy-duty food processor. (I like to spoon the seeds into a measuring cup and transfer them that way. When I have about 70g of seeds left on the pan I will use the parchment paper to 'funnel' the remaining seeds into the processor.)

4. Process the seeds for a few minutes, stopping to scrape down the bowl every minute. They will look dry and powdery at this stage. (If your food processor has a feed tube, leave it open to allow steam to escape.)

5. Add the coconut oil and process for a couple of minutes more. The butter will clump together into a large ball and start rattling around for a bit. The ball will eventually break down into butter again. Stop to scrape down the bowl as needed.

6. Add in the ground sugar, salt and cinnamon (if using). Process for a few minutes more, until smooth. With the motor running, slowly stream in the vanilla extract. Add the vanilla bean seeds, if using. You can add a touch more oil if you need to thin out the butter (but do not add water or liquid sweetener because it will make the butter seize up). I process for a total of 9 to 12 minutes, but timing will vary based on your food processor and texture preference. Some machines may need to run for upward of 15 minutes to get the seed butter smooth enough.

(recipe continues)

7. Transfer the sunflower seed butter to an airtight container and refrigerate. It'll keep for about 2 months, and it will remain 'spreadable' even when chilled.

Tip If for some reason your seeds aren't breaking down after the specified times, add a touch more coconut oil, a teaspoon at a time. Some machines just might need to run a bit longer though, so be patient!

Sun-Dried Tomato and Garlic Super-Seed Crackers

VEGAN, GLUTEN-FREE, NUT-FREE, SOYA-FREE, OIL-FREE, KID-FRIENDLY
OPTION, FREEZER-FRIENDLY

MAKES 35 (5CM SQUARE) CRACKERS

PREP TIME: **20 MINUTES**

BAKE TIME: **53 TO 55 MINUTES**

These elegant, chewy crackers are fit for a high-end bakery! Infused with sun-dried tomatoes, oregano, garlic, oats and a slew of nutritious seeds, they taste like pizza, but they're full of health benefits. The combination of seeds is rich in healthy fatty acids and antioxidants, and the recipe is both gluten-free and tree nut-free. They may look intimidating to make, but they come together incredibly fast and easily. If you've ever been intimidated by rolling out cracker dough, you have to try this recipe; the dough doesn't even require a rolling pin. Simply spread it out with your hands! Try the crackers with my Roasted Garlic and Sun-Dried Tomato Hummus (page 85), Every Day Lemon-Garlic Hummus (page 91), or simply on their own. If you aren't a sun-dried tomato fan, be sure to try out the 9-spice variation or my Endurance Crackers (page 89) instead.

1. Preheat the oven to 300°F (150°C). Line two standard baking sheets (32 × 40cm) or one extra-large baking sheet (38 × 53cm) with parchment paper.

2. Place the sun-dried tomatoes in a bowl and cover with the boiling water. Set aside to soak for 5 to 10 minutes.

3. In a large bowl, stir together the remaining ingredients.

4. With a slotted spoon, scoop the softened sun-dried tomatoes out of the soaking water and transfer to a mini food processor, reserving the soaking water. Process the tomatoes until minced. Alternatively, you can chop the tomatoes by hand—just be sure to chop them very fine so the crackers are easy to slice. Scoop the tomatoes into the bowl with the seed mixture.

5. Add the tomato-soaking water to the bowl with the seed mixture. Stir for about a minute, until the water has been mostly absorbed by the seed mixture and is no longer pooling on the bottom of the bowl.

6. Transfer half the seed mixture to each baking sheet (or if using one extra-large baking sheet, spoon all of it onto the sheet). With your hands, spread the mixture starting in the centre and pushing outward, until you form a large, misshapen rectangle, no more than 5mm thick. The mixture will be very wet, but this is normal. Be sure that the dough is uniform in thickness and the corners aren't too thick.

(recipe continues)

20g sun-dried tomatoes (dry, not oil-packed)

375ml boiling water

140g raw hulled sunflower seeds

85g gluten-free rolled oats

40g hemp hearts

35g raw (pumpkin seeds)

35g white sesame seeds

2 tablespoons (30g) black sesame seeds or more white sesame seeds

2 tablespoons whole chia seeds

3 tablespoons ground chia seeds

1¼ teaspoons garlic powder

1 large clove garlic, grated on a Microplane

2 teaspoons dried oregano

1 teaspoon coconut sugar or natural cane sugar

1 teaspoon dried basil

¾ teaspoon fine sea salt, or to taste

⅛ teaspoon cayenne pepper, or to taste (optional)

7. Bake for 30 minutes. Remove the baking sheet(s) and using a pizza slicer, carefully slice the dough into large crackers. Carefully flip each cracker using a spatula or your hands. Don't worry if a couple break here and there! If for some reason the crackers are sticking to the parchment paper, just leave them as they are and remove them after the second bake.

8. Return the baking sheet(s) to the oven and bake for 23 to 25 minutes more, until the crackers are golden. Watch closely during the last 5 to 10 minutes of baking to ensure they don't burn. Remove from the oven and let cool on the baking sheet(s) for 5 minutes. Transfer the crackers to a couple of cooling racks and let cool completely. Store the cooled crackers in a paper bag on the counter for up to 1 week. You can also store them in an airtight container in the fridge for up to 1 week or in a freezer-safe zip-top bag in the freezer for 3 to 4 weeks. If the crackers soften while storing (this can happen in humid environments), toast in the oven at 300°F (150°C) for 5 to 7 minutes, then let cool completely. This is usually enough to return them to their former crispness!

Tip To make ground chia seed, in a high-speed blender, grind 40g chia seeds on high until a fine powder forms. Store any unused ground chia seed in the fridge in an airtight container.

Make it kid-friendly Serve my Roasted Garlic and Sun-Dried Tomato Hummus (page 85) with these crackers for dipping.

For 9-Spice Super-Seed Crackers Omit the sun-dried tomatoes and use 375ml room-temperature water (it doesn't have to be boiling since we're not soaking the tomatoes any more). Swap the garlic powder, garlic clove, oregano, basil, salt and cayenne for 1 batch (about 2 tablespoons) of my 9-Spice Mix (page 258). Proceed as directed.

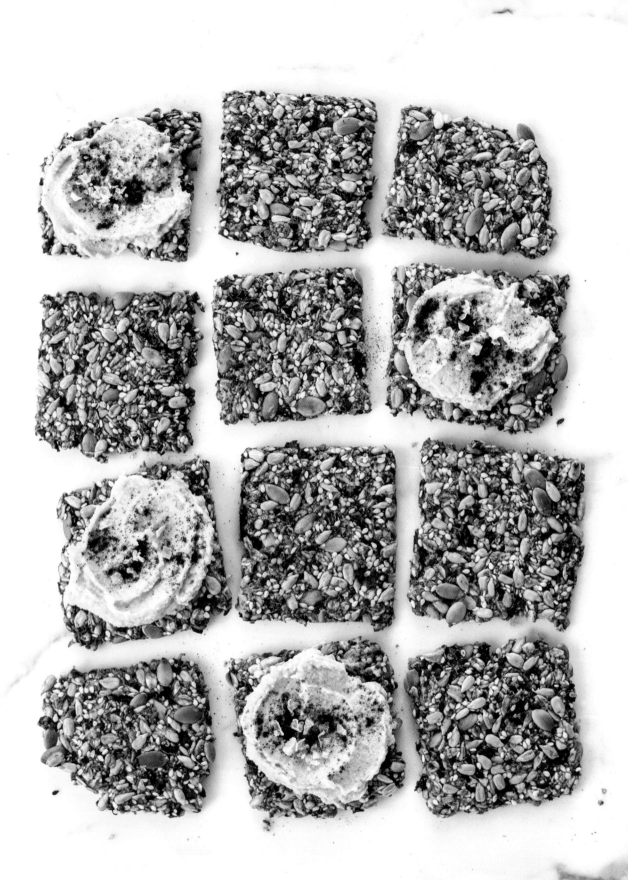

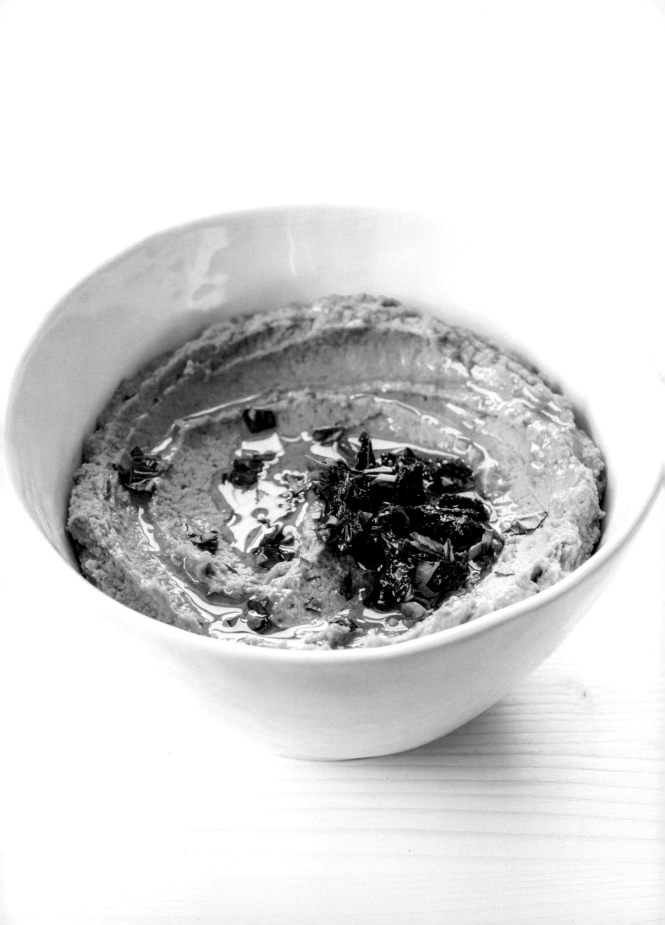

Roasted Garlic and Sun-Dried Tomato Hummus

VEGAN, GLUTEN-FREE, NUT-FREE, SOYA-FREE, GRAIN-FREE, KID-FRIENDLY

MAKES 500ML

PREP TIME: **15 MINUTES**

COOK TIME: **35 TO 40 MINUTES**

This hummus recipe combines a magical flavour combination—roasted garlic and sun-dried tomatoes. When tomatoes are sun-dried, their flavour concentrates and intensifies, producing a salty and slightly sweet, intense tomato flavour. Roasting removes garlic's pungent, sharp bite and leaves behind a sweet, caramelized, buttery flavour that's great on garlic bread or mixed into pasta sauces, hummus, soups and more. When you roast garlic, you can also eat much more of it without digestive upset (for those who are sensitive to it when consumed raw). Serve this creamy hummus with pitta bread, Sun-Dried Tomato and Garlic Super-Seed Crackers (page 81), or crudités. It's also lovely on a wrap or sandwich!

1. Preheat the oven to 425°F (220°C).

2. Peel off the outer layers of skin from the garlic heads, leaving the skin on the individual cloves. Slice off 5mm to 1cm from the top of each head to expose the individual cloves. If your knife misses a couple of cloves, just use a paring knife to cut the tips off.

3. Set each head on its own piece of aluminium foil and drizzle about ½ teaspoon of the extra-virgin olive oil on top of each, making sure to cover each exposed clove. Wrap the garlic heads in the foil and place them directly on the oven rack or on a small baking sheet.

4. Roast in the oven for 35 to 40 minutes, until the cloves are golden and very soft.

5. Let cool slightly, then carefully unwrap and let cool further. Once cool enough to handle, gently squeeze the garlic cloves out of the skins. You should have a scant 60ml of roasted garlic cloves.

6. In a food processor, mince the sun-dried tomatoes. Add half the roasted garlic cloves, olive oil, lemon juice, tahini and chickpeas. Process again, scraping down the bowl as necessary. Taste and add the remaining roasted garlic cloves if desired (you know I do!).

7. Add the water as needed to thin the hummus to your desired consistency, and finally add the salt and cayenne (if using). Process again. Let the machine run for at least a minute to get the hummus really smooth.

8. Spoon into a serving bowl and garnish with a drizzle of olive oil, fresh basil and finely chopped sun-dried tomatoes. Serve with crackers, crudités, or fresh bread.

FOR THE HUMMUS

2 medium garlic heads

1 teaspoon extra-virgin olive oil

15g oil-packed sun-dried tomatoes, drained

2 tablespoons sun-dried tomato olive oil or light-tasting olive oil

2 tablespoons plus 1 teaspoon fresh lemon juice, or to taste

2 tablespoons tahini

1 400g can chickpeas, drained and rinsed, or 250g cooked chickpeas

2 to 3 tablespoons water, or as needed to thin

½ to ¾ teaspoon fine sea salt, to taste

Dash of cayenne pepper (optional)

FOR SERVING

Olive oil, for drizzling

Finely chopped oil-packed sun-dried tomatoes

Minced fresh basil leaves, or a pinch of dried basil (optional)

Crackers, crudités or fresh bread

Tip I love Mediterranean Organic brand jarred, oil-packed sun-dried tomatoes.

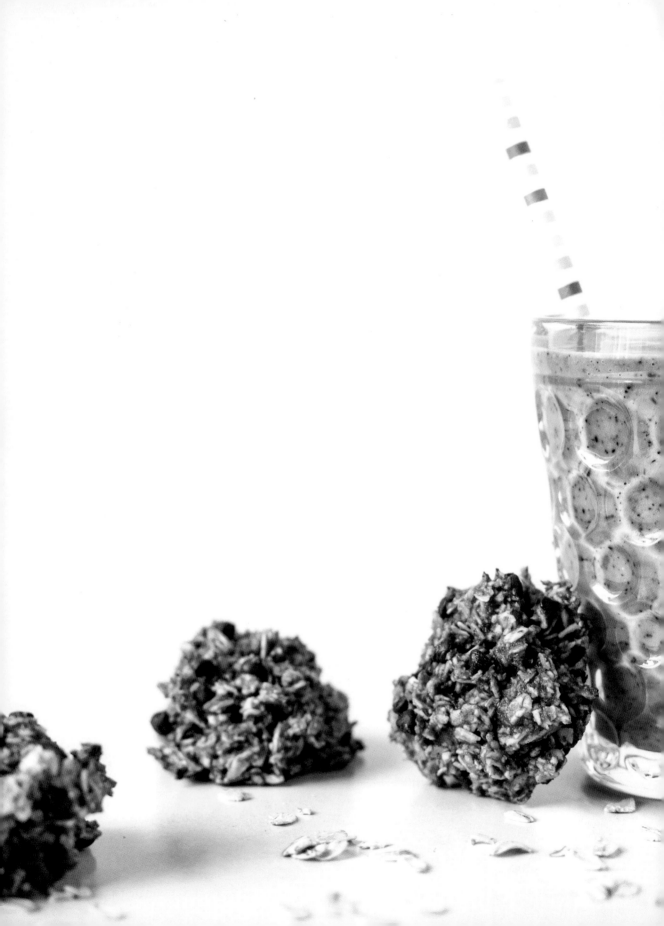

Banana Bread Muffin Tops

VEGAN, GLUTEN-FREE, NUT-FREE OPTION, SOYA-FREE OPTION,
KID-FRIENDLY, FREEZER-FRIENDLY

MAKES 10 MUFFIN TOPS

PREP TIME: **10 MINUTES**

COOK TIME: **17 TO 19 MINUTES**

Dense, moist, and chewy, these banana bread muffin tops are what I make when I'm craving banana bread but want something quick and healthy. Sweetened with banana and dates, these muffin tops contain no added sugars (aside from chocolate chips, but you can easily swap them for walnuts if you prefer). I use Enjoy Life mini chocolate chips—I love this brand because the chips are mini and you don't have to use as many of them when you bake. Try the muffin tops warm, served with a pat of vegan butter, nut butter, coconut oil or coconut butter.

1. Preheat the oven to 350°F (180°C). Line a large baking sheet with parchment paper.

2. In a food processor, combine the bananas, dates, coconut oil and vanilla and process until smooth. (I let it run for a minute or so to ensure it gets very smooth.)

3. Add the cinnamon, baking powder, and salt and process again until combined.

4. Add 130g of the rolled oats and process for only 4 to 5 seconds, just long enough to roughly chop the oats.

5. Remove the processor bowl from the base. Remove the blade and set aside. Carefully stir in the remaining 40g rolled oats and the chocolate chips. (If your food processor is small, you can transfer the dough into a bowl before mixing.)

6. Spoon the dough in large portions (about 3 tablespoons) onto the prepared baking sheet. Do not press down on the dough to flatten—simply leave it in mounds on the baking sheet.

7. Bake for 10 minutes, rotate the pan, and bake for 7 to 9 minutes more, until golden on the bottom.

8. Immediately transfer the baking sheet to a cooling rack and let cool for 10 minutes. Then lift off the muffin tops and place on the rack to cool completely. They will be quite moist even after baking (this is normal!). Store any leftover muffins tops in an airtight container in the fridge for 2 to 3 days, or in freezer-safe bags with the air pressed out in the freezer for 2 to 3 weeks.

Tip Make sure you use very soft Medjool dates. If you are using firm dates, be sure to soak them in boiling water for 20 to 30 minutes until softened and then drain before proceeding with the recipe.

2 large very ripe bananas (340g with peel)

125g pitted Medjool dates

60ml virgin coconut oil, softened

1 teaspoon pure vanilla extract

1 teaspoon ground cinnamon, or more to taste

1 teaspoon baking powder

¼ teaspoon plus ⅛ teaspoon fine sea salt

170g gluten-free rolled oats

40g non-dairy mini chocolate chips or chopped toasted walnuts

Make it nut-free Use non-dairy chocolate chips instead of walnuts.

Make it soya-free Use soya-free non-dairy chocolate chips, such as Enjoy Life brand.

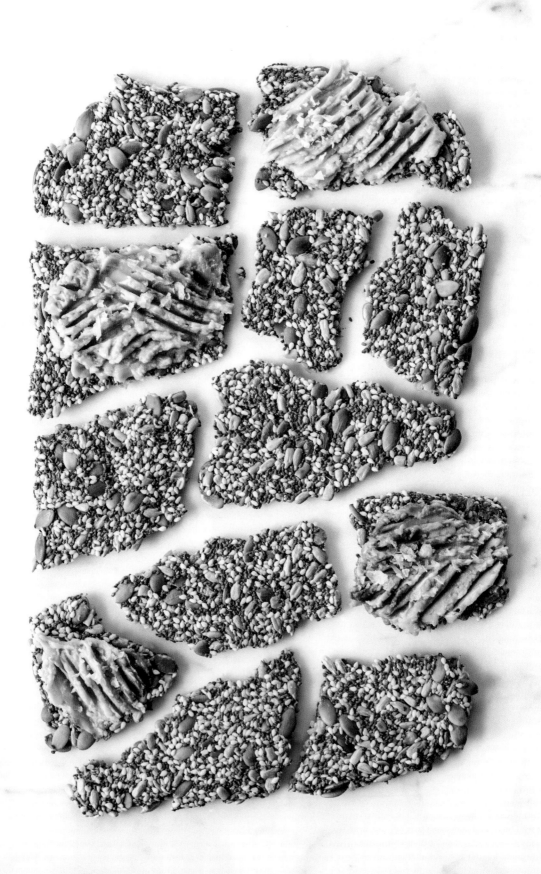

Endurance Crackers

VEGAN, GLUTEN-FREE, NUT-FREE, SOYA-FREE, GRAIN-FREE, OIL-FREE, FREEZER-FRIENDLY

MAKES 25 TO 30 CRACKERS

PREP TIME: **10 MINUTES**

COOK TIME: **60 TO 70 MINUTES**

These crackers are one of the most popular snack recipes on my blog, so I knew they had to go in this book. After being wowed by the crispy texture and light flavour of the raw seed crackers from the ChocolaTree Organic Oasis restaurant in Sedona, Arizona, I became determined to make my own version at home. I call them 'endurance crackers' because the healthy fats in the chia, sunflower, sesame and pumpkin seeds will help to keep you satisfied and energized for hours after you eat. Nevertheless, the crackers are also extremely light and crispy, which makes them easy to transport and nibble on at any time of day. I purposely left the flavour very light, so the crackers will work with a variety of dips and spreads. Feel free to change up the seasonings and spices as you wish; sometimes I like to add a tablespoon or two of my 9-Spice Mix (page 258) for variety.

1. Preheat the oven to 300°F (150°C). Line a large baking sheet with parchment paper.

2. In a large bowl, combine the chia seeds, sunflower seeds, pepitas, and sesame seeds.

3. Add the water, garlic, and Herbamare. Stir with a spatula until combined. Allow the mixture to sit for a couple of minutes until the chia seeds absorb the water. After the 2-minute rest, when you stir the mixture, you shouldn't see a pool of water on the bottom of the bowl.

4. With the spatula (and a hand, if necessary), spread the mixture onto the prepared baking sheet in two small rectangles, each about 30 × 18cm and 3 to 5mm thick. Sprinkle additional Herbamare on top.

5. Bake for 35 minutes. Remove from the oven and carefully flip each rectangle with a spatula. Bake for 25 to 35 minutes more, until lightly golden around the edges. Watch closely near the end to make sure they don't burn. Let cool for 10 to 15 minutes on the pan and then break the rectangles into crackers and let cool completely on the pan. Store in an airtight container or jar on the counter for up to 2 weeks. You can also freeze the crackers in freezer bags for up to 1 month. If the crackers soften while storing (this can happen in humid environments), toast in the oven at 300°F (150°C) for 5 to 7 minutes, then let cool completely. This is usually enough to restore them to their former crispness!

80g chia seeds

210g raw hulled sunflower seeds

65g raw (pumpkin seeds)

75g raw white sesame seeds

250ml water

1 large clove garlic, finely grated

¼ teaspoon Herbamare (see page 307) or fine sea salt, plus more as needed

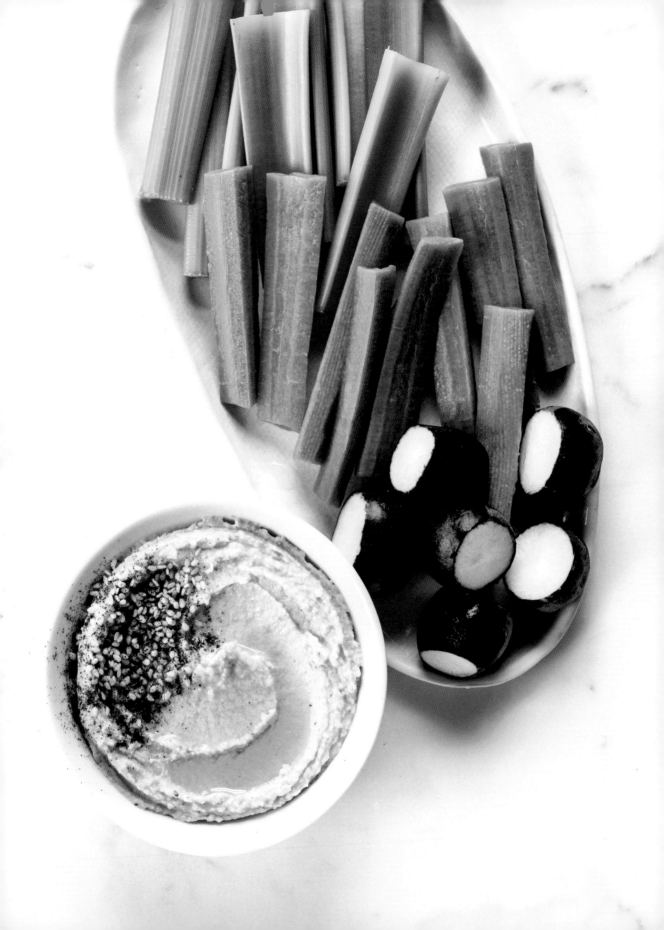

Every Day Lemon-Garlic Hummus

VEGAN, GLUTEN-FREE, NUT-FREE, SOYA-FREE, GRAIN-FREE

MAKES 375ML

CHILL TIME: **A FEW HOURS OR OVERNIGHT (OPTIONAL)**

This flavourful hummus pairs well with so many dishes, including my beloved 9-Spice Avocado Hummus Toast (page 39), The Big Tabbouleh Bowl (page 157), Endurance Crackers (page 89) and Every Day Glow salad (page 115). I suggest using refined avocado oil or a light-tasting olive oil in this hummus, which helps the flavours of garlic and lemon remain bright, and gives it an unbelievably light and smooth texture (a strong-tasting oil will overpower this hummus). Serve it with crudités. Thank you to Christine Burke for inspiring this hummus recipe.

1. Mince the garlic in a food processor.

2. Set aside 1 to 2 tablespoons of the chickpeas for garnish and add the remainder to the food processor, along with the lemon juice and tahini. Process until combined. Scrape down the processor bowl.

3. With the motor running, stream in the avocado oil and process for a good minute or two, until the hummus is very smooth. Add salt to taste and the pepper and process again.

4. Spoon the hummus into a container, cover, and refrigerate for a few hours or overnight (this allows the garlic flavour to settle and the flavours to meld), or enjoy it immediately if you dare!

5. Serve with a drizzle of olive oil and a sprinkle of paprika. Scatter the sesame seeds (if using) and reserved chickpeas on top.

Tip If you aren't a huge garlic fan, I recommend starting with just one small clove. You can always add more later if you wish.

2 small/medium cloves garlic (about 7g; see Tip)

1 400g can chickpeas, drained and rinsed, 250g cooked chickpeas

3 to 4 tablespoons fresh lemon juice (from 1 large lemon), to taste

1 tablespoon tahini

3 to 4 tablespoons refined avocado oil or light-tasting olive oil, to taste, plus more for serving

¾ to 1 teaspoon fine sea salt, to taste

¼ teaspoon freshly ground black pepper

Sweet paprika, for garnish

Sesame seeds, for garnish (optional)

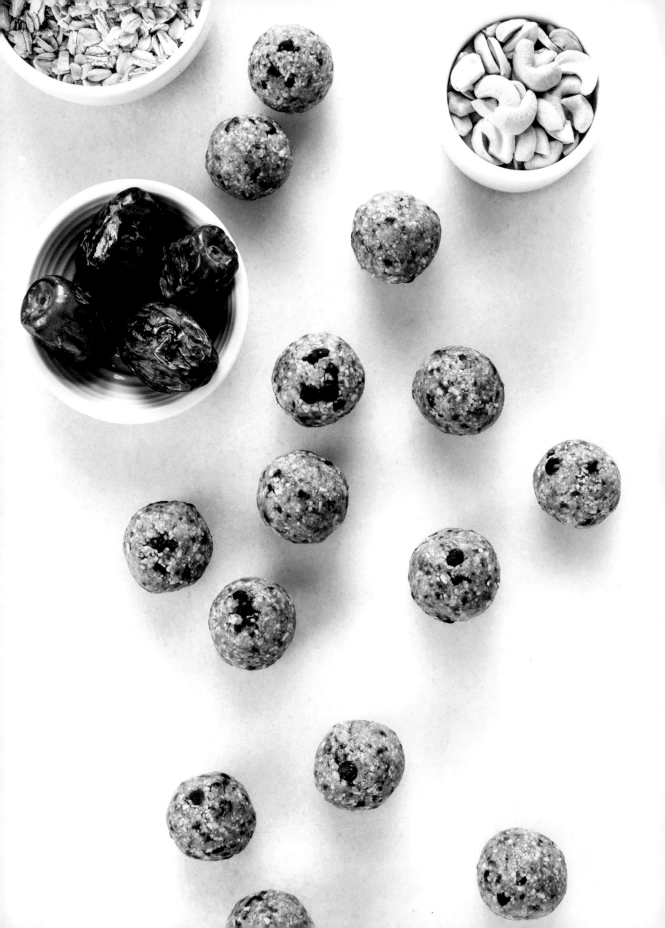

Cookie Dough Balls V

VEGAN, GLUTEN-FREE, SOYA-FREE OPTION, OIL-FREE, KID-FRIENDLY OPTION, FREEZER-FRIENDLY

MAKES 15 BALLS

PREP TIME: **10 MINUTES**

FREEZE TIME: **30 MINUTES**

If you've been following my blog for a while, then it's no secret that I have a thing for making healthier versions of cookie dough — healthy enough for them to pass as an energy-dense snack! Well, this is my fifth version to date, and it's definitely my new favourite. The base is made from cashews and rolled oats, and it's sweetened with Medjool dates and a splash of maple syrup. I like to use a tablespoon of Raw Cashew Butter (see page 75) because it gives these a distinctly buttery, cookie dough flavour, but feel free to swap it for almond or peanut butter if you wish. The latter will make these balls taste like peanut butter chocolate chip cookies — and there's nothing wrong with that! Keep these stashed in your freezer for a portable snack anytime. I love to pop one or two before a workout when I'm running out the door.

1. In a food processor, combine the cashews and oats and process until a fine flour forms, 30 to 60 seconds. Be sure not to process too long or the oils will be released and the cashews will turn into butter.

2. Add the dates and process again until the dates are finely chopped.

3. Add the maple syrup, cashew butter, vanilla and salt. Process until combined. The dough should stick together when you press it between your fingers. If it's too dry, add a teaspoon of water and process again.

4. Pulse in the chocolate chips until combined.

5. Line a large plate with parchment paper. Remove the blade from the food processor. Using your hand, grab a tablespoon of dough and roll it between your hands into a ball. Set the ball on the lined plate and repeat with the rest of the dough.

6. Chill the dough balls in the freezer for about 30 minutes. This just firms them up a bit, but you can enjoy them at room temperature, too. Store any leftovers in an airtight container in the fridge for up to 1 week or in a freezer-safe bag in the freezer for up to 1 month.

Tip These cookie dough balls work best with very soft and fresh Medjool dates. If your dates are dry or firm, soak them in a bowl of boiled water for 20 to 30 minutes. Drain well before use.

130g raw cashews

45g gluten-free rolled oats

70g pitted Medjool dates (see Tip)

1 tablespoon pure maple syrup

1 tablespoon Raw Cashew Butter (see page 75)

½ teaspoon pure vanilla extract

¼ teaspoon fine sea salt, or to taste

2 tablespoons non-dairy mini chocolate chips (I use Enjoy Life brand)

Make it soya-free Use soya-free non-dairy chocolate chips, such as Enjoy Life brand.

Make it kid-friendly Cookie dough balls can pose a choking hazard for little ones. As an alternative option, you can press the dough into a square pan and slice them into tiny, bite-size squares.

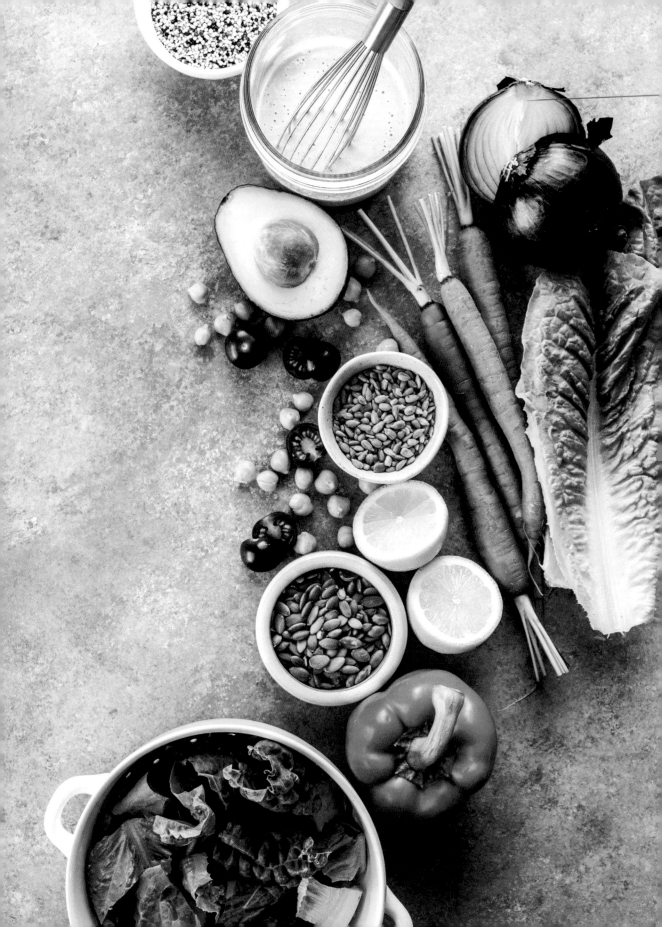

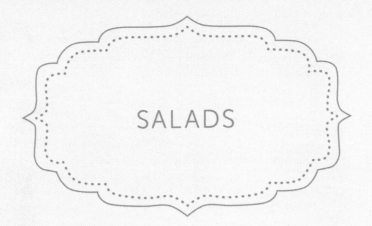

SALADS

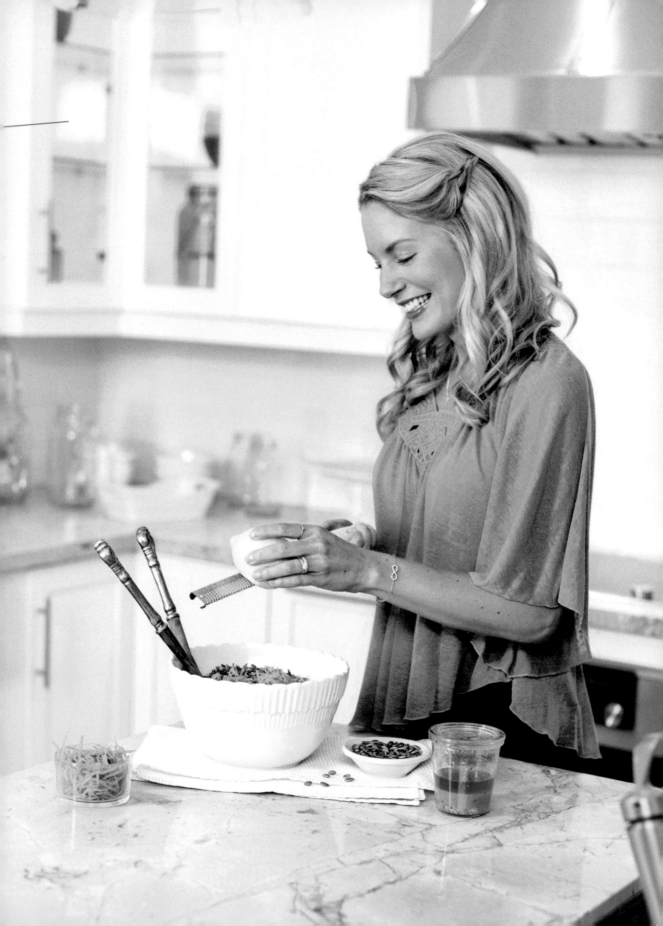

I'M THAT GIRL who brings a salad with me wherever I go, whether it's to a family gathering or a friend's barbecue down the street. I love to share salads that defy the mundane reputation that salads commonly have. Salads can be so much more than a boring blend of lettuce and tomato! Friends and family have come to expect hearty, satisfying, and flavourful creations from me, served both warm and chilled. Selfishly, I don't think I'll ever tire of hearing the words, 'I didn't think I liked kale! Uncle Jerry, you HAVE to try this!!' (see: Crowd-Pleasing Caesar Salad), or 'I could eat this every day for the rest of my life' (see: Thai Crunch Salad). Be careful: the salads in this chapter might steal the spotlight from the main course!

Of course, this chapter wouldn't be complete without sharing my go-to Every Day Glow salad — it doesn't seem like anything unusual at first glance, but when you try it, you'll understand my obsession. The simple ingredients just work. Tried-and-true salads should never be 'too easy' for a cookbook. I hope you'll enjoy this chapter's mix of potluck-inspired salads like my Protein Power Rainbow Quinoa Salad, and filling workday salads like my Curried Chickpea Salad, which will keep in the fridge for a few days.

Make it kid-friendly It can be difficult for some children to chew kale. If this is the case for your little one, swap some of the kale for an equal amount of an easier-to-chew green, such as finely chopped spinach.

Protein Power Rainbow Quinoa Salad

VEGAN, GLUTEN-FREE, NUT-FREE, SOYA-FREE, KID-FRIENDLY OPTION

MAKES 1.5L

PREP TIME: **30 MINUTES**

COOK TIME: **13 TO 16 MINUTES**

This makes a great potluck and workday salad because it's so portable. It's also packed with protein thanks to the quinoa, chickpeas, hemp hearts and kale, so it will leave you feeling full for hours! I like to use lacinato kale (also called dinosaur kale) in this salad because of its smooth texture, but regular curly kale will work, too. Just be sure to finely chop the kale (think *shredded*) so the greens are delicate and easy to chew. The ingredients are generously coated in a red wine vinaigrette, which provides so much flavour. I like my salad dressings to have an acidic bite, but if you don't like the tart flavour as much as I do, feel free to add a bit more maple syrup to the dressing—you can totally customize it to your own preferences. Once this salad has been sitting for longer than an hour, I find the flavours tend to mellow quite a bit. If you are bringing this salad to an event, you can bring the dressing separately and mix it just before serving or reawaken the flavors by adding a splash of red wine vinegar, lemon juice and/or lemon zest along with a splash of olive oil. This salad is also great in The Big Tabbouleh Bowl (page 157).

1. Make the salad Rinse the quinoa in a fine-mesh sieve. Combine the quinoa, water, and a pinch of salt in a medium pot and stir. Bring to a boil over medium to high heat, then reduce the heat to low, cover, and simmer for 13 to 16 minutes, until the water has been absorbed and the quinoa is fluffy. Remove from the heat, uncover, fluff with fork, and let cool slightly.

2. Meanwhile, place the chickpeas in an extra-large bowl. Add the kale, carrot, spring onion, parsley and tomatoes (if using) to the serving bowl along with the chickpeas.

3. Make the red wine vinaigrette In a small bowl, whisk together the vinegar, Dijon mustard, and garlic. While whisking, slowly stream in the oil. Whisk in the salt, pepper, maple syrup and lemon zest, adjusting to taste if desired.

4. Add the cooked quinoa to the bowl along with the veggies. Pour on all the dressing and toss well to combine. Season generously with salt and pepper. Sprinkle with the seeds and serve. Store any leftovers in an airtight container in the fridge for 3 to 5 days.

Tip 1. To toast the pumpkin seeds, preheat the oven to 300°F (150°C). Spread the seeds on a small baking sheet and toast in the oven for 9 to 12 minutes, until they start to puff up slightly and are lightly golden in some places.
2. If you need to serve a larger crowd, this recipe also doubles beautifully!

FOR THE SALAD

170g uncooked rainbow quinoa or regular quinoa, or 185g cooked quinoa

375ml water

1 400g can chickpeas, drained and rinsed, or 250g cooked chickpeas

300g de-stemmed lacinato kale, finely chopped

3 medium carrots, julienned and chopped into bite-size pieces (185g)

50g chopped spring onion

15g fresh parsley leaves, finely chopped

15g oil-packed sun-dried tomatoes, drained and finely chopped (optional, but recommended)

FOR THE RED WINE VINAIGRETTE

60ml red wine vinegar

2 teaspoons Dijon mustard

1 large clove garlic, minced

60ml extra-virgin olive oil

1/4 teaspoon fine sea salt

Freshly ground black pepper

1 teaspoon pure maple syrup, or to taste

Zest of 1 medium lemon (about 1 tablespoon)

FOR THE GARNISH

Fine sea salt and freshly ground black pepper

160g toasted pumpkin seeds

1 tablespoon hemp hearts

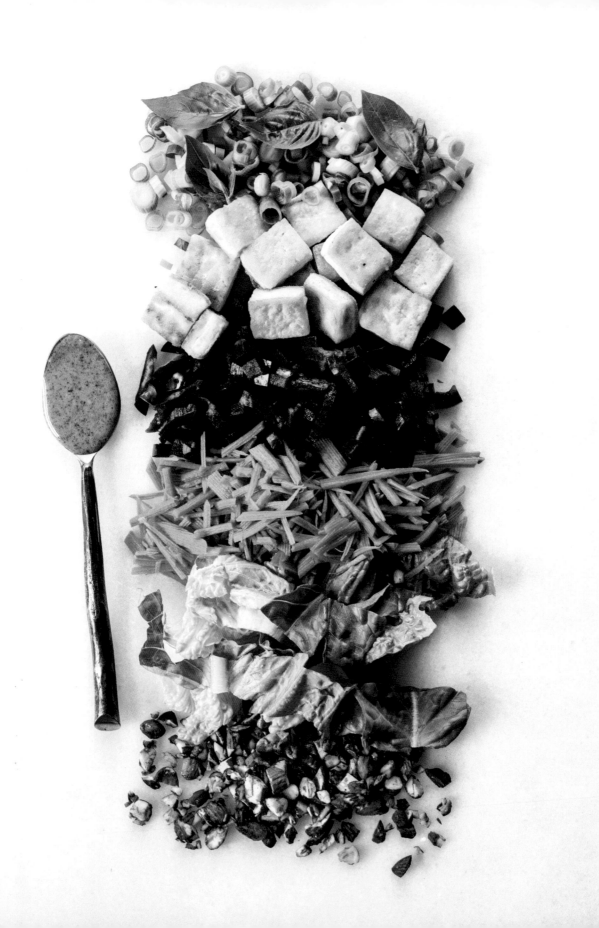

Thai Crunch Salad

VEGAN, GLUTEN-FREE, GRAIN-FREE, ADVANCE PREP REQUIRED
SERVES 4

PREP TIME: **30 MINUTES**

COOK TIME: **20 TO 25 MINUTES**

This salad is a show-stopper! The combination of Roasted Tamari Almonds (page 263), Cast-Iron Tofu (page 137), and fresh vegetables gives it plenty of contrast in texture, not to mention nutritional variety. In my personal opinion, though, the highlight of this salad is the creamy Thai Almond Butter Sauce (page 249), which I challenge you not to eat on its own with a spoon! Yes, the sauce is irresistibly rich and decadent, and it showcases the traditional Thai flavours of ginger, garlic lime, and tamari. The dressing can easily double as a dip for summer rolls, baked tofu or crudités, too. If you'd like to turn this salad into a heartier entrée, try swapping the romaine lettuce for cooked soba noodles for even more staying power.

1. Place the romaine in a large salad bowl, or divide it among four individual bowls.

2. Add the carrot, bell pepper, spring onion, coriander, tofu and almonds.

3. Serve the Thai Almond Butter Sauce on the side and drizzle it over the salads just before serving.

Tip If you don't have a julienne peeler, you can use a regular peeler to create thin carrot 'ribbons' or you can grate the carrot on a box grater. If you use a box grater, I would probably reduce the amount of carrots to 110g so they don't overwhelm the salad. (For my tips on how to julienne carrots, see page xvi.)

1 medium head romaine lettuce, chopped

3 medium carrots, julienned and chopped into bite-size pieces (185g)

1 medium red bell pepper, seeded and diced or 188g diced cucumber

4 spring onions, thinly sliced

15g chopped fresh coriander or basil leaves

Cast-Iron Tofu (page 137)

Roasted Tamari Almonds (page 263)

Thai Almond Butter Sauce (page 249)

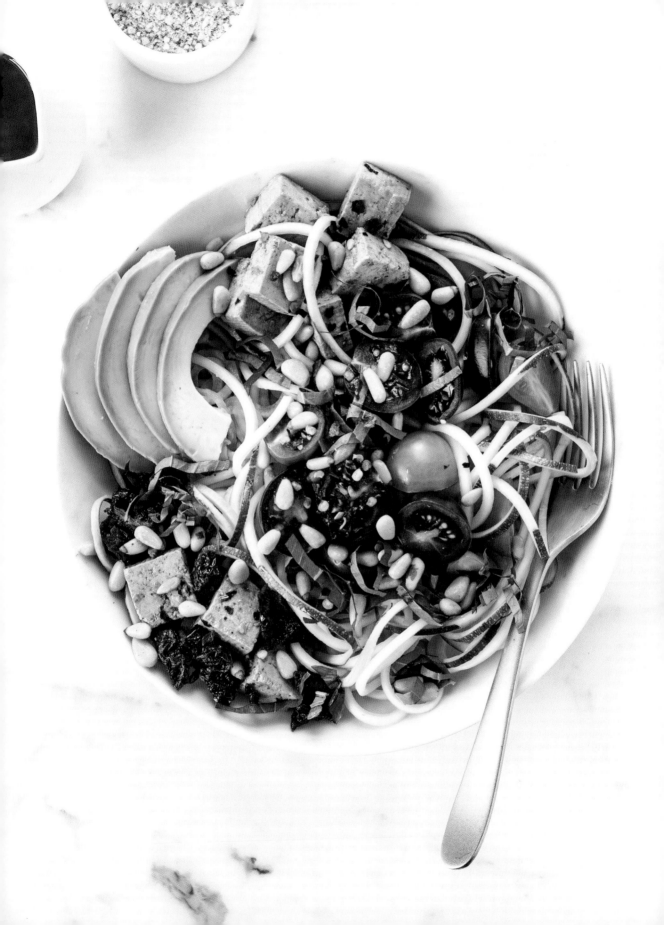

Spiralized Courgette Summer Salad

VEGAN, GLUTEN-FREE, NUT-FREE OPTION, GRAIN-FREE,
ADVANCE PREP REQUIRED, KID-FRIENDLY

SERVES 2

PREP TIME: **10 MINUTES**

MARINATING TIME: **30 MINUTES OR
OVERNIGHT**

When the weather is too hot for me to contemplate turning on the oven, this is the light and energizing salad I turn to. Though it's a dish made with spiralized courgette, which is a light, grain-free alternative to pasta, it's still very rich in protein, thanks to the flavourful Italian tofu. As soon as your tofu has marinated, this dish will come together in just a few minutes! It's also a big hit with adults and kids alike. See my tips on page xvi for the tools I use to spiralize courgettes.

1. Prepare the tofu, adding the tomatoes to the marinade along with the tofu, and toss until combined. Marinate for at least 30 minutes, or up to 8 to 12 hours. If the marinade partially solidifies while chilling (this can happen due to the olive oil), simply let it sit at room temperature before serving until it liquefies again.

2. Spiralize the courgette and roughly chop it (if desired). Divide the courgette between two large bowls.

3. Top each bowl of courgette with a generous portion of the marinated tofu and tomatoes, as well as a few spoonfuls of the marinade (this acts as a dressing). Add the sliced avocado, basil, a couple of spoonfuls of cashew Vegan Parmesan Cheese and, if desired, top with sun-dried tomatoes, red pepper flakes and pine nuts.

Make it nut-free Use Pumpkin Seed Parmesan Cheese (see page 267) instead of the Cashew Parmesan Cheese, and use sesame seeds instead of pine nuts.

Marinated Italian Tofu (page 135)

150g cherry or grape tomatoes, halved

1 medium courgette, spiralized

1 avocado, pitted and sliced

10g fresh basil leaves, thinly sliced

Vegan Parmesan Cheese (page 267), made with cashews

1 to 2 tablespoons oil-packed sun-dried tomatoes, drained and chopped, to taste (optional)

Red pepper flakes (optional)

Handful of pine nuts or sesame seeds, toasted (optional)

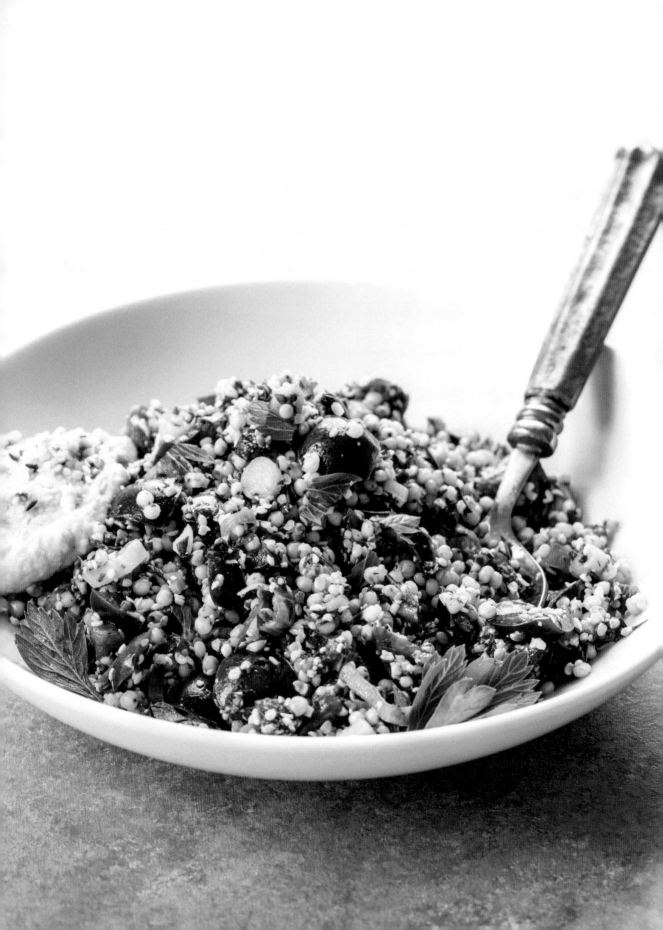

Hemp Heart and Sorghum Tabbouleh

VEGAN, GLUTEN-FREE, NUT-FREE, SOYA-FREE, KID-FRIENDLY

SERVES 5

PREP TIME: **20 MINUTES**

COOK TIME: **40 TO 60 MINUTES**

Packed with protein-rich hemp hearts and fiber-rich sorghum, this is a tabbouleh with some staying power! It features traditional tabbouleh ingredients, including parsley, spring onions and tomatoes, but I throw in mint for a fresh twist, and I use nutrient-dense hemp hearts and sorghum in place of bulgur, for an unbelievably chewy, satisfying texture. This tabbouleh makes a great snack or light summery lunch, and I also love to pair it with hummus in a wrap or with pitta wedges and cucumber slices. For even more protein, try adding chickpeas to this dish. If you prepare it in advance, I suggest waiting to mix in the dressing until just before serving because the flavours tend to dissipate as it sits.

1. **Make the tabbouleh** If desired, soak the sorghum overnight in a bowl of water. This reduces the cook time slightly, but it's optional. Drain.

2. Put the sorghum in a medium pot and add water to cover by 5 to 8cm. Bring the mixture to a boil over medium-high heat, then reduce the heat to medium and simmer, uncovered, for 40 to 45 minutes if you soaked the grains overnight, or 50 to 60 minutes if you did not soak. When the sorghum is soft and tender with a bit of chewiness, it's ready. Drain off any excess water and transfer the sorghum to a large bowl.

3. In a food processor, combine the parsley, mint and garlic and process until finely chopped. (You can also chop it by hand.) Transfer the herbs to the bowl with the sorghum and add the hemp hearts, tomatoes and spring onions. Stir.

4. **Make the dressing** In a small bowl, whisk together the lemon zest, lemon juice, oil, vinegar and maple syrup. Add the dressing to the tabbouleh and stir well until combined.

5. Season the tabbouleh with salt and pepper and mix again. Sprinkle on a bit of Herbamare, if desired. Leftovers will keep in an airtight container in the fridge for up to 3 days. The flavours tend to dissipate with time, so you can reawaken the dressing by adding a splash of fresh lemon juice or red wine vinegar and a pinch of salt, if desired.

Tip Look for sorghum in the gluten-free or organic section at your grocery store, or in ethnic grocery stores.

FOR THE TABBOULEH

50g uncooked sorghum

60g fresh parsley leaves

15g packed fresh mint leaves

2 medium cloves garlic, minced

80g hemp hearts

270g diced cherry tomatoes

4 spring onions, thinly sliced (about 60g)

FOR THE DRESSING

Fresh lemon zest (I add about 1 teaspoon)

2 tablespoons fresh lemon juice

2 tablespoons extra-virgin olive oil, or to taste

1 teaspoon red wine vinegar (optional)

1 teaspoon pure maple syrup, or more to taste

FOR THE GARNISH

½ teaspoon fine sea salt, or to taste

Freshly ground black pepper

Herbamare (see page 307; optional)

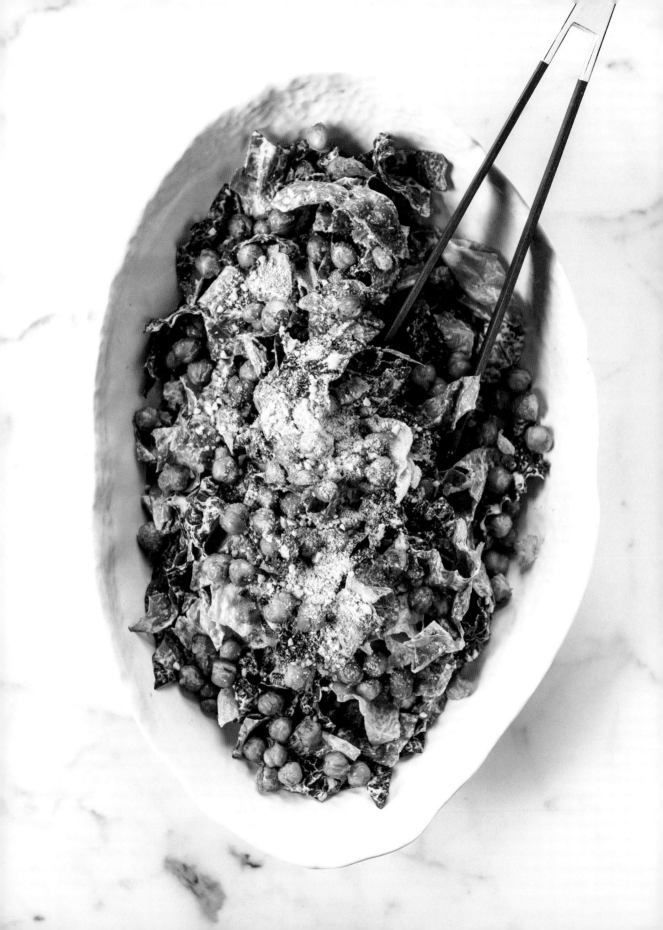

Crowd-Pleasing Caesar Salad

VEGAN, GLUTEN-FREE OPTION, GRAIN-FREE, ADVANCE PREP REQUIRED

SERVES 6

SOAK TIME: 1 TO 2 HOURS, OR OVERNIGHT

PREP TIME: 35 TO 40 MINUTES

COOK TIME: 35 MINUTES

This is one of the most popular salad recipes on my website, and once you try it, you'll understand why. I start with a creamy, tart dressing that's close in flavour and texture to a traditional Caesar. (My magic ingredients? Vegan Worcestershire sauce and capers, which give the dressing the traditional briny quality we find in Caesars, and raw cashews for creaminess.) In place of croutons, I use crispy (and nutritious!) roasted chickpeas. I top the salad with an addictive vegan 'parmesan', which you can use in pastas and other salads, too. The dressing will keep in the fridge in a sealed container for at least 5 days, and you can easily double it for a larger group. It thickens up a lot when chilled, so be sure to let it sit at room temperature to soften before using. If you'd like a more traditional alternative to the roasted chickpea croutons, feel free to use my Easiest Garlic Croutons (page 257) instead. A big thanks to the folks at Vega for inspiring this dressing recipe!

1. **Make the dressing** Place the cashews in a bowl and add water to cover by a couple of inches. Soak for 1 to 2 hours or overnight. Drain and rinse.

2. Transfer the cashews to a high-speed blender and add the remaining dressing ingredients except the salt. Blend on high until the dressing is super smooth. You can add an additional splash of water if necessary to get it blending. Add salt and adjust the other seasonings, if desired, and blend briefly to combine. Set aside.

3. **Make the garlic roasted chickpeas** Preheat the oven to 400°F (200°C). Line a large baking sheet with parchment paper. Place the chickpeas in a dishcloth and rub dry (it's okay if some skins fall off). Spread the chickpeas out on the baking sheet. Drizzle with the oil and roll the chickpeas around with your hands to coat. Sprinkle on the garlic powder, salt, and cayenne (if using) and gently shake the pan until combined. Roast for 15 minutes, then gently roll the chickpeas around on the baking sheet and roast for 15 to 20 minutes more, until lightly golden. Remove from the oven and let cool for about 10 minutes. The chickpeas will be soft coming out of the oven, but they will firm up as they cool.

(recipe continues)

FOR THE DRESSING

65g raw cashews

60ml water

2 tablespoons extra-virgin olive oil

1 tablespoon fresh lemon juice

1½ teaspoons Dijon mustard

1 or 2 cloves garlic, to taste

¼ to ½ teaspoon garlic powder, to taste

1½ teaspoons vegan Worcestershire sauce

2½ teaspoons capers

½ teaspoon freshly ground black pepper, or to taste

½ teaspoon fine sea salt, or to taste

FOR THE GARLIC ROASTED CHICKPEAS

1 400g can chickpeas, drained and rinsed, or 250g cooked chickpeas

1 teaspoon extra-virgin olive oil

½ teaspoon garlic powder

½ teaspoon fine sea salt

⅛ to ¼ teaspoon cayenne pepper, to taste (optional)

2 small heads romaine lettuce, chopped (about 750g chopped)

1 small/medium bunch lacinato kale, stemmed and leaves finely chopped, or more romaine (500g)

1 batch Vegan Parmesan Cheese (page 267), made with cashews

Freshly ground black pepper

4. Make the salad Place the romaine and kale in an extra-large bowl. Add all the dressing and toss until fully coated. Sprinkle on the roasted chickpeas and the Parmesan cheese. Garnish with freshly ground black pepper. Serve immediately.

Tip For a quick-soak method, cover the cashews with boiling water and soak for 30 to 60 minutes.

Make it gluten-free Use a certified gluten-free brand of Worcestershire sauce, such as Wizard's Gluten-Free Organic Worcestershire Sauce or Whole Foods' 365 Worcestershire Sauce.

Stuffed Avocado Salad

VEGAN, GLUTEN-FREE OPTION, NUT-FREE, SOYA-FREE, KID-FRIENDLY OPTION

SERVES 6

SOAK TIME: **OVERNIGHT (OPTIONAL)**

PREP TIME: **30 MINUTES**

COOK TIME: **20 TO 40 MINUTES**

If you're looking to prepare a salad that's hearty and filling—something that can stand on its own as a light meal—this is the salad for you. Creamy avocado provides heart-healthy fats, while the spelt berries and black beans add plenty of protein and fibre to the dish. The salad is delightfully crunchy and chewy—the perfect complement to the buttery avocado base. I love the combination of smoky cumin and bright, refreshing lime juice, and I'll often make a double batch of the dressing to use on other salads. This recipe will make enough to serve six (which is why it calls for three avocados—half an avocado per person), but if you don't plan on serving that many people, simply reduce the amount of avocado (since the avocados are best served fresh). If you have some on hand, my Fresh Cherry Tomato Salsa (page 63) is lovely spooned on top!

1. **Make the black bean salad** If desired, soak the spelt berries overnight in a large bowl of water. This simply reduces the cooking time, but it's totally optional. Drain and rinse.

2. Put the spelt berries in a medium pot and add water to cover. Bring to a boil over medium to high heat, reduce the heat to medium, and simmer for 20 minutes if you soaked the spelt berries, or up to 40 minutes if you did not soak them, until tender but still chewy. Drain, rinse, and let cool for 5 to 10 minutes.

3. Transfer the spelt berries to a large bowl and add the black beans, coriander, spring onion, bell pepper, and corn. Stir to combine.

4. **Make the dressing** In a small bowl, whisk together the lime juice, olive oil, minced garlic, cumin, maple syrup, salt, and black pepper.

5. Pour the dressing on top of the black bean salad and stir well. Taste and add more dressing, if desired. I usually add another ¼ teaspoon salt, more black pepper and cumin, a squeeze of lime juice, and a few shakes of cayenne pepper for some heat until everything pops. You can serve the salad immediately or transfer it to the fridge for 30 to 60 minutes to allow the flavours to meld.

(recipe continues)

FOR THE BLACK BEAN SALAD

180g uncooked spelt berries or wheat berries

1 400g can black beans, drained and rinsed, or 255g cooked black beans

25g fresh coriander leaves, finely chopped

115g finely chopped spring onion

1 medium/large red bell pepper, finely chopped (175g)

130g fresh sweetcorn kernels (from about 1 small cob)

FOR THE CUMIN-LIME DRESSING

60ml fresh lime juice (from about 2 large limes)

2 to 3 tablespoons extra-virgin olive oil, to taste

2 to 3 medium cloves garlic, minced

1 teaspoon ground cumin

1½ teaspoons pure maple syrup, or more to taste

½ teaspoon fine sea salt, plus more to taste

Freshly ground black pepper

Cayenne pepper (optional)

3 large ripe avocados

Lemon-Tahini Dressing (page 265; optional)

6. Assemble the avocados Halve and pit each avocado. Carefully scoop out the flesh so it remains intact. Place the avocado half on a plate, and 'stuff' or top with the black bean salad. Allow the black bean salad to spill out onto the plate. Repeat for the rest of the avocados. You can top the salad with a drizzle of Lemon-Tahini Dressing, if desired. Black bean salad leftovers can be stored in the fridge in an airtight container for 3 to 5 days. The avocado is best served fresh, though. Stir the salad before serving each time to redistribute the dressing. If the dressing mellows a bit, you can liven it up with a squeeze of lime juice, a pinch of salt and a dash of the spices.

Tip Not a fan of avocado? Simply enjoy the black bean salad on its own or as a side dish, or serve it in a wrap or pitta with hummus.

Make it gluten-free Swap 190g uncooked sorghum for the spelt berries and follow the cooking instructions on page 287. If you don't have sorghum, you can use 170g uncooked quinoa. The quinoa will absorb the flavours of the dressing much more than the spelt berries, so I recommend freshening the dressing (with a squeeze of lime juice, pinch of salt and drizzle of olive oil, to taste) if the salad sits for any length of time.

Make it kid-friendly Lightly mash the beans with the back of a fork. Serve the salad alongside tortilla chips or pitta chips for scooping!

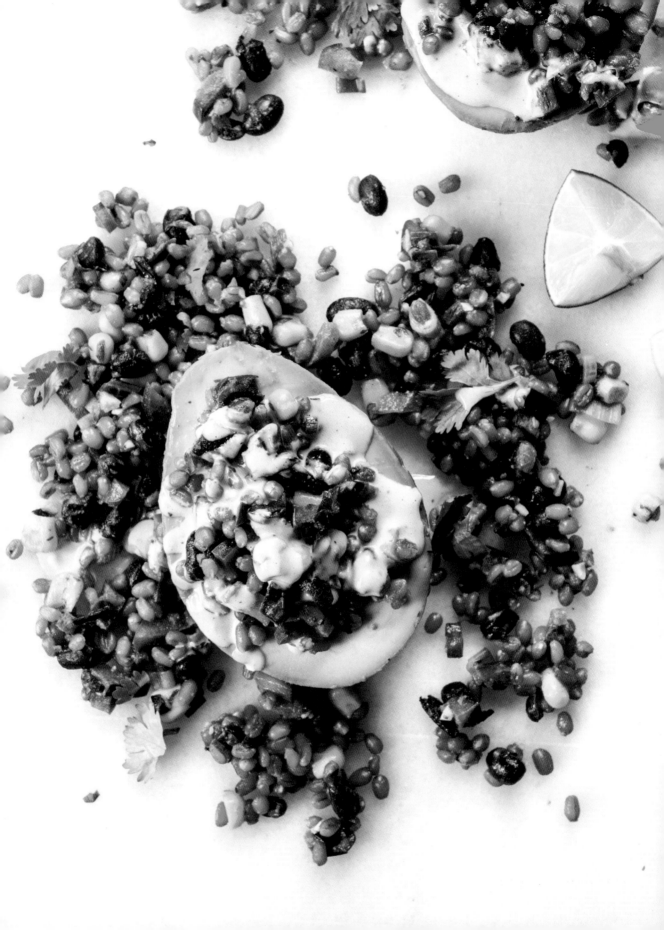

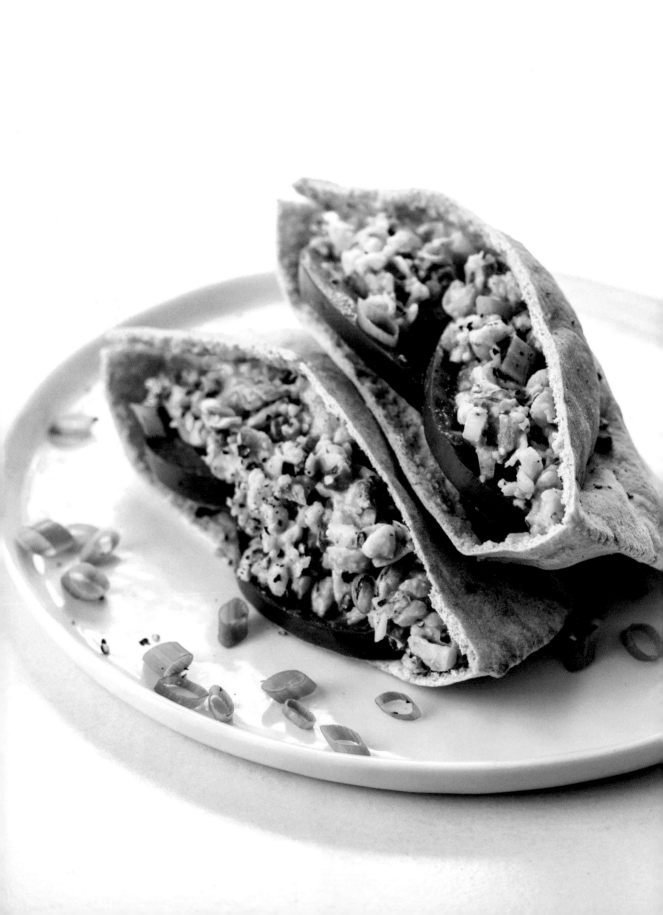

Curried Chickpea Salad

VEGAN, GLUTEN-FREE, NUT-FREE, SOYA-FREE OPTION, GRAIN-FREE, FREEZER-FRIENDLY

SERVES 3

PREP TIME: **15 MINUTES**

This chickpea salad is lightly spiced with curry flavours—just enough to give it character without overpowering the salad. Feel free to tweak all the spices to your own tastes by adding more or less ginger, curry powder or turmeric. You can serve this salad scooped into pieces of Boston or Bibb lettuce, stuffed in a wholemeal pitta, or with Endurance Crackers (page 89). If you have a picnic or road trip in your future, you'll be happy to know that it packs well, too. It keeps in the fridge for three to four days, so feel free to double the recipe if you'd like leftovers for the workweek!

1. In a large bowl, mash the chickpeas with a potato masher until flaked in texture.

2. Stir in the spring onions, bell pepper, coriander, mayonnaise, garlic, ginger, turmeric and curry powder until combined.

3. Stir in the lemon juice, salt and black pepper, adjusting the quantities to taste. Add a dash or two of cayenne if you want some heat.

4. Serve with toasted bread, with crackers, on wholemeal wraps, or on top of a basic leafy green salad. The salad will keep in an airtight container in the fridge for 3 to 4 days. Stir well before serving. You can also transfer the salad to a freezer-safe zip-top bag, press out all the air, and freeze for up to 1 month.

Make it soya-free If you'd like a soya-free version of this salad, be sure to use soya-free vegan mayonnaise. Vegenaise make a great soya-free version.

For Lemon-Dill Chickpea Salad Omit the coriander, ginger, turmeric and curry powder. Replace it with 1½ teaspoons yellow mustard and 2 teaspoons minced fresh dill, and increase the lemon juice to 1½ to 3 teaspoons, to taste.

1 400g can chickpeas, drained and rinsed, or 250g cooked chickpeas

3 spring onions, thinly sliced

90g finely chopped red bell pepper

15g fresh coriander leaves, finely chopped

3 tablespoons Homemade Vegan Mayo (page 269) or store-bought

1 clove garlic, minced

½ teaspoon grated fresh ginger, or to taste

½ teaspoon ground turmeric

¼ teaspoon curry powder, or more to taste

1 to 1½ teaspoons fresh lemon juice, to taste

¼ teaspoon plus ⅛ teaspoon fine sea salt, or to taste

Freshly ground black pepper

Cayenne pepper (optional)

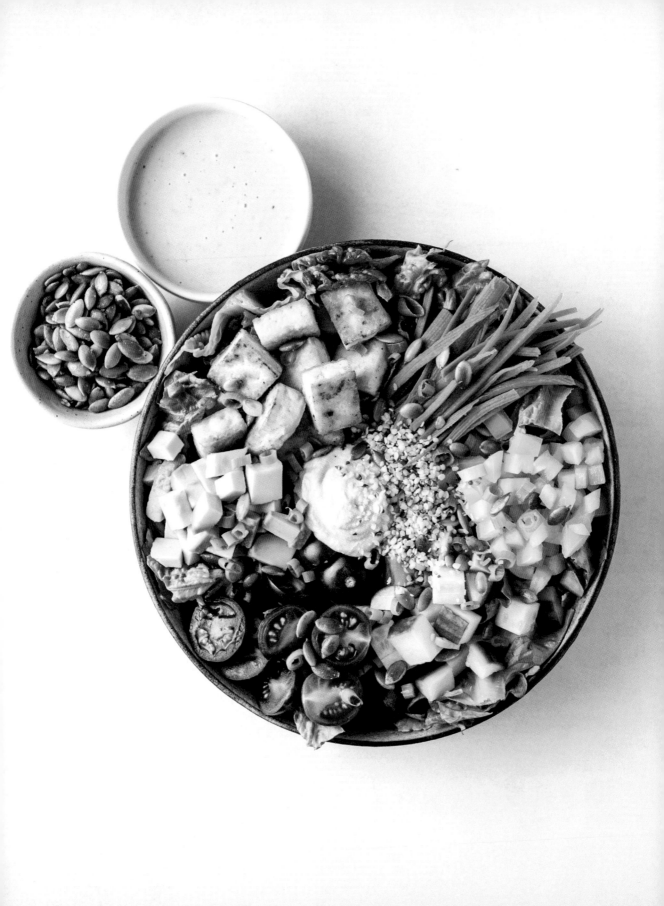

Every Day Glow

VEGAN, GLUTEN-FREE, NUT-FREE, SOYA-FREE OPTION, GRAIN-FREE, ADVANCE PREP REQUIRED

SERVES 2

PREP TIME: **20 MINUTES**

This is a handy, everyday salad, and it never fails to energize me! It packs some of my favourite vegetables and my go-to Lemon-Tahini Dressing. I always try to keep these veggies stocked in my crisper so I can make this salad at the drop of a hat. That said, part of the joy of this salad is changing it up by varying the greens, veggies, toppings and/or dressing. The hemp hearts provide a nice boost of protein, but if you'd like to amp up the protein even more, I highly recommend adding Marinated Italian Tofu, The Best Marinated Lentils, or Cast-Iron Tofu on top. If I have some on hand, I'll also often add a handful of bean sprouts and Roasted Tamari Almonds (page 263).

1. Place the lettuce in a large bowl. Arrange the chopped vegetables on top, followed by the hemp hearts and pumpkin seeds. Add a protein, if desired. Add a spoonful of hummus on top and then drizzle with the dressing. Serve immediately.

Make it soya-free Leave out the tofu, and instead use one of the other protein options listed.

300g chopped romaine lettuce or greens of your choice

75g cherry or grape tomatoes, halved

40g diced cucumber

90g diced yellow, orange, or red bell pepper

60g julienned or grated carrot

½ avocado, pitted and sliced or chopped

2 spring onions, thinly sliced

2 tablespoons hemp hearts

2 tablespoons pumpkin seeds, toasted

Optional protein additions: Cast-Iron Tofu (page 137), The Best Marinated Lentils (page 129), Curried Chickpea Salad (page 113), Marinated Italian Tofu (page 135), or cooked chickpeas or other beans

Spoonful of Every Day Lemon-Garlic Hummus (page 91) or prepared hummus

Lemon-Tahini Dressing (page 265)

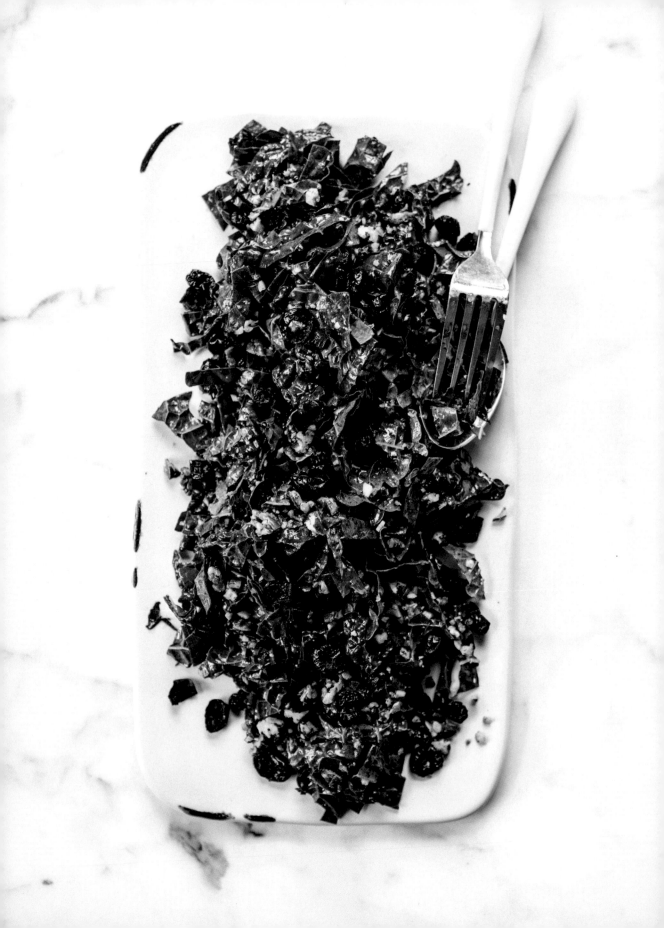

The Best Shredded Kale Salad

VEGAN, GLUTEN-FREE, NUT-FREE OPTION, SOYA-FREE, GRAIN-FREE
SERVES 4

PREP TIME: **25 MINUTES**

COOK TIME: **8 TO 12 MINUTES**

If you're a salad lover, then you've probably tried your fair share of kale salads. Trust me when I say that, no matter how many kale salads you've enjoyed, this one is a game changer. The key to this salad is finely chopping or shredding the kale. The lemon-garlic dressing will coat each and every tiny piece of kale, working its magical softening powers and infusing it with so much flavour. Instead of cheese, I top the salad with my homemade toasted pecan Parmesan, which adds a delectable, nutty, savoury flavour. Two bunches of kale might seem like a lot, but once it's shredded, it only makes about 800g, and then it further reduces in volume by almost half as it marinates. If you are making this salad for more than four people, I suggest doubling the entire recipe. The salad can be served with soup for a light dinner, or paired with roasted root vegetables and chickpeas for a hearty autumn meal.

1. **Make the toasted pecan Parmesan** Preheat the oven to 300°F (150°C). Chop the pecans into pieces roughly the size of peas. Spread the pecans over a baking sheet and toast in the oven for 8 to 12 minutes, until fragrant and lightly golden.

2. Transfer the pecans to a medium bowl, add the garlic, nutritional yeast, oil and salt, and stir well until combined. Set aside.

3. **Make the salad and dressing** Finely chop the kale leaves into thin 5mm strands 2.5 to 5cm in length. You should have about 800g chopped kale. Place it in a large bowl.

4. In a mini food processor, process the garlic until minced. Add the lemon, oil, salt and pepper and process until combined.

5. Pour the dressing onto the kale and massage the dressing into the kale with your hands. Keep massaging for 30 seconds or so to ensure that everything is coated perfectly. Taste the salad and add the maple syrup, if a sweeter dressing is desired.

6. Sprinkle the pecan parmesan all over the kale. Toss on a handful or two of dried cranberries. Cover and refrigerate for 30 to 60 minutes to soften, or serve immediately.

Make it nut-free Swap the Pecan Parmesan for my Pumpkin Seed Parmesan Cheese (see page 267).

FOR THE TOASTED PECAN PARMESAN

125g raw pecans

1 large clove garlic, grated on a Microplane

3 to 4 teaspoons nutritional yeast, to taste

4½ teaspoons extra-virgin olive oil

¼ teaspoon fine sea salt

FOR THE SALAD AND DRESSING

2 large bunches lacinato kale, de-stemmed

2 large cloves garlic

60ml fresh lemon juice (from 1 extra-large lemon)

3 to 4 tablespoons extra-virgin olive oil, to taste

¼ teaspoon fine sea salt

¼ teaspoon freshly ground black pepper (just eyeball it)

1 teaspoon pure maple syrup, or to taste (optional)

1 to 2 handfuls dried cranberries or dried cherries, for garnish

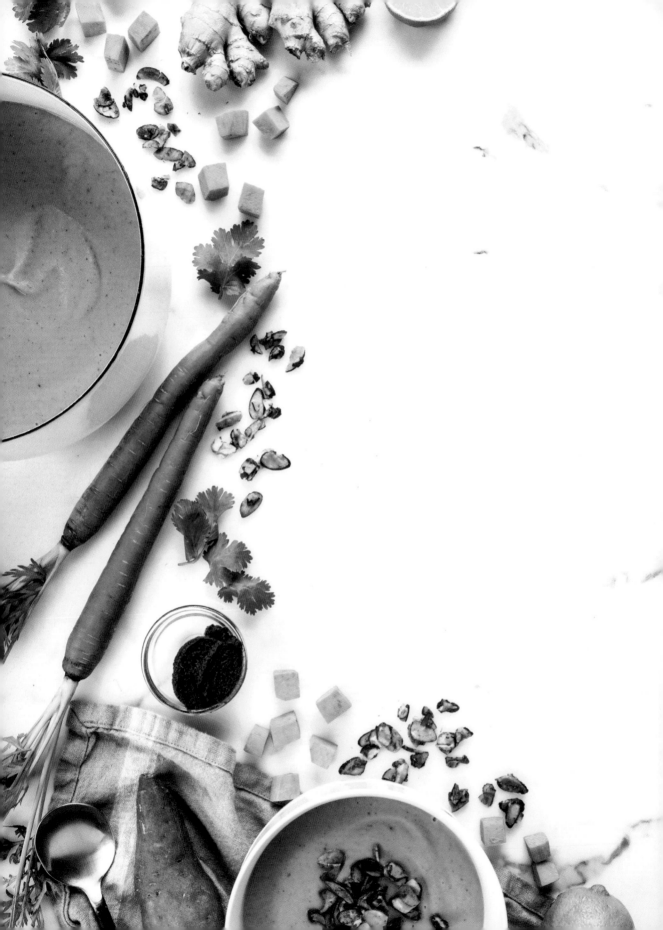

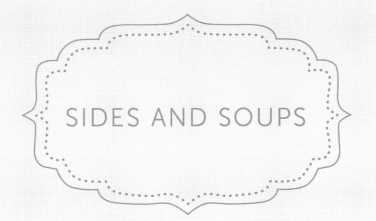

SIDES AND SOUPS

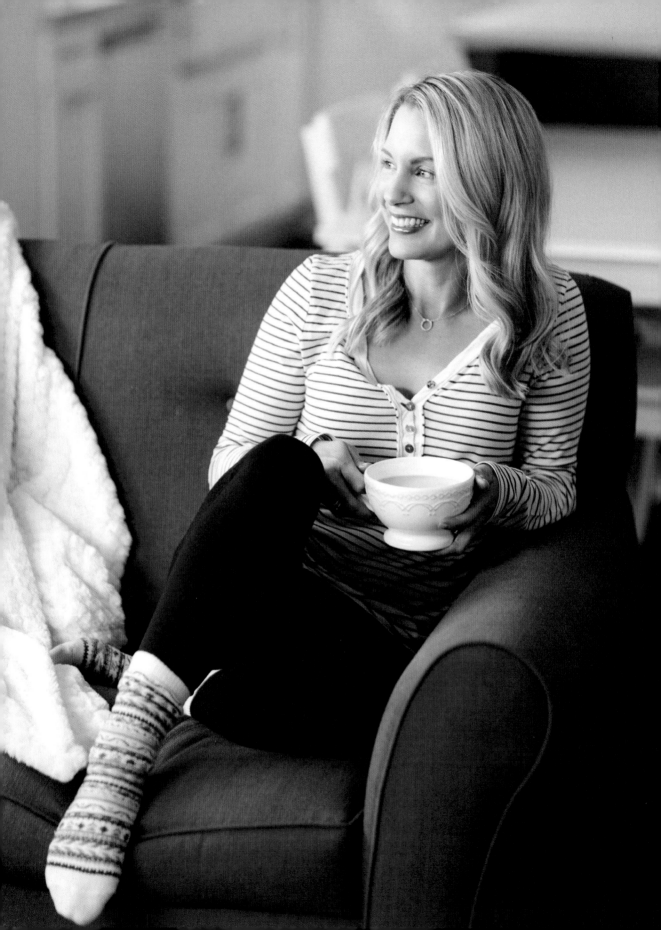

THIS CHAPTER WILL give you building blocks for creating a wide variety of meals. Return to this chapter whenever you need to mix and match recipes, or if you're looking for a way to turn an entrée or a salad into a complete meal. During the cooler fall and winter months, dishes like my Roasted Garlic Basil Pesto Potatoes, Sweet Potato Casserole, Roasted Brussels Sprouts and Coconut 'Bacon' and Crispy Smashed Potatoes are all warm and comforting to the max. During the warmer months, my Go-To Gazpacho and The Best Marinated Lentils are on a weekly rotation in our house. I made Eric a believer in chilled soup with the gazpacho recipe, and I hope to do the same for you! Be sure to also check out my Garlic Cauliflower Mashed Potatoes (page 187) in the entrée chapter; they make a lovely side to a number of meals, and they are the ultimate comfort food!

Soups are ideal for mixing and matching: served with a simple salad, they make for a perfect, light dinner or lunch, and they can also be paired with an entrée for a super-nutritious and hearty meal. I've included a handful of new soup recipes in this chapter. If you are looking to hit the reset button after indulgent holiday eating, my Metabolism-Revving Spicy Cabbage Soup will help you get back on track. (It'll also change your mind if you think you're not a fan of cabbage soup!) We love making a pot of Creamy Thai Carrot Sweet Potato Soup and Golden French Lentil Stew for an easy weeknight meal that's healthy and super satisfying. Soup also freezes beautifully, so you can make a double batch and savour the leftovers at another time.

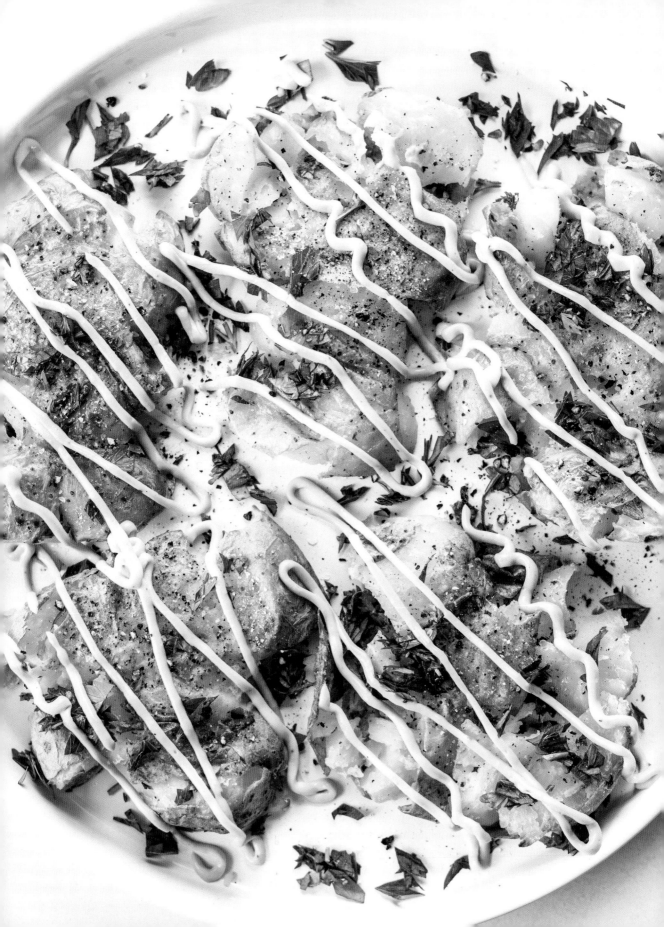

Crispy Smashed Potatoes

VEGAN, GLUTEN-FREE, NUT-FREE, SOYA-FREE OPTION, GRAIN-FREE,
KID-FRIENDLY

MAKES 6 TO 8 MEDIUM POTATOES (3 OR 4 SERVINGS)

PREP TIME: **20 MINUTES**

COOK TIME: **45 TO 55 MINUTES**

This is one of my all-time favourite ways to enjoy Yukon Gold potatoes: smashed, crispy, and served with an addictive avocado garlic aioli sauce. You'll also love the brightness that fresh parsley and lemon add to this otherwise hearty, comfort-food dish. These smashed potatoes make a killer side dish, and everyone, kids and adults alike, will gobble them up. Eric, Adriana and I usually manage to polish off the batch just between the three of us, so I suggest doubling the recipe (including the sauce) if you're serving a group. If you have leftovers, you can reheat the potatoes in the oven until warmed through (just be sure to prepare and serve the sauce fresh, as the colour will change if it sits for too long). If you don't have Yukon Gold potatoes on hand, feel free to use red or new potatoes. I advise against using baking potatoes, as their texture is too dry. Try to select organic potatoes if possible, since conventional potatoes are on the Environmental Working Group's Dirty Dozen list.

1. **Make the potatoes** Put the potatoes into a large pot (no need to peel the potatoes—I actually prefer the texture with the peel on) and add water to cover. Bring the water to a boil over high heat, then reduce the heat slightly and simmer for 20 to 25 minutes, until the potatoes are fork-tender. Drain in a colander and let cool for 10 minutes.

2. Preheat the oven to 450°F (230°C). Place the potatoes on a large lightly greased baking sheet. (I skip the parchment paper here because I find the potatoes get a bit crispier if they roast directly on the baking sheet, but feel free to use parchment paper if your pan tends to stick.) With the base of a mug or metal measuring cup, 'smash' or press down on each potato until it's somewhat flattened. The potatoes will be about 1cm thick after smashing. Some potatoes might break apart a little, but this is normal.

3. Drizzle each potato with about 1 teaspoon of the oil and sprinkle with a generous amount of salt and pepper. Finally, sprinkle on some garlic powder.

(recipe continues)

FOR THE POTATOES

900g Yukon Gold, red or new potatoes

2 to 3 tablespoons extra-virgin olive oil or avocado oil

Fine sea salt and freshly ground black pepper

Garlic powder

20g to 30g fresh parsley leaves, minced

FOR THE AVOCADO GARLIC AIOLI

1 large or 2 small cloves garlic

1 large ripe avocado, halved and pitted

1½ teaspoons fresh lemon juice

60ml Homemade Vegan Mayo (page 269), or store-bought

Fine sea salt and freshly ground black pepper

4. Roast the potatoes for 25 to 30 minutes until crispy, golden, and browned on the bottom. Keep an eye on them, as the cook time will vary depending on the size of the potatoes. Remove from the oven and sprinkle with the parsley. Season with more sea salt and pepper.

5. Meanwhile, make the avocado garlic aioli In a food processor, pulse the garlic until minced. Add the rest of the aioli ingredients and process until smooth, scraping down the bowl as needed. Add salt and pepper to taste.

6. Serve the potatoes immediately with avocado garlic aioli. You can add a big dollop of aioli on top of each potato or transfer the aioli to a plastic bag, snip off one corner, and pipe it on top.

Make it soya-free Use soya-free mayonnaise.

Roasted Garlic Basil Pesto Potatoes with Rocket

VEGAN, GLUTEN-FREE, NUT-FREE, SOYA-FREE, GRAIN-FREE, KID-FRIENDLY

SERVES 4

PREP TIME: **15 MINUTES**

COOK TIME: **40 MINUTES**

This is one of those amazing side dishes that disappears incredibly fast! It's a fancy, restaurant-worthy recipe that is sure to impress special guests. (If you are serving a large crowd, I recommend doubling the recipe since it only serves four as a side.) If you've been sceptical about rocket in the past, I encourage you to give this recipe a try; the spicy, peppery-tasting green pairs beautifully with a bold and bright pesto. If you can't find small-leaf rocket, be sure to chop small-leaf rocket into bite-size pieces so it's easier to eat. Hemp hearts add a kick of protein and omega-3 fatty acids for a nutritional boost. This dish is amazing served warm, but the chilled leftovers taste great as well.

1. Preheat the oven to 400°F (200°C). Line an extra-large baking sheet (38 × 53cm) with parchment paper.

2. Make the potatoes Place the potatoes on the baking sheet and toss with the olive oil until thoroughly coated. Spread the potatoes into an even layer. Season with a couple of pinches of salt and pepper.

3. Make the roasted garlic Slice the top off the garlic bulb so all the individual garlic cloves are trimmed. Place garlic bulb on a square of aluminium foil (about 20cm square) and drizzle the top of the cloves with the olive oil. Wrap the garlic bulb entirely in the foil and place it on the baking sheet with the potatoes.

4. Roast the potatoes and garlic for 20 minutes, then remove the pan from the oven and flip the potatoes with a spatula. Return the potatoes and garlic to the oven and continue roasting for 15 to 20 minutes more, until the potatoes are golden and fork-tender.

5. Make the pesto In a food processor, combine the pesto ingredients and process until mostly smooth, stopping to scrape down the bowl as necessary. Keep the pesto in the processor because we will add the roasted garlic as the final step.

6. Remove the potatoes and garlic from the oven. Carefully unwrap the garlic bulb and let cool for 5 to 10 minutes, until it's cool enough to handle.

(recipe continues)

FOR THE POTATOES

900g Yukon Gold or red potatoes, unpeeled, chopped into 2.5cm cubes

1 tablespoon plus 1½ teaspoons extra-virgin olive oil

Fine sea salt and freshly ground black pepper

FOR THE ROASTED GARLIC

1 large garlic head

½ teaspoon extra-virgin olive oil

FOR THE PESTO

20g fresh basil leaves

3 to 4 tablespoons hemp hearts

60ml extra-virgin olive oil

2 tablespoons fresh lemon juice, or to taste

¼ teaspoon fine sea salt

Freshly ground black pepper

FOR THE SALAD

75g baby leaf rocket, chopped

Fresh lemon juice, for serving (optional)

1 tablespoon hemp hearts, for garnish

7. Turn off the oven and return the potatoes to the oven with the door ajar so they stay warm. (You can also put the potatoes into an oven-safe casserole dish so the dish stays warm when serving.) Squeeze the roasted garlic cloves out of the bulb. You should have about 2 packed tablespoons of roasted garlic. Add it into the food processor with the pesto. Process until mostly smooth—you can add a touch more oil if necessary to get it going.

8. Assemble the salad This is the important part where you need to act fast; I like to assemble the salad very quickly so that it's warm when I serve it. Grab a large serving bowl and place the rocket in the bottom of the bowl. You can break it up into smaller pieces with your hands. Then, remove the potatoes from the oven and quickly place them into the serving bowl on top of the rocket. Toss the potatoes and rocket with the pesto until thoroughly combined. Taste and season with salt and pepper. Sometimes I add another drizzle of lemon juice if I feel the dish needs more acidity. Sprinkle on the hemp hearts and serve immediately.

Tip On the rare chance that you have any leftovers, I've discovered that this side works well as a cold potato salad. Just serve it straight from the fridge!

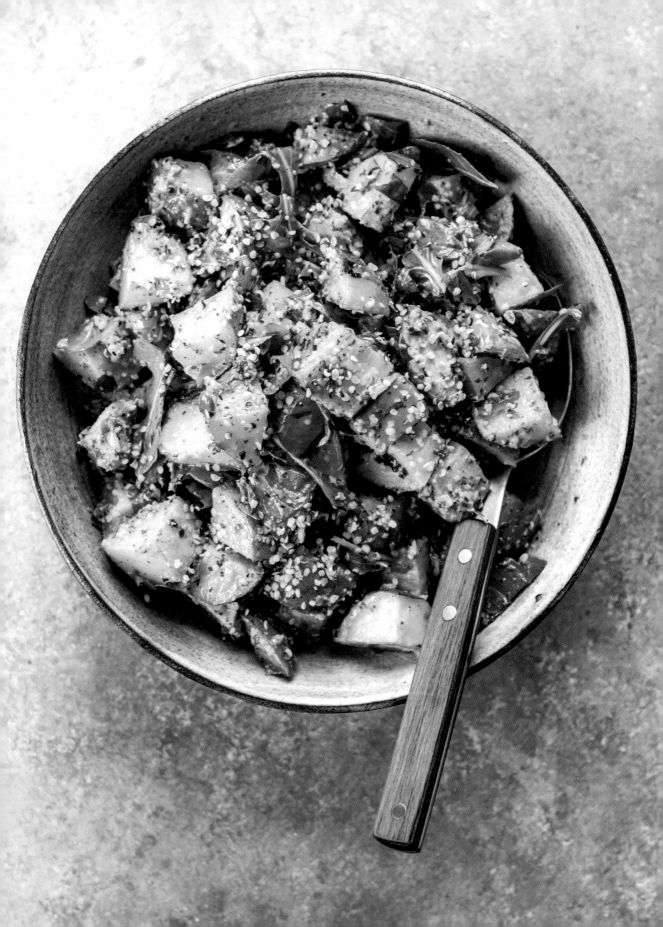

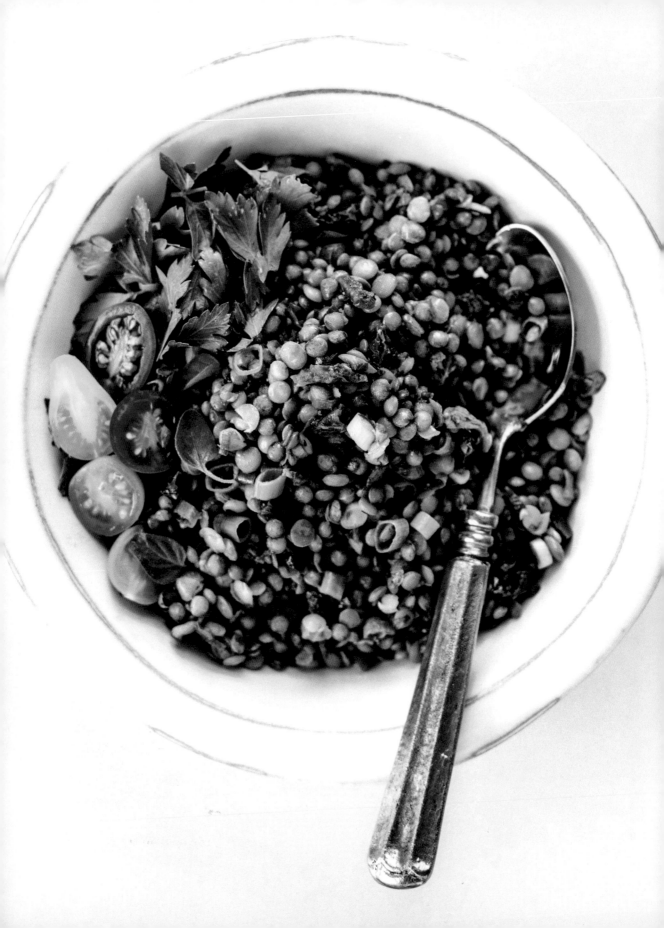

The Best Marinated Lentils

VEGAN, GLUTEN-FREE, NUT-FREE, SOYA-FREE, GRAIN-FREE,
FREEZER-FRIENDLY

MAKES 300g

PREP TIME: 15 MINUTES

COOK TIME: 20 TO 25 MINUTES

Every plant-based eater needs a quick, satisfying, versatile and protein-heavy side dish to rely on at a moment's notice. I created this lentil dish because I was looking for something that could be thrown together in less than a half hour and that I could store in the fridge for the whole workweek. Sun-dried tomatoes add umami and depth of flavour, while the tart, mustardy vinaigrette adds brightness and acidity to the earthy lentils. It's delicious on top of salads, stuffed into lettuce cups, thrown into wraps or pittas, or simply served as the main protein source for any meal. I like to serve it alongside a quick-and-easy stir-fry of seasonal vegetables. For the best texture, I recommend cooking the lentils from scratch (as opposed to using canned lentils). If you already have cooked lentils on hand, you'll need about 265g for this recipe.

1. Pick over the lentils, discarding any debris. Rinse and drain the lentils and put them in a medium saucepan along with 1l of water. Bring to a boil over medium to high heat, then reduce the heat to medium. Simmer, uncovered, for 20 to 25 minutes, until tender.

2. In a large bowl, whisk together the oil, vinegar, lemon juice, mustard, maple syrup, salt, and pepper. Stir in the spring onions, parsley and tomatoes.

3. Drain the lentils very well. Spoon them into the bowl with the other ingredients (it's okay if they are still warm) and stir well. Season with additional salt and pepper.

4. Serve immediately, or let cool slightly and then cover and marinate in the fridge for a couple of hours or overnight. Stir well before serving. This dish will keep in an airtight container in the fridge for up to 1 week, or you can freeze it in a freezer-safe zip-top bag with the air pressed out for up to 1 month. After thawing, I recommend adding extra dressing and salt to liven it up again.

200g uncooked French green lentils

100g uncooked green or brown lentils

2 tablespoons extra-virgin olive oil

2 tablespoons plus 1½ teaspoons red wine vinegar, or to taste

1 tablespoon fresh lemon juice

1½ teaspoons Dijon mustard

1½ teaspoons pure maple syrup

1 teaspoon fine sea salt, or to taste

¼ teaspoon freshly ground black pepper

100g to 150g thinly sliced spring onions (about 1 medium bunch), dark and light green parts only

20g fresh parsley leaves, minced

65g oil-packed sun-dried tomatoes, drained and finely chopped

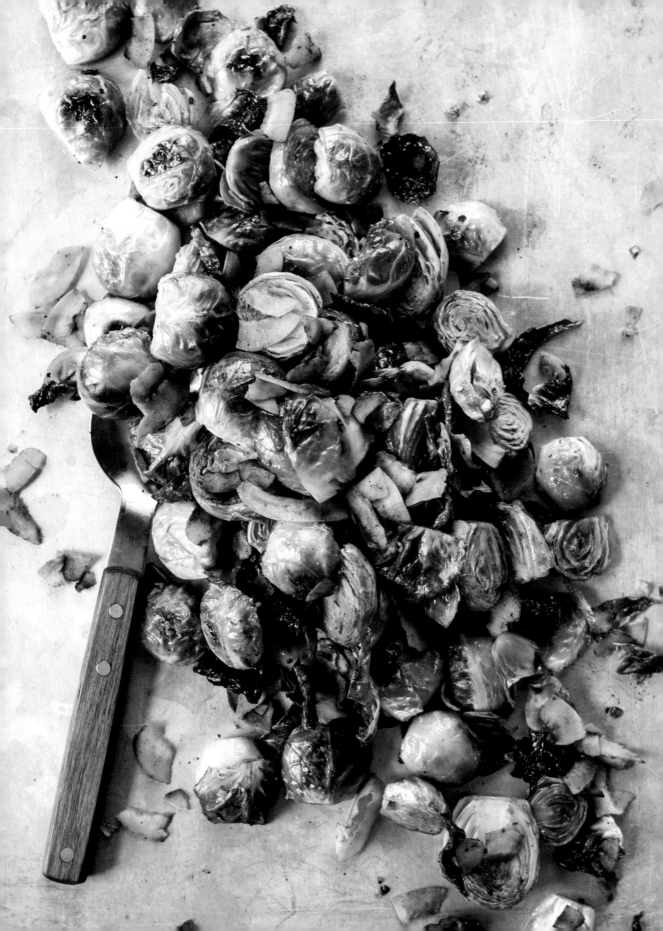

Roasted Brussels Sprouts and Coconut 'Bacon'

VEGAN, GLUTEN-FREE, NUT-FREE, SOYA-FREE OPTION, GRAIN-FREE

SERVES 4

PREP TIME: **20 MINUTES**

COOK TIME: **25 TO 30 MINUTES**

This dish is a fun, plant-based take on traditional bacon and Brussels sprouts, with all the smoky-sweet flavors of the original dish. The salty, fragrant, and slightly sweet coconut bacon doesn't taste *exactly* like bacon (I'm not a miracle worker here!), but it's delicious in its own right! To make the coconut bacon, you want to use large-flake unsweetened coconut (also known as 'coconut chips'), not shredded coconut. In the rare event that you have leftovers, I recommend spreading them over a parchment paper-lined baking sheet and reheating them in the oven at 350°F (180°C) until warmed through.

1. **Make the Brussels sprouts** Preheat the oven to 400°F (200°C). Line a large baking sheet with parchment paper.

2. Place the Brussels sprouts in a large bowl. Add the oil and maple syrup and toss to coat. Sprinkle on the garlic and toss again to coat. Season with salt, black pepper, cayenne (if using) and garlic granules. Spread the Brussels sprouts over the prepared baking sheet in an even layer.

3. Roast for 15 minutes, then gently stir/flip the Brussels sprouts and roast for 10 to 20 minutes more, until lightly charred in some spots and fork-tender. I prefer to char them for a better flavour, but watch closely so they don't scorch.

4. **Meanwhile, make the coconut bacon** In a bowl, stir together the large-flake coconut, coconut aminos, maple syrup, salt, paprika, cayenne, and liquid smoke (if using). Scoop the coconut mixture into a large skillet and toast the coconut over medium heat, stirring frequently, for 5 to 10 minutes. You may want to turn on the cooker's fan and open a window while it cooks, as the smoked aroma is quite powerful! Immediately remove the coconut from the pan and place it on a parchment paper-lined plate so it doesn't stick to the skillet as it dries.

5. Spoon the Brussels sprouts into a serving dish. Sprinkle the coconut bacon on top. Season with additional salt, pepper and garlic granules. Serve immediately.

Make it soya-free Use coconut aminos instead of tamari.

FOR THE BRUSSELS SPROUTS

900g Brussels sprouts, trimmed and halved

1 tablespoon extra-virgin olive oil

1 tablespoon pure maple syrup

2 cloves garlic, minced or grated on a Microplane

Fine sea salt and freshly ground black pepper

$1/8$ teaspoon cayenne pepper, or $1/4$ teaspoon red pepper flakes (optional)

$1/8$ to $1/4$ teaspoon garlic granules or powder, to taste

FOR THE COCONUT BACON

40g unsweetened large-flake coconut (not shredded coconut)

$1 1/2$ teaspoons coconut aminos or low-sodium tamari

$1/2$ teaspoon pure maple syrup

$1/8$ teaspoon fine sea salt

$1/8$ teaspoon smoked paprika

Pinch of cayenne pepper

$1/8$ teaspoon liquid smoke (optional)

Fine sea salt and freshly ground black pepper

$1/8$ to $1/4$ teaspoon garlic granules, to taste

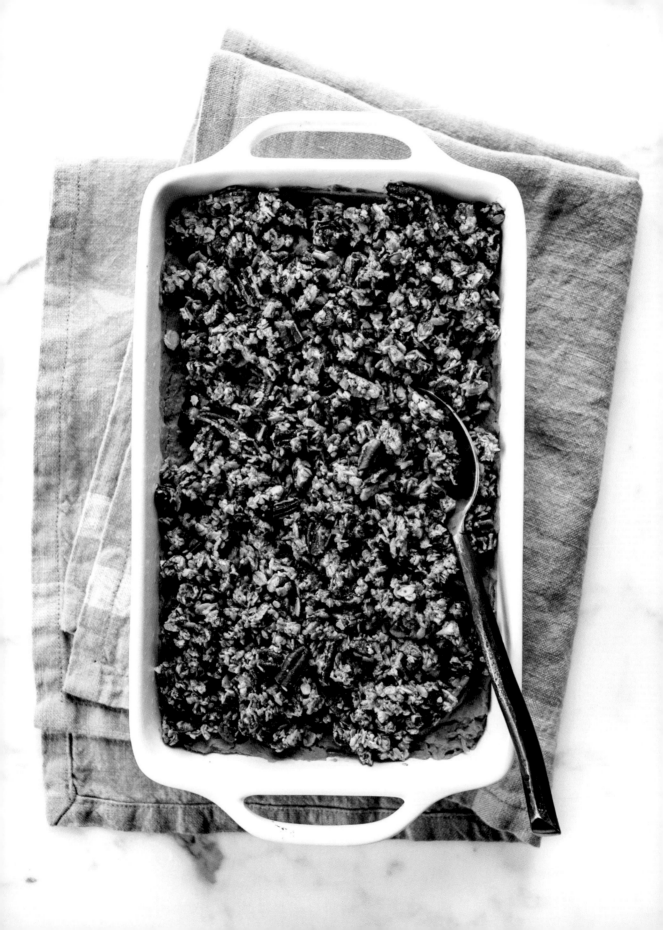

Sweet Potato Casserole

VEGAN, GLUTEN-FREE, SOYA-FREE OPTION, KID-FRIENDLY, FREEZER-FRIENDLY

SERVES 8

PREP TIME: 35 MINUTES

COOK TIME: 29 TO 38 MINUTES

You'll want this side dish to adorn your holiday dinner table! The crunchy nut crumble tastes just like an oatmeal cookie, and the creamy sweet potato filling has hints of cinnamon and vanilla to help complement the recipe's natural sweetness. I recommend adding a pat of dairy-free spread or coconut oil on top of each serving to take the dish over the top. For an even more decadent twist, try serving it with Coconut Whipped Cream (page 275).

1. Preheat the oven to 375°F (190°C). Lightly grease a 2.5l casserole dish with coconut oil or dairy-free spread.

2. **Make the sweet potato mash** Place the sweet potatoes in a large pot and add water to cover. Bring to a boil over high heat, reduce the heat to medium-high, and gently boil for 15 to 20 minutes, until the potatoes are fork-tender. Drain and transfer back into the pot.

3. Add the spread and coconut oil and mash until smooth. Stir in the maple syrup, vanilla, cinnamon, nutmeg and salt. Taste and adjust the seasonings, if desired. If you'd like to thin it out a bit so it's easy to spread, add some almond milk and stir again. Spoon the mixture into the prepared casserole dish and smooth out the top.

4. **Make the crunchy pecan crumble** In a food processor, pulse the oats until coarsely chopped. Do not grind them into a flour, as you want to retain some texture. In a medium bowl, stir together the oats, chopped pecans, almond meal/flour, cinnamon and salt. Pour on the melted spread, melted coconut oil and maple syrup. Stir until thoroughly combined.

5. Sprinkle the crumble topping all over the sweet potato mixture in an even layer.

6. Bake for 14 to 18 minutes, until the dish is hot throughout. The topping will still be quite light in colour. Plate and serve immediately with a pat of dairy-free spread or coconut oil on top. The casserole will keep wrapped up in the fridge for 4 to 5 days, or you can freeze it for up to 1 month. Sometimes I will prepare this casserole in 2 small oven-safe dishes, cook one of them and freeze the other for another time.

Tip If you don't want a light coconut flavour, be sure to use refined coconut oil.

Make it soya-free Use soya-free, dairy-free spread.

FOR THE SWEET POTATO MASH

2 to 2.25kg sweet potatoes (4 or 5 large), peeled and chopped into 2.5cm chunks

4 teaspoons dairy-free spread

4 teaspoons virgin coconut oil (or more dairy-free spread)

37ml pure maple syrup, or to taste

1 teaspoon pure vanilla extract

¾ teaspoon ground cinnamon

⅛ teaspoon ground nutmeg

½ to ¾ teaspoon fine sea salt, to taste

Almond milk, as needed

FOR THE CRUNCHY PECAN CRUMBLE

85g gluten-free rolled oats

190g pecan halves, chopped

25g ground almonds or almond flour

1 teaspoon ground cinnamon

¼ teaspoon fine sea salt

2 tablespoons dairy-free spread melted

2 tablespoons virgin coconut oil (or more dairy-free spread), melted

2 tablespoons plus 1½ teaspoons pure maple syrup

Dairy-free spread or coconut oil, for serving

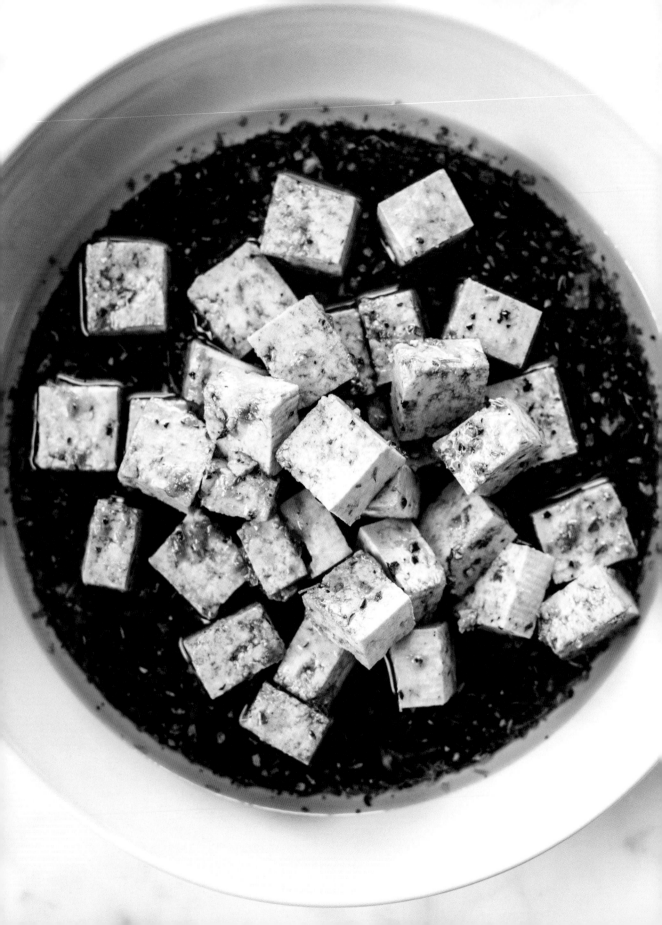

Marinated Italian Tofu

VEGAN, GLUTEN-FREE, NUT-FREE, GRAIN-FREE, ADVANCE PREP REQUIRED, KID-FRIENDLY

SERVES 4

PREP TIME: **10 MINUTES**

MARINATE TIME: **30 MINUTES OR OVERNIGHT**

This is a quick-and-easy, no-oven-required method of adding a ton of flavour to tofu. Tofu tastes very neutral when it's served plain, but it absorbs flavour really well. A great marinade can be the difference between tofu that's bland and tofu that's show-stopping! This marinade has a great sweet-and-sour flavour from the balsamic vinegar, which is enhanced by a generous amount of garlic and herbs. Once I came up with it, I was absolutely hooked. These marinated cubes make the perfect salad topper in the summer, and the fact that you won't have to turn on your oven to enjoy them is a big plus in hot months. If you prefer your tofu warm, you can sear the cubes lightly in a frying pan. Otherwise, just toss the tofu in the marinade and let it sit for as long as you have—thirty minutes or up to overnight, your choice. I even keep leftovers in the fridge (soaking in the marinade) for up to a few days. The marinade is a perfect base for tweaking and creating different flavours—feel free to experiment with your favourite spices or herbs (fresh or dry). Try the marinated tofu in a wrap, stir-fry, or salad for an easy, flavourful boost of protein!

1 340 to 450g block firm or extra-firm tofu, drained and patted dry

75ml extra-virgin olive oil

75ml balsamic vinegar

2 tablespoons low-sodium tamari

4 medium cloves garlic, grated on a Microplane

1 teaspoon pure maple syrup, or more to taste

1 teaspoon lemon zest

1/2 teaspoon dried basil

1/2 teaspoon dried oregano

1/4 teaspoon dried thyme

1/4 teaspoon fine sea salt

1/8 teaspoon freshly ground black pepper

1. Slice the tofu into about 64 1cm cubes (I slice the entire block in half crosswise, then slice four long columns, and then eight rows across in each piece; see page 311 for a photo tutorial). Place the tofu cubes in a large container with a lid or a large zip-top bag.

2. Add the oil, vinegar, tamari, garlic, maple syrup, lemon zest, basil, oregano, thyme, salt and pepper and secure the lid (or seal the bag). Toss until the tofu is thoroughly coated in the marinade.

3. Marinate the tofu in the fridge for at least 30 minutes, but longer if you have the time. Sometimes I marinate it for an hour, other times I marinate it overnight. The flavour just keeps getting better! Store any leftovers in the fridge for 3 to 4 days. The marinade tends to solidify when chilled due to the olive oil; if this happens, simply leave the container/bag on the counter at room temperature and it will liquefy once again.

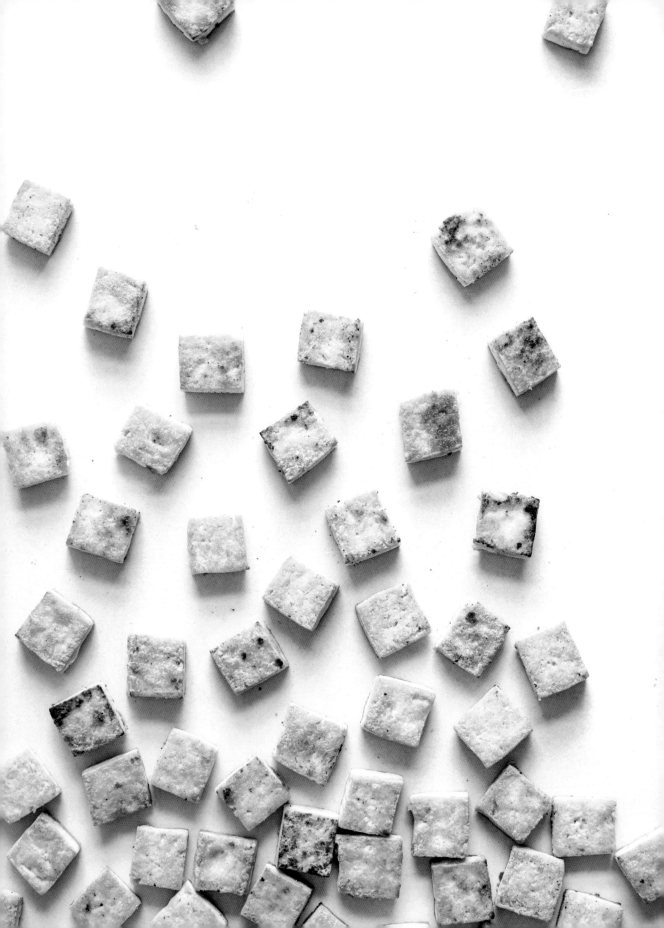

Cast-Iron Tofu

VEGAN, GLUTEN-FREE, NUT-FREE, GRAIN-FREE, ADVANCE PREP REQUIRED, KID-FRIENDLY

SERVES 4

PREP TIME: **10 MINUTES**

PRESS TIME: **30 MINUTES OR OVERNIGHT**

COOK TIME: **8 TO 12 MINUTES**

A lot of people find the texture of tofu to be too mushy or soft. This cooking method creates crispy, lightly flavored tofu that works well in a variety of dishes and may just win over the tofu haters in your life. I purposely kept the flavour of this tofu light, so that it can take on the flavours in any dish that you add it to. Try it folded into my Lemon-Tahini Dressing (page 265) and as a topping on the Every Day Glow salad (page 115), or as an easy protein source in my Soba Noodle Salad (page 183). The recipe is designed for a cast-iron skillet, as it will intensify the crispy shell of the tofu. If you don't have a cast-iron skillet, you can use a regular frying pan—just note that the tofu won't get quite as crispy.

1 340 to 450g block firm or extra-firm tofu

3 teaspoons avocado oil, grapeseed oil or olive oil

1 teaspoon garlic powder

¼ teaspoon fine sea salt

¼ teaspoon onion powder (optional)

1. Following the instructions on page 271, press the tofu overnight, or for at least 30 minutes.

2. Slice the pressed tofu into 9 or 10 rectangles 1cm thick and then slice each rectangle into 6 squares, to make a total of 54 to 60 tofu pieces.

3. Heat a large cast-iron (or non-stick) frying pan over medium-high heat for several minutes.

4. In a large bowl, combine the tofu with 1½ teaspoons of the oil. Gently stir until all the tofu is coated. Stir in the garlic powder, salt, and onion powder (if using).

5. When a drop of water gently sizzles on the frying pan, it is hot enough. Carefully add the remaining 1½ teaspoons oil and tilt the pan to coat it evenly with the oil. Add the tofu to the pan in a single layer (be careful, as the oil might splatter—use a splatter guard, if desired), making sure all the pieces lay flat. If yours is too small to cook all the tofu at once, work in batches.

6. Cook the tofu on one side for 4 to 7 minutes, until you have a golden crust with some speckled brown spots (the crust should be about 1.5mm in thickness). With a fork, flip each piece (yes, this step is a bit arduous) and cook for 4 to 5 minutes more, until golden. Serve immediately; the tofu crust will soften as it cools.

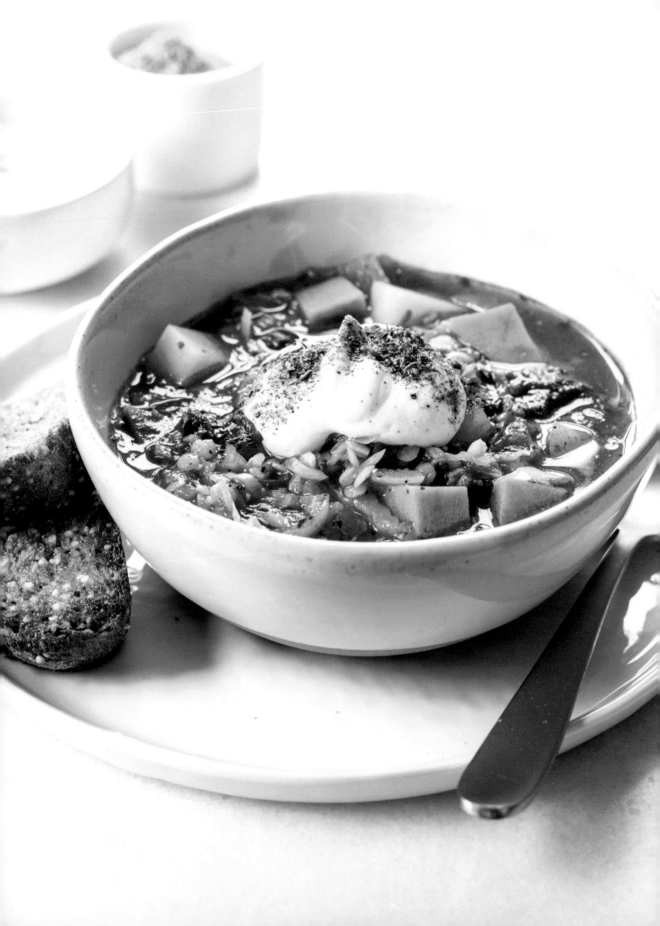

Metabolism-Revving Spicy Cabbage Soup

VEGAN, GLUTEN-FREE, NUT-FREE OPTION, SOYA-FREE, GRAIN-FREE,
FREEZER-FRIENDLY

MAKES 2L (4 SERVINGS)

PREP TIME: **20 TO 25 MINUTES**

COOK TIME: **25 TO 30 MINUTES**

Cabbage isn't particularly high on my veggie excitement totem pole, and it's probably not very high on yours, either. But this soup changes my mind about humble cabbage each and every time. It's the ultimate get-your-diet-back-on-track soup, yet it manages not to taste like diet food. I eat this soup religiously all winter long, as it helps balance out all the indulgent holiday eating that tends to go on.

Because traditional cabbage soup recipes tend to be a little bland and lacking in protein, I decided to kick things up a few notches by using my 9-Spice Mix for flavour and some red lentils to boost the protein. The result is a flavourful, spicy bowl of cabbage soup that's full of protein and fibre, and its flavour only intensifies as the leftovers sit. Thanks to the lentils, this soup can stand alone as a meal, especially if you pair it with a hunk of bread on the side.

1. In a large stockpot, heat the oil over medium heat. Add the onion and garlic and sauté for 5 to 6 minutes, until the onion is softened. Stir in 2 tablespoons of 9-Spice Mix and cook for a minute or so, until fragrant.

2. Add the cabbage and diced tomatoes with their juices. Simmer over medium to high heat for about 5 minutes.

3. Add the broth, red lentils and potatoes. Stir. Cover and simmer over medium heat for 15 to 20 minutes, or until the lentils and potatoes are tender.

4. Season with salt and pepper to taste. You can also add 1 to 1½ teaspoons more 9-Spice Mix if you'd like it a bit spicier.

5. Serve with a dollop of Cashew Sour Cream (if using). The cashew cream will quickly blend into the soup, resulting in a creamy broth. This soup will keep in the fridge for up to a week, and it freezes well for 1 to 2 months.

Tip It's important to chop the potatoes small so they cook quickly. Cutting them into 1cm pieces is perfect.

Make it nut-free Leave out the cashew cream for serving.

4 teaspoons extra-virgin olive oil

1 large sweet onion, chopped

3 cloves garlic, minced

2 tablespoons 9-Spice Mix (page 258), or more to taste

450g green cabbage (¼ large head), cored and finely shredded

1 400g can diced tomatoes, with juices

1l low-sodium vegetable broth

100g uncooked red lentils

2 medium Yukon Gold potatoes or 1 small peeled sweet potato (225g), chopped into 1cm cubes

½ to 1 teaspoon fine sea salt

Freshly ground black pepper

Cashew Sour Cream (page 261), for serving (optional)

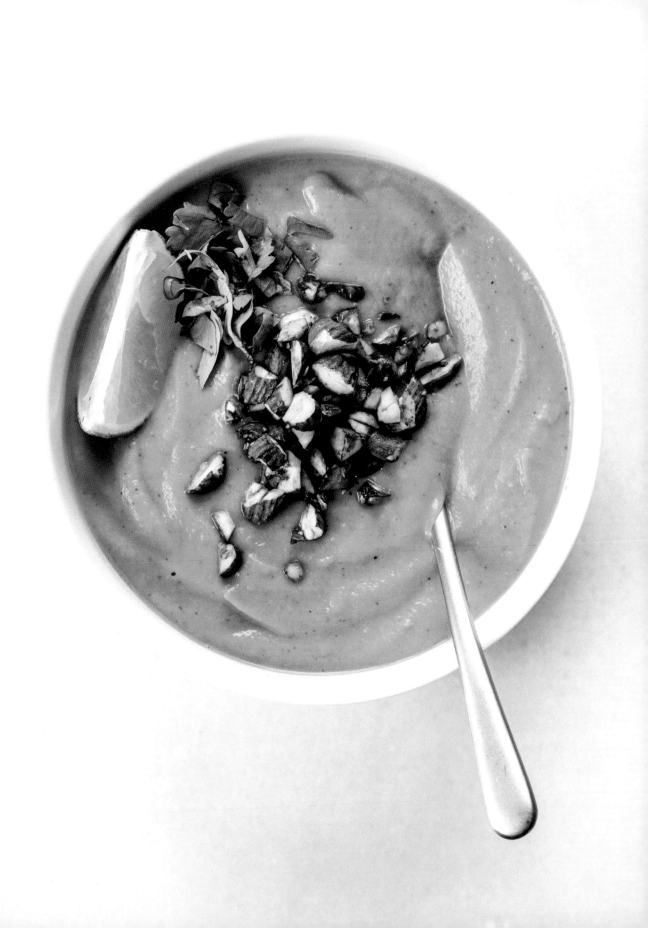

Creamy Thai Carrot Sweet Potato Soup

VEGAN, GLUTEN-FREE, SOYA-FREE OPTION, GRAIN-FREE, FREEZER-FRIENDLY

MAKES 2L (4 SERVINGS)

PREP: **25 MINUTES**

COOK TIME: **20 TO 26 MINUTES**

This is my favourite blended soup, and we've been making it once a week during the fall and winter seasons. It's 'in the vault', as we like to say! The soup shows off the flavour of red curry paste, an authentic Thai ingredient. It's warm and spicy, but not overpowering, and it's usually enhanced with notes of lemongrass, garlic, ginger and chilli. It works wonders in this soup, creating rich and full-blown flavour in an instant! The soup also boasts a rich, thick texture, which makes it very comforting as the weather turns cooler. If you don't have any almond butter, feel free to use peanut butter instead. It's also fantastic served with a scoop of cooked rice on the bottom of the bowl to make it heartier. A big thanks to my friend Angela Simpson, the blogger behind eat-spin-run-repeat.com, for inspiring this delicious recipe!

1. In a large pot, melt the coconut oil over medium heat.

2. Add the onion, garlic, and ginger and sauté for 5 to 6 minutes, until the onion is translucent.

3. Stir in the curry paste.

4. In a small bowl, whisk together some of the broth with the almond butter until smooth. Add the mixture to the pot, along with the remaining broth, carrots, sweet potatoes, salt, and cayenne (if using). Stir until combined.

5. Bring the soup to a low boil over medium-high heat and then reduce the heat to medium-low. Cover and simmer for 15 to 20 minutes, until the potatoes and carrots are fork-tender.

6. Ladle the soup carefully into a blender. You will likely have to do this in a couple of batches, depending on the size of your blender. With the lid slightly ajar to allow steam to escape, blend on low and slowly increase the speed until the soup is completely smooth. (Alternatively, you can use a stick blender and blend the soup directly in the pot.)

7. Return the soup to the pot and season with salt and black pepper. If desired, you can thin the soup out with a bit more broth if it's too thick for your preference. Reheat if necessary.

8. Ladle the soup into bowls and top with minced coriander, almonds, and a squeeze of lime juice, if desired. This soup will keep in the fridge for up to a week, and freezes well for 1 to 2 months.

FOR THE SOUP

1 tablespoon virgin coconut oil

300g diced sweet onion

2 cloves garlic, minced

1 tablespoon minced fresh ginger

2 tablespoons red curry paste

1l low-sodium vegetable broth, plus more if needed

60ml raw almond butter

450g diced peeled carrots (1cm dice)

600g diced peeled sweet potatoes (1cm dice)

½ teaspoon fine sea salt, plus more to taste

¼ teaspoon cayenne pepper (optional)

Freshly ground black pepper

TOPPING SUGGESTIONS

Minced fresh coriander

Roasted Tamari Almonds (page 263)

Fresh lime juice

Make it soya-free Prepare the Roasted Tamari Almonds with coconut aminos instead of tamari.

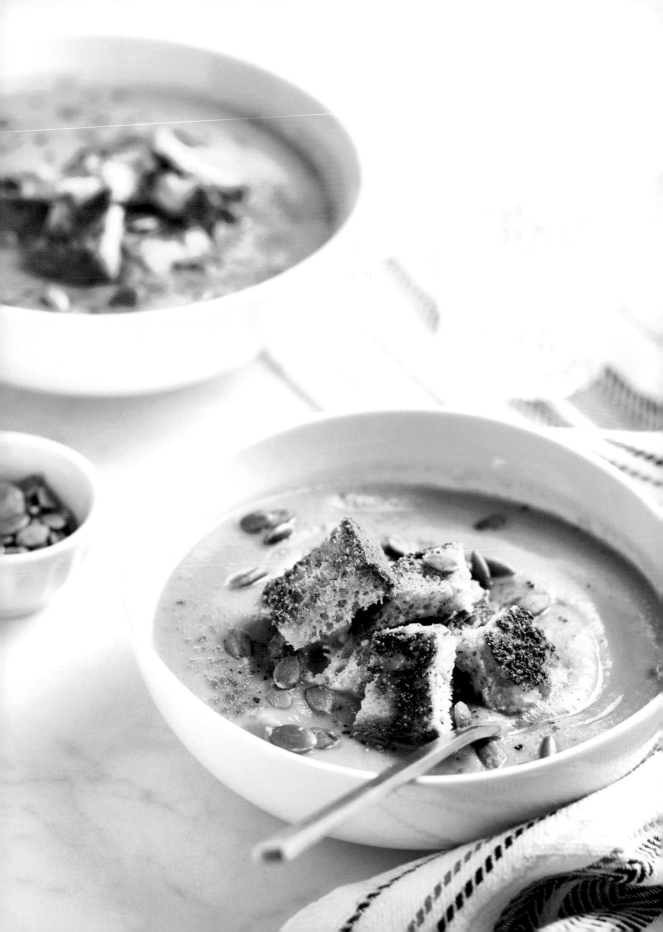

6 Vegetable and 'Cheese' Soup

VEGAN, GLUTEN-FREE, NUT-FREE, SOYA-FREE, GRAIN-FREE OPTION,
REFINED SUGAR-FREE

MAKES 2 TO 2.5L (4 SERVINGS)

PREP TIME: 25 MINUTES

COOK TIME: 20 MINUTES

Silky smooth and bursting with six healthy vegetables, this luxurious soup is an easy, everyday soup to enjoy all fall and winter long. The nutritional yeast gives this soup a bit of a 'cheese-like' flavour, and I keep the spices simple to allow the flavours of the vegetables to shine. The beauty of making a puréed soup is that you don't have to fuss over chopping the vegetables too precisely since it'll be blended anyway; this results in a faster prep time. To give this creamy soup some texture, try topping it with my Easiest Garlic Croutons (page 257) and toasted pumpkin seeds for a little crunch.

1. In a large pot, heat the oil over medium heat. Add the onion, garlic, and a couple pinches of salt and sauté over medium heat for 3 to 4 minutes until the onion is softened.

2. Add the celery, carrots, broccoli, and sweet potato. Continue to sauté over medium heat for about 5 minutes. Stir frequently.

3. Add the broth and stir. Bring the soup to a low boil. Cover and simmer over medium-low heat for 12 to 15 minutes, or until the vegetables are fork-tender.

4. Turn off the heat and remove the lid. Allow the soup to cool slightly for 5 minutes or so.

5. Carefully scoop the soup into a blender (you might have to do this in a couple of batches depending on the size of your blender). Add 3 tablespoons of nutritional yeast, ½ teaspoon of salt, and cayenne (if using). Alternatively, you can use a stick blender.

6. With the blender lid ajar (to allow the steam to escape), carefully blend the mixture starting at a low speed and increasing the speed until the soup is smooth.

7. Pour the puréed soup back into the pot. Stir and add more salt, to taste. Then, add more nutritional yeast (if desired), black pepper, and vinegar, to taste.

8. Ladle the soup into bowls. Garnish with toasted pumpkin seeds and croutons, if desired.

9. Transfer leftovers into a Mason jar and allow to cool before securing the lid and storing in the fridge for 5 to 7 days. To freeze, add cooled soup into a container or Mason jar, leaving an inch (2.5cm) at the top for expansion. Secure lid and freeze for 1 to 2 months.

2 tablespoons extra-virgin olive oil

1 medium-large onion, chopped (about 300 to 375g)

3 large cloves garlic, minced

225g celery, chopped (about 2 to 3 stalks)

150g carrots, peeled and chopped (about 2 small-medium carrots)

1050g broccoli florets (about 1 large broccoli head)

400g sweet potato, peeled and chopped (about 1 small sweet potato)

1.25 to 1.5ml low-sodium vegetable broth, as needed

3 to 4 tablespoons nutritional yeast, to taste

Salt and pepper, to taste (I use about 1 teaspoon)

¼ teaspoon cayenne pepper (optional)

White wine vinegar or fresh lemon juice, to taste (I usually add 1 to 2 teaspoons of white wine vinegar for flavour)

Toasted pumpkin seeds, for serving

Easiest Garlic Croutons (page 257), for serving

Make it grain-free Serve this soup without the Easiest Garlic Croutons.

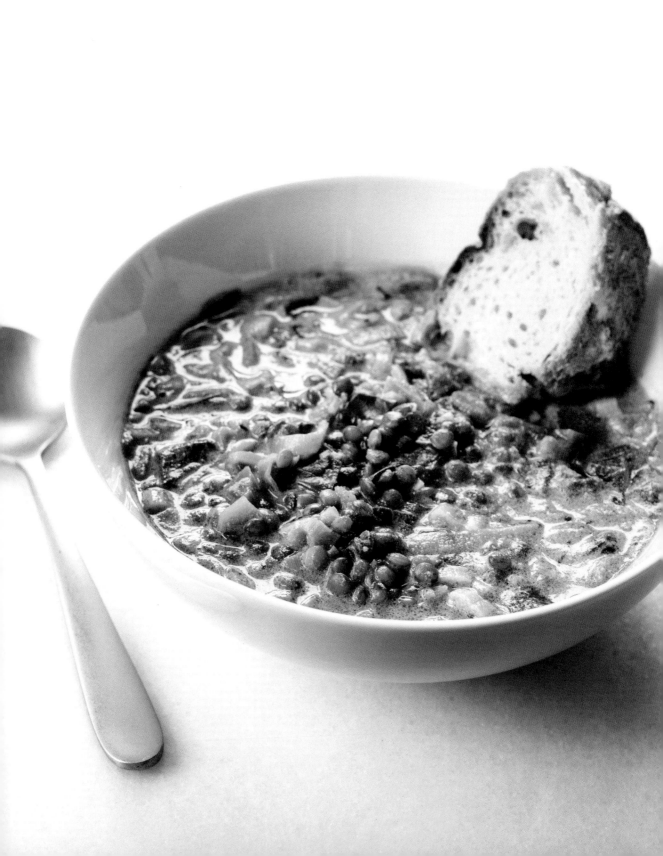

Golden French Lentil Stew

VEGAN, GLUTEN-FREE, NUT-FREE OPTION, SOYA-FREE, GRAIN-FREE,
ADVANCE PREP REQUIRED, KID-FRIENDLY OPTION, FREEZER-FRIENDLY

MAKES 2L (4 SERVINGS)

SOAK TIME: **1 TO 2 HOURS, OR OVERNIGHT**

PREP TIME: **20 TO 25 MINUTES**

COOK TIME: **36 TO 43 MINUTES**

This golden-hued stew is remarkably rich and creamy, thanks to the addition of a dairy-free cream base that can be either nut- or seed-based. Turmeric gives this stew its joyful, rich colour, not to mention anti-inflammatory benefits; curcumin, one of the compounds in turmeric, has been shown to help reduce swelling and inflammation. When I was developing this recipe, I tested the stew with both cashew and sunflower seed cream, and both versions work beautifully. It's a friendly recipe for those with tree nut allergies (providing you can still eat sunflower seeds). The stew is spiced with dried thyme and cumin, and it packs a hefty portion of greens (Swiss chard or kale—your choice!) and other hearty vegetables like carrot and celery. The French green lentils hold their shape well and add a lovely, chewy element, but feel free to use green or brown lentils if that's all you can find. The stew will just be thicker, since green and brown lentils break down a bit more.

1. Put the cashews in a bowl and cover with a couple of inches of water. Soak for 1 to 2 hours or overnight. (For a quick-soak method, cover with boiling water and soak for 30 to 60 minutes.) Drain and rinse. Transfer the cashews to a high-speed blender along with 125ml of the water. Blend on high until super smooth and creamy in texture. Set the cashew cream aside.

2. In a large Dutch oven or stockpot, heat the oil over medium heat. Stir in the onion, garlic, and a couple pinches of salt, and sauté until the onion is softened, 4 to 6 minutes.

3. Stir in the carrots and celery, and cook for another few minutes or so. Stir in the cumin, thyme, and turmeric until combined.

4. Add the diced tomatoes with their juices, lentils, broth, and remaining water. Increase the heat to high and bring to a low boil. Reduce the heat to medium and simmer, uncovered, for 30 to 35 minutes, until the lentils are tender.

(recipe continues)

- 65g raw cashews or 45g raw sunflower seeds
- 500ml water
- 2 tablespoons extra-virgin olive oil
- 1 large brown or sweet onion, diced, or 2 leeks, cleaned and thinly sliced (about 300g)
- 4 large cloves garlic, minced (2 tablespoons)
- 1 to 1½ teaspoons fine sea salt, to taste, plus a couple of pinches
- 2 medium carrots, diced (150g)
- 2 stalks celery, diced (170g)
- 2 teaspoons ground cumin
- 1½ teaspoons dried thyme
- 1 teaspoon ground turmeric
- 1 400g can of chopped tomatoes, with juices
- 50g uncooked French green lentils, picked over and rinsed
- 1l low-sodium vegetable broth
- 300g de-stemmed and chopped Swiss chard or kale leaves
- Freshly ground black pepper
- 1 to 2 teaspoons white wine vinegar, to taste

5. Stir in the cashew cream and chard. Add salt, pepper, and vinegar to taste. (The vinegar's role is to lend brightness to the soup; add a little bit at a time and keep tasting, as it can quickly overwhelm.) Cook for a couple of minutes over low-medium heat, until the chard is wilted, and then serve. This stew will keep in an airtight container in the fridge for up to 5 days, or you can freeze it for 1 to 2 months (always let it cool completely before storing). The stew will thicken after sitting in the fridge; you can thin it out with a bit of broth when you reheat it, if desired, or simply serve it thick with some crusty bread.

Tip When the cashew (or sunflower seed) cream is mixed into the soup, the broth can take on a speckled appearance due to it reacting with the vinegar. This is totally normal and does not affect the delicious flavor of the soup!

Make it nut-free Use sunflower seed cream rather than cashew cream.

Make it kid-friendly This soup has a lot of nutrient-packed ingredients, which can mean a lot of chewing for little ones. You can purée their servings in a blender and serve with my Easiest Garlic Croutons (page 257) cut into strips for dipping.

Go-To Gazpacho

VEGAN, GLUTEN-FREE, NUT-FREE, SOYA-FREE, GRAIN-FREE, OIL-FREE, FREEZER-FRIENDLY

MAKES 2L (4 SERVINGS)

PREP TIME: **10 MINUTES**

This is the perfect soup to serve on a hot summer's day—bonus points if you are eating al fresco! Gazpacho can seem like an intimidating soup to get right, or at least it was for me in the beginning. The flavours were difficult to balance. After a lot of trial and error, I came up with my perfect version, and this recipe never lets me down! It's my favourite way to use in-season tomatoes; I make this gazpacho about once a week in the summer. Look for smaller tomatoes, like Roma (plum) tomatoes, as they are the most flavourful. Also be aware that this recipe makes a lot—almost two litres' worth. I find that the ingredients just fit in my 2l Vitamix. If you are using a smaller blender, I recommend blending in batches before mixing it all together at the end, or simply use the food processor method (detailed below) for a chunky soup. Don't worry about the yield, though: You'll gobble up the flavourful, fresh soup quickly, and leftovers deepen in flavour over the course of a few days. I can often be found guzzling it straight from a big Mason jar! That doesn't surprise you, though, I'm sure. To change up the flavours, try adding a couple of tablespoons of fresh basil, coriander or parsley into the mix.

1. **For smooth gazpacho** In a blender, combine the tomatoes, bell pepper, cucumber, onion, garlic, vegetable cocktail and lime juice and blend on low speed until the desired texture is achieved. Season to taste with salt, vinegar, black pepper, and cayenne (if using) and blend again briefly to combine. Note that the intensity of the red colour will vary based on the tomatoes and ingredients used.

2. **For chunky gazpacho** Mince the garlic in a food processor. Add the tomatoes, bell pepper, cucumber and onion and pulse until the desired texture is reached. Transfer the vegetables to a large bowl or extra-large mason jar and stir in the rest of the ingredients.

3. Transfer to a jar or bowl, cover, and chill for 3 to 4 hours, or overnight.

675g ripe tomatoes (6 or 7 small), cored and roughly chopped

1 large red bell pepper, seeded and roughly chopped

1 cucumber (about 450g), peeled and roughly chopped

40g chopped sweet onion

1 large clove garlic

500ml vegetable cocktail or tomato juice (see Tip)

1 tablespoon fresh lime juice

Fine sea salt

4 teaspoons to 3 tablespoons red wine vinegar, sherry vinegar or balsamic vinegar to taste

Freshly ground black pepper

Cayenne pepper (optional)

TOPPING SUGGESTIONS

Chopped avocado

Drizzle of extra-virgin olive oil

Easiest Garlic Croutons (page 257)

Diced cucumber and red bell pepper

Chopped fresh basil, parsley or coriander

(recipe continues)

4. Portion into bowls and top with your desired garnishes. This soup will keep in the fridge for 3 days and freezes well for 1 to 2 months. Stir (or shake, if storing in a jar) before serving, as the soup tends to separate.

Tip 1. I love using R. W. Knudsen Family 'Very Veggie' Low-Sodium Vegetable Cocktail in this soup. I find using a vegetable cocktail adds a lot of flavour; however, feel free to use plain tomato juice if you prefer. 2. If you blend the gazpacho smooth, you can sip it from a glass just like a vegetable cocktail! I love to throw some into a Mason jar and pack it in the cooler for a quick refreshing drink that's packed with veggies.

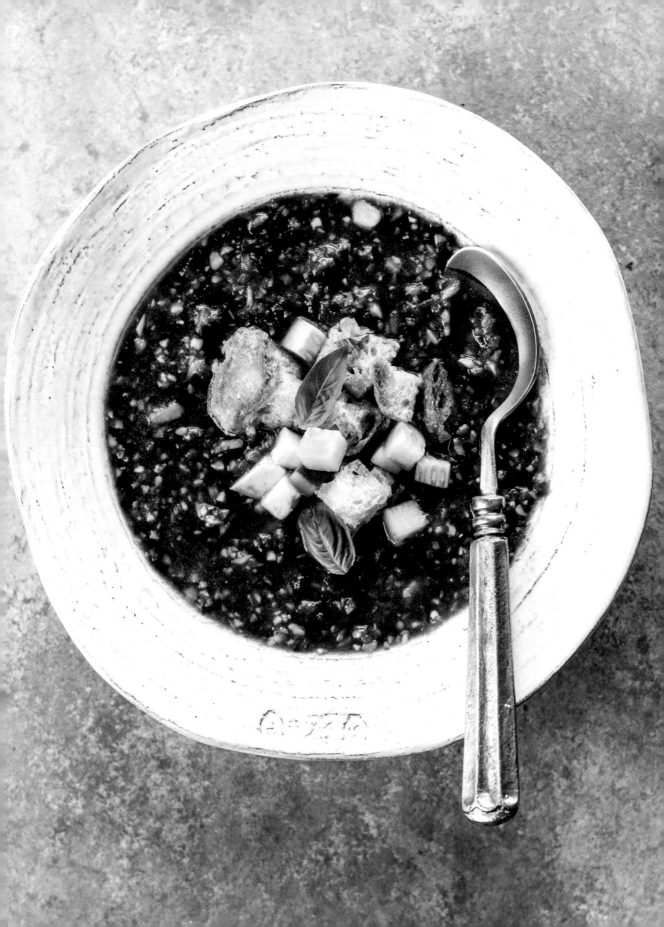

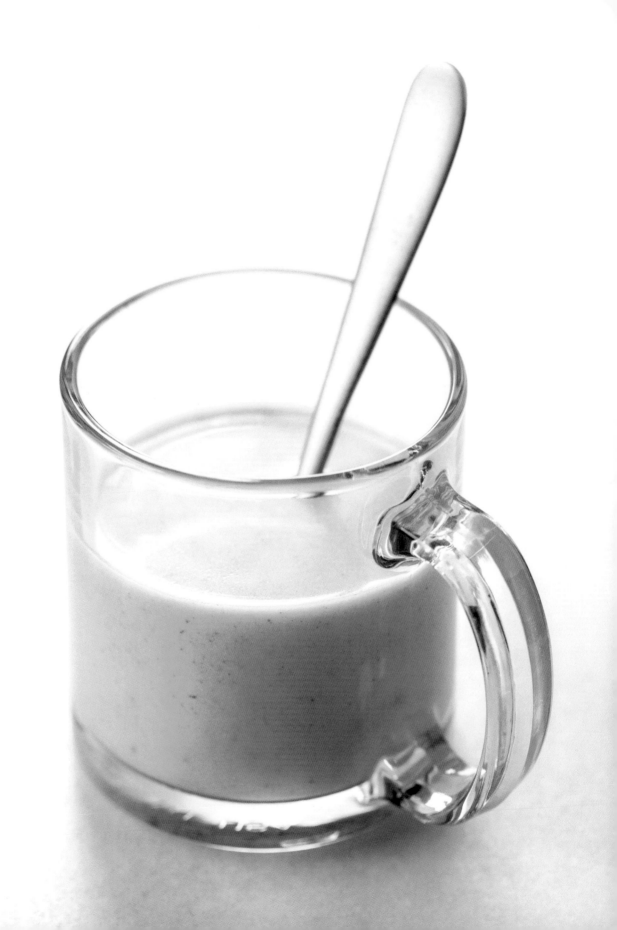

Miracle Healing Broth

VEGAN, GLUTEN-FREE, NUT-FREE, SOYA-FREE, GRAIN-FREE, FREEZER-FRIENDLY

MAKES (1 OR 2 SERVINGS)

PREP TIME: **5 TO 10 MINUTES**

COOK TIME: **10 MINUTES**

One day, I was feeling run down and looking for something I could prepare effortlessly in just a few minutes. I made a list of my favourite healing foods, and then I started tossing things into a pot! Well, on my very first attempt, this broth blew me away. I still can't believe how amazing this healing broth tastes, and how incredibly nutritious it is at the same time. It's packed with fresh garlic, which is great for the immune system, as well as anti-inflammatory and antibacterial fresh ginger. The base incorporates coconut milk, so the broth has a super-luxurious, creamy texture that just feels so decadent. I strain the soup for an even smoother texture. A bit of fresh lemon juice and cayenne pepper provide an extra boost of immune-enhancing properties, as well as a kick of tart, spicy flavour! Make this healing broth whenever you need a serious energy boost, or when you are trying to recover from a cold.

1. In a medium pot, melt the oil over low-medium heat.

2. Add the onion, garlic and ginger and stir to combine. Sauté over medium heat, stirring frequently, for about 5 minutes, or until the onion is softened.

3. Stir in the turmeric until combined, followed by the coconut milk. Bring to a low simmer over medium-high heat.

4. Add the salt, pepper, cayenne, and lemon juice to taste. Simmer over medium heat for 3 to 4 minutes, or longer, if desired.

5. Place a fine-mesh sieve over a bowl. Carefully pour the broth into the sieve. With a spoon, press down gently on the solids to release a bit more broth. Compost the solids.

6. Pour the broth into one or two mugs and sip away! Leftovers can be stored an airtight container in the fridge for a couple of days or it can be frozen for 1 to 2 months. To reheat, place the broth into a small pot over medium heat, whisk to combine, and gently warm.

Tip I like to grate the garlic cloves on a Microplane because grated garlic infuses the broth with so much flavour. If you don't have a Microplane, you can mince the garlic cloves in a mini food processor or with a knife. Go slowly when you are grating garlic; it's easy to take some skin off your fingers!

1 tablespoon virgin coconut oil

225g diced onion

6 medium/large cloves garlic, grated on a Microplane (1 heaped table-spoon; see Tip)

1 tablespoon grated fresh ginger

1/2 teaspoon ground turmeric, or to taste

1 400ml can light coconut milk

1/4 teaspoon fine sea salt, or to taste

1/8 teaspoon freshly ground black pepper, or to taste

Up to 1/8 teaspoon cayenne pepper, to taste

1/2 teaspoon fresh lemon juice, or to taste

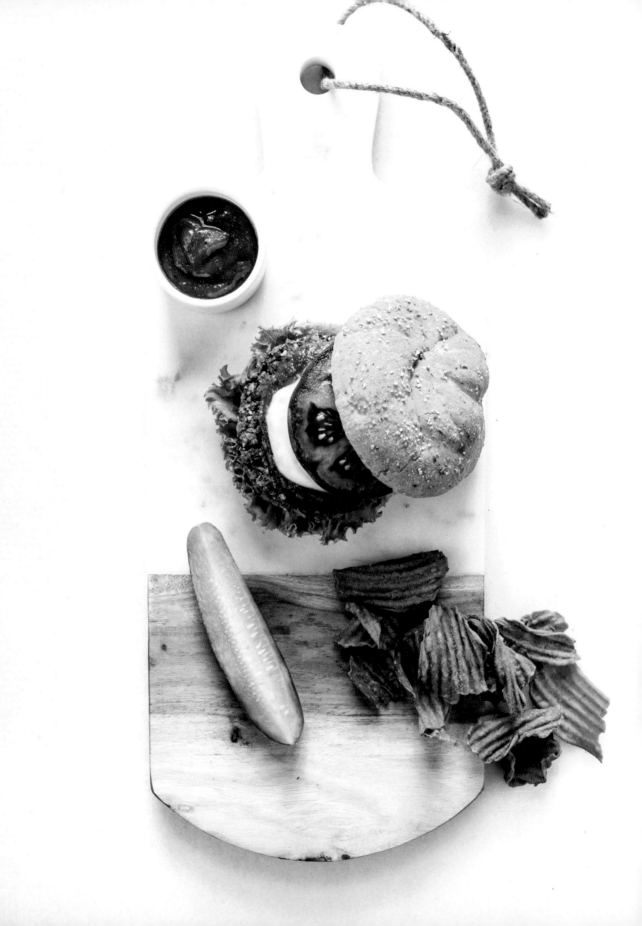

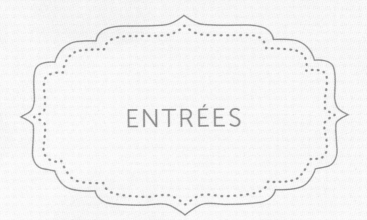

ENTRÉES

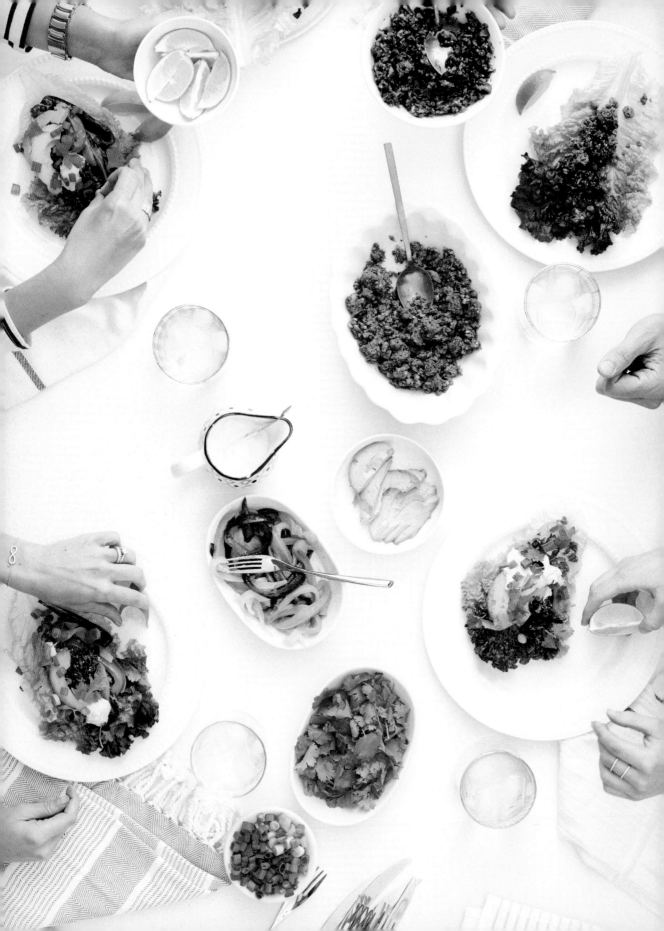

AS BUSINESS OWNERS with long work hours, Eric and I didn't always make time to sit down for meals, but Adriana gave us the motivation to bring this ritual back into our lives on a regular basis and put extra effort into making sure that our meals are balanced. This chapter has some of our favorite go-to weeknight dinners, such as Fusilli Lentil-Mushroom Bolognese, Loaded Sweet Potatoes and Sun-Dried Tomato Pasta. We also frequently enjoy making meals out of a couple of sides or a hearty soup, such as my Golden French Lentil Stew (page 145) with some crusty bread, so keep that chapter in mind when planning dinner recipes. If you have a special occasion or some extra time on the weekend, try my Ultimate Green Taco Wraps, Chilli Cheese Nachos or Shepherd's Pie; these recipes take longer to prepare, but they are truly show-stoppers! Freezer-friendly meals are always handy and my Oh Em Gee Veggie Burgers, Fail-Proof Marinara Sauce, Fusilli Lentil-Mushroom Bolognese, and Comforting Red Lentil and Chickpea Curry are great make-ahead and freeze options. Rest assured that these are recipes your whole family will devour; based on the feedback from my recipe testers, family and friends, these easy meals will satisfy plant-based eaters and meat-eaters alike!

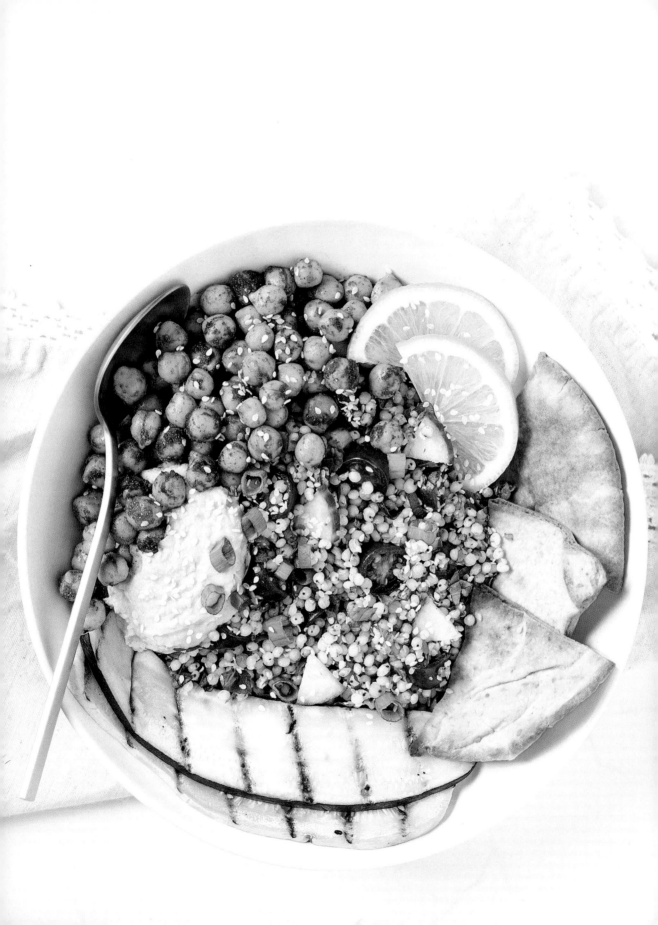

The Big Tabbouleh Bowl

VEGAN, GLUTEN-FREE, NUT-FREE, SOYA-FREE

SERVES 4 OR 5

PREP TIME: 45 MINUTES
(INCLUDES ALL RECIPE COMPONENTS)

COOK TIME: 50 TO 60 MINUTES
(INCLUDES ALL RECIPE COMPONENTS)

This bowl ranks right up there among the food of my dreams! The recipe combines many of my favourite side dishes, including my Hemp Heart and Sorghum Tabbouleh, Every Day Lemon-Garlic Hummus, Lemon-Tahini Dressing, and Falafel-Spiced Chickpeas. This is why the prep time is longer, but if you have some of these ingredients already prepared, the recipe comes together quite fast. It's a great way to use up leftover dressing or hummus. Serve it with fresh pitta bread (or for a crunchy twist, serve it with my Endurance Crackers, page 89), olives (if you are a fan), grilled courgettes, fresh herbs and sesame seeds. Or simply mix and match the recipes with what you have on hand. It's awesome countless ways, and it'll leave you feeling energized, happy and satisfied!

1. Prepare the tabbouleh, hummus and dressing, preferably in advance so they are ready to go.

2. **Make the falafel-spiced chickpea** In a large bowl, combine the chickpeas and oil, and stir well to coat. Add the remaining ingredients and stir until thoroughly combined.

3. Heat a grill to low-medium heat (or heat a grill pan over medium heat). Brush each courgette slice with oil on both sides and then place on the bottom rack of the grill (or on the grill pan). Grill for a few minutes per side, or until the courgettes are tender and have char lines.

4. In each bowl, add your desired amounts of tabbouleh, hummus, chickpeas, courgettes, pitta bread, and olives (if using), and drizzle it all with the dressing. Garnish with sesame seeds, fresh herbs and lemon wedges, if desired.

FOR THE BOWL

Hemp Heart and Sorghum Tabbouleh (page 105)

Every Day Lemon-Garlic Hummus (page 91)

Lemon-Tahini Dressing (page 265)

FOR THE FALAFEL-SPICED CHICKPEAS

1 400g can chickpeas, drained and rinsed or 250g cooked chickpeas

1 teaspoon extra-virgin olive oil

½ teaspoon garlic powder

½ teaspoon onion powder

½ teaspoon ground cumin

½ teaspoon ground coriander

½ teaspoon smoked or sweet paprika

½ teaspoon fine sea salt

FOR ASSEMBLY

2 medium courgettes or more if desired, sliced

Oil, for grilling

Pitta bread, cut into triangles

Olives (optional)

Sesame seeds (optional)

Minced fresh herbs (such as parsley, mint or coriander–optional)

Lemon wedges (optional)

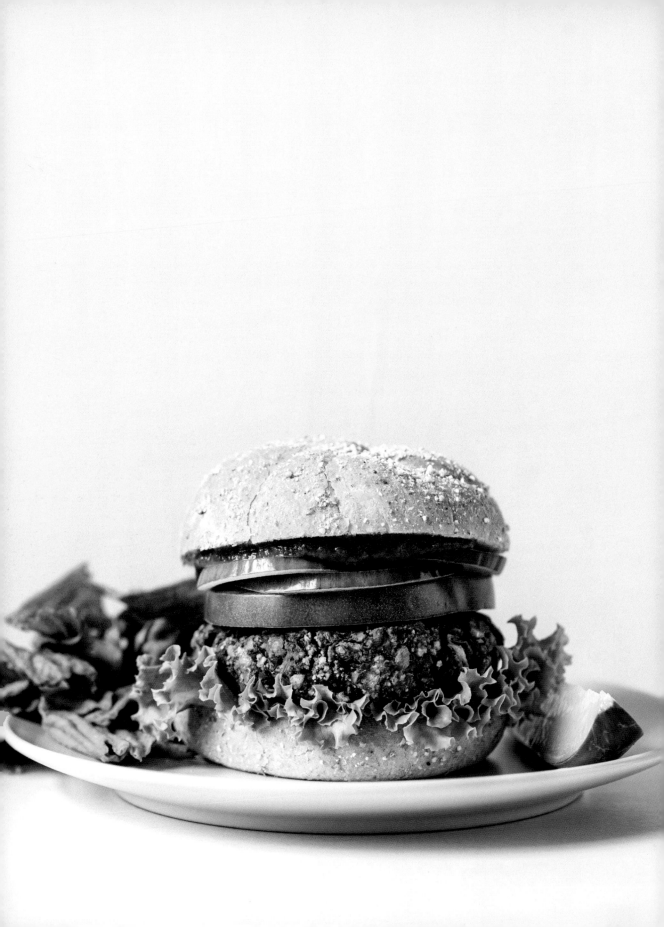

Oh Em Gee Veggie Burgers

VEGAN, GLUTEN-FREE OPTION, NUT-FREE OPTION, SOYA-FREE,
ADVANCE PREP REQUIRED, KID-FRIENDLY OPTION, FREEZER-FRIENDLY

MAKES 11 OR 12 MEDIUM PATTIES (11 OR 12 SERVINGS)

PREP TIME: **40 MINUTES**

COOK TIME: **25 TO 35 MINUTES**

This is my family's new favorite veggie burger recipe! I must have tested twenty-five veggie burger recipes for this cookbook, and I finally came up with a version that everyone went crazy over. Packed with sweet potato (or butternut squash—your choice), black beans, barbecue sauce, garlic, and an array of flavourful spices, the burger bakes up perfectly and holds together very well. The texture is spot-on. My favorite toppings to pair with this burger are barbecue sauce, vegan mayo, avocado, tomato, and salt and pepper. Try it out yourself!

I'll admit these veggie burgers are a bit involved to prepare, but trust me when I say that the work is worth it, because this recipe makes a huge batch, enough for 11 or 12 patties, which you can freeze after cooking and cooling. To save time, I recommend roasting the sweet potato and making the 9-Spice Mix the day before. Also, be sure to chop all the ingredients very finely and evenly, as this will help the patties hold together. I always recommend that you read the entire recipe before you begin, but this is especially true here since there are so many steps.

1. Preheat the oven to 375°F (190°C). Line two large baking sheets with parchment paper.

2. Peel the sweet potato and cut it into 1cm cubes (or peel, seed, and cube the butternut squash). You should have 800g of chopped sweet potato. Spread the cubes over one prepared baking sheet and toss with 1 tablespoon of the oil. Season with a pinch of salt. Roast for 15 minutes, then flip and roast for 15 to 20 minutes more, until fork-tender. Let cool on the pan for 5 to 10 minutes and set aside.

3. In a large frying pan, toast the walnuts over medium heat for 5 to 6 minutes, until fragrant and lightly golden. Transfer the walnuts to an extra-large bowl.

4. Wipe out the pan, if necessary, and heat the remaining 2 teaspoons oil over medium heat. Add the onion and garlic, stir to combine, and sauté for 3 to 5 minutes, until softened. Transfer to the bowl with the walnuts and stir to combine.

FOR THE BURGERS

565g sweet potato or butternut squash (see Tip)

25ml extra-virgin olive oil

¼ to ½ teaspoon fine sea salt, or to taste, plus a pinch

100g walnuts, finely chopped, or 70g hulled sunflower seeds

75g finely chopped onion

3 tablespoons minced garlic (6 or 7 large cloves)

2 400g cans black beans, drained and rinsed

2 to 3 tablespoons 9-Spice Mix (page 258), to taste

15g fresh flat-leaf parsley, finely chopped

75ml Easy Barbecue Sauce (page 255), or store-bought

90g spelt breadcrumbs or bread-crumbs of your choice

2 tablespoons gluten-free oat flour

Buns, for serving

TOPPING SUGGESTIONS

Homemade Vegan Mayo (page 269), or store-bought

Easy Barbecue Sauce (page 255), or store-bought

Sliced avocado

Sliced red onion

Sliced tomato

(recipe continues)

5. In a food processor, pulse the beans until you have a mixture of bean paste, chopped beans, and fully intact beans. Be careful not to overprocess them, as you still want a bit of texture. Transfer the beans to the bowl.

6. Measure out 400g of the roasted sweet potato and transfer to the large bowl. With a fork, lightly mash the potato into the other ingredients in the bowl.

7. Add the 9-Spice Mix, salt, parsley, barbecue sauce, bread crumbs and oat flour to the bowl. Stir until thoroughly combined. You can knead the dough together with your hands if that's easier, or just keep stirring. Taste and adjust the seasonings, if desired.

8. Scoop a handful of the dough and shape it into a round, uniform patty, packing it tightly as you rotate the patty in your hands. Place the patty on the lined baking sheet (I use the baking sheet I roasted the potato on). Repeat to make 11 or 12 patties in total, setting them at least 2.5cm apart on the baking sheet.

9. Bake for 15 minutes, gently flip with a spatula, and bake for 10 to 20 minutes more, until firm and lightly golden. With a spatula, gently transfer the patties to a cooling rack and let cool for about 20 minutes before serving (this helps them firm up). Serve the patty in a bun along with your desired toppings.

10. Let any leftover patties cool completely before storing in an airtight container in the fridge for up to 3 days. You can also wrap the patties individually in aluminium foil, place in a freezer bag with the air sucked out, and freeze for 3 to 4 weeks. Thaw completely on the counter or in the fridge before reheating in a greased skillet over medium-high heat for a few minutes on each side.

Tip You will need 400g of roasted sweet potato (or butternut squash) for this burger recipe. Any leftover roasted potato or squash can be served alongside the burgers, so feel free to make extra.

Make it gluten-free Use gluten-free breadcrumbs instead of spelt breadcrumbs.

Make it nut-free Use hulled sunflower seeds instead of walnuts.

Make it kid-friendly Shape small patties and serve them on slider buns. They are the perfect size for precious hands!

Fusilli Lentil-Mushroom Bolognese

VEGAN, GLUTEN-FREE OPTION, NUT-FREE, SOYA-FREE, KID-FRIENDLY OPTION, FREEZER-FRIENDLY

SERVES 6 TO 8

PREP TIME: **15 MINUTES**

COOK TIME: **15 TO 20 MINUTES**

I came up with this recipe one rainy fall evening. We were looking for comfort food, something that came together quickly and would 'stick to our bones'. Well, comfort food this certainly is, and it turned out to be one of the biggest hits of all the recipes I've created, adored by adults, kids, toddlers and teenagers alike! This pasta dish makes a huge pot and we always enjoy the leftovers—straight from the fridge or warmed up—the next day. Traditional bolognese is a meat-based sauce, but my version uses lentils for a high-fibre, plant-based twist. The 'secret' ingredient—tahini—gives it an unexpected, but delicious, creaminess. Try serving it with a simple side salad of marinated greens (try my Shake-and-Go Balsamic Vinaigrette, page 273) and some crusty bread to complete the meal. It's just divine and so simple, but it'll impress the heck out of your guests, too. This pasta is also great served with a scoop of some warmed-up All-Purpose Cheese Sauce (page 251) for a luxurious, cheesy twist. Get ready to make this recipe time and time again!

1. Bring a large pot of water to a boil for the pasta.

2. In a large Dutch oven or saucepan, heat the oil over medium heat. Add the onion, garlic, and a pinch of salt and stir. Sauté for 4 to 5 minutes, until the onion is softened.

3. Stir in the mushrooms, oregano, basil and thyme and cook for 7 to 8 minutes over medium-high heat, until most of the water cooks off.

4. When the water for the pasta boils, add the pasta and cook until al dente, following package directions.

5. Into the pot with the mushrooms, stir in the marinara sauce, lentils, roasted red pepper and tahini until combined. Make sure you stir well to fully incorporate the tahini. Simmer over medium heat, uncovered, for a few more minutes.

(recipe continues)

2 tablespoons extra-virgin olive oil

1 medium sweet onion, diced (about 300g)

3 large cloves garlic, minced

¼ to ¾ teaspoon fine sea salt, to taste, plus a pinch

450g sliced chestnut mushrooms

1 teaspoon dried oregano, or to taste

1 teaspoon dried basil, or to taste

1 teaspoon dried thyme

400g fusilli pasta (about 550g uncooked pasta)

750ml Fail-Proof Tomato Sauce (page 175) or store-bought chunky tomato sauce

1 400g can lentils, drained and rinsed, or 300g cooked lentils

60g jarred roasted red pepper, drained and chopped

2 tablespoons 'runny' tahini (see Tip)

½ teaspoon freshly ground black pepper

½ teaspoon red pepper flakes (optional, but recommended)

6. Drain the pasta and rinse it with cold water to halt the cooking process. Stir the pasta into the lentil-veggie mixture until thoroughly combined. Taste and season with salt, black pepper, and red pepper flakes (if using). Heat for a couple of minutes, or until heated throughout. Serve and enjoy. Leftovers can be stored in an airtight container in the fridge for up to 5 days. The leftovers are even delicious chilled, straight from the fridge! You can also freeze the cooled pasta in an airtight container or a freezer-safe zip-top bag with the air pressed out for 2 to 3 weeks. After thawing, add a splash of tomato sauce and seasonings to the pasta while reheating to freshen it up.

Tip 1. I recommend using a 'runny' tahini so it mixes easily into the pasta. Avoid using the firm and dry tahini you often find at the bottom of a jar.
2. To save on prep time, you can buy pre-sliced mushrooms.

Make it gluten-free Use gluten-free pasta.

Make it kid-friendly Reduce the mushrooms by half and chop them very small (think smaller than pea size) so they disappear into the pasta. The mushrooms will be undetectable, but your meal will still retain its immunity-boosting benefits!

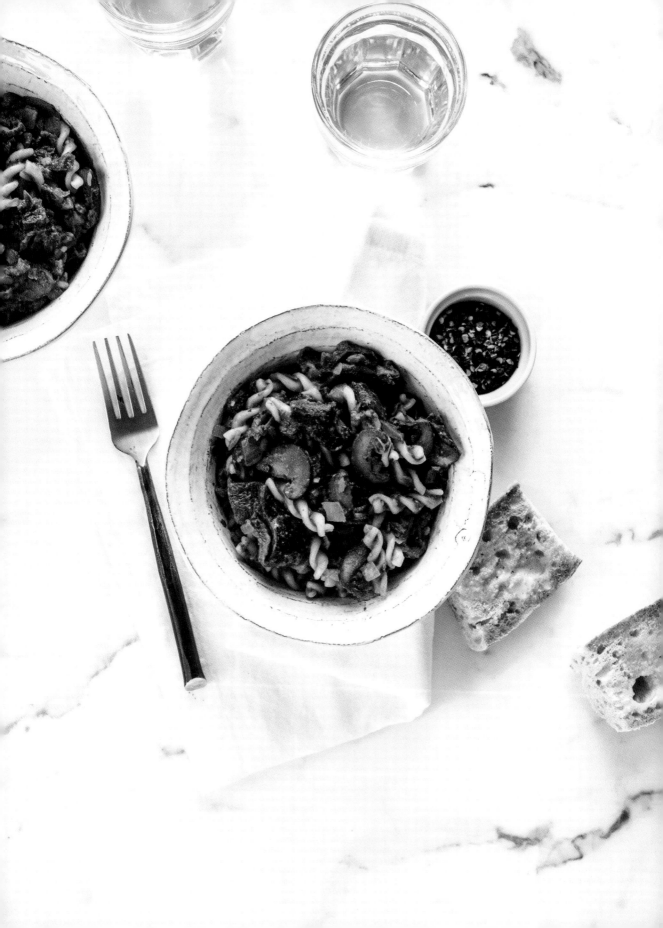

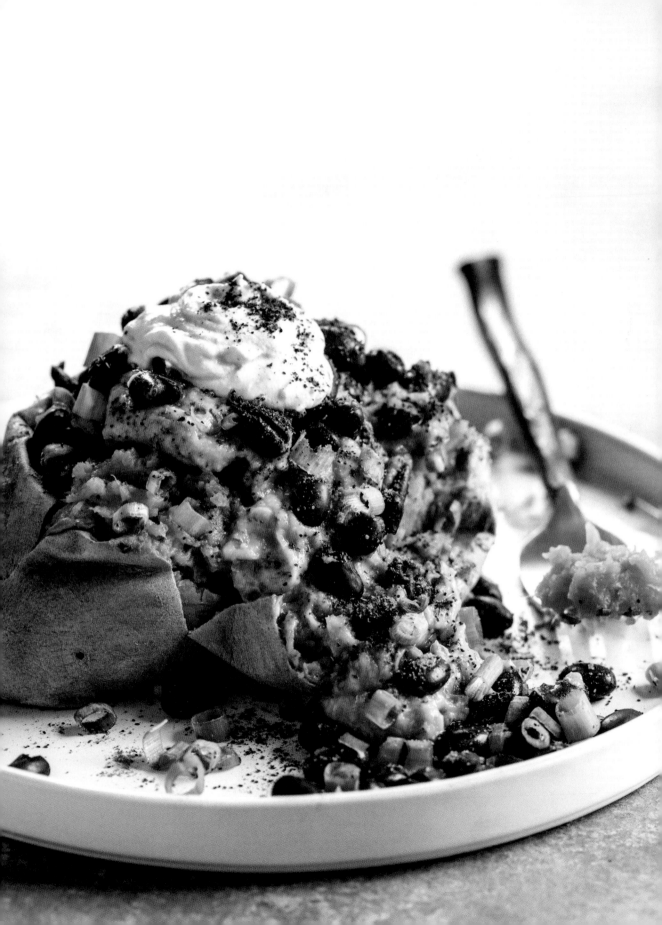

Loaded Sweet Potatoes

VEGAN, GLUTEN-FREE, NUT-FREE, SOYA-FREE, GRAIN-FREE,
KID-FRIENDLY OPTION

SERVES 2 AS A MAIN COURSE OR 4 AS A SIDE

PREP TIME: 20 MINUTES

COOK TIME: 45 TO 75 MINUTES

This is one of my easiest go-to weeknight meals. I throw the sweet potatoes in the oven, and I whip up the avocado crema and toppings about fifteen minutes before they are finished roasting. It does take a while for the potatoes to roast, but almost all this time is inactive, so you can be away from the kitchen taking care of other end-of-the-day tasks. If you're in a real rush to get dinner on the table, feel free to chop the sweet potatoes into small cubes and roast them at 400°F (200°C) for 20 to 35 minutes, flipping once halfway through, and then top them with the fixings. Green salad, rice and/or corn on the cob make perfect side dishes for this comforting dish, but it's satisfying all on its own too. A fun way to vary this recipe is to swap the baked sweet potato for baked russet potatoes and the avocado coriander crema for my All-Purpose Cheese Sauce (page 251).

1. Preheat the oven to 400°F (200°C). Line a baking sheet with parchment paper.

2. With a fork, poke several holes into each potato. Place on a baking sheet and roast for 45 to 75 minutes (timing depends on the size), until the flesh is tender and you can easily slide a knife through the center. After baking, let the potatoes cool for 5 to 10 minutes.

3. Make the avocado coriander crema In a food processor, process the coriander and garlic until minced. Add the rest of the ingredients and process until mostly smooth. There might be small bits of coriander, but this is okay.

4. In a medium frying pan, heat the oil over medium heat. Add the onion and garlic and sauté for 3 to 5 minutes, until softened. Stir in the chilli powder, cumin and black beans and cook for another minute or two. Add the salt, pepper, and lime juice and stir again to combine.

5. Assemble the sweet potatoes Slice each potato in half lengthwise. With a knife, score the flesh in a crisscross pattern. Gently mash the flesh with a fork to fluff. Sprinkle on some sea salt and pepper to season.

6. Layer the avocado crema and black beans by the spoonful across each potato half. Garnish each with spring onion, a pinch of chilli powder and cumin, and a sprinkle of salt and pepper. Serve immediately.

2 medium sweet potatoes

FOR THE AVOCADO CORIANDER CREMA

25g fresh coriander, large stems removed

1 small clove garlic

1 medium/large ripe avocado, pitted

4 teaspoons fresh lime juice, or to taste

1 tablespoon water

¼ teaspoon fine sea salt, or to taste

FOR THE LOADED SWEET POTATOES

1 tablespoon extra-virgin olive oil

150g diced sweet onion

2 medium cloves garlic, minced

¼ teaspoon chilli powder, plus more for serving

¼ teaspoon ground cumin, plus more for serving

1 400g can black beans, drained and rinsed, or 260g cooked black beans

Fine sea salt and freshly ground black pepper

Fresh lime juice

2 spring onions, thinly sliced

Tip If you have leftover black beans, you can freeze them for a later use (such as in my Black Bean Rancheros, page 51).

Make it kid-friendly Top the potatoes with chopped avocado instead of the avocado coriander crema.

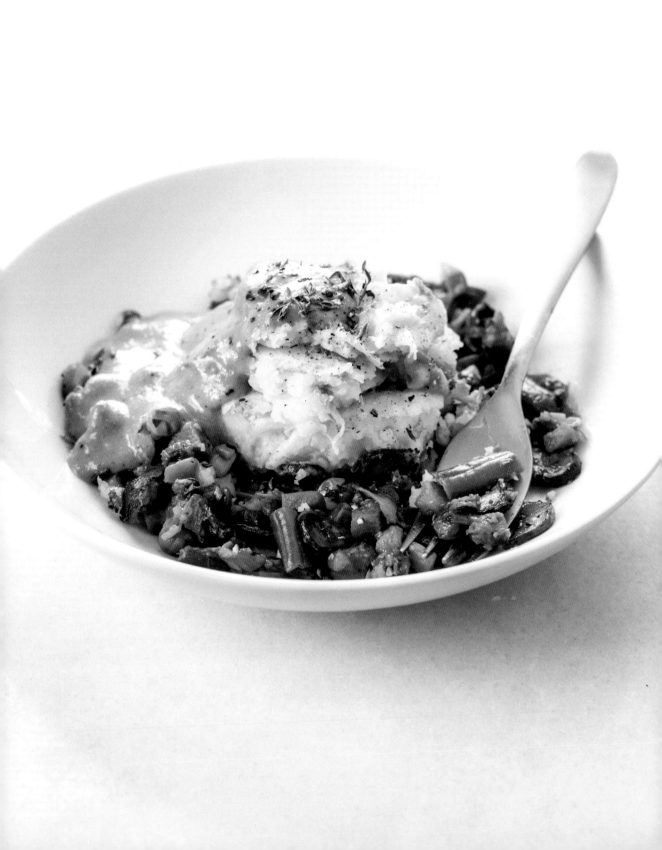

Shepherd's Pie

VEGAN, GLUTEN-FREE, NUT-FREE, SOYA-FREE OPTION, GRAIN-FREE OPTION, ADVANCE PREP REQUIRED, KID-FRIENDLY OPTION

SERVES 8

PREP TIME: **30 MINUTES**

COOK TIME: **40 MINUTES**

This is one of those special occasion recipes that requires a bit more prep time than usual, but it's so worth it when you are feeding a crowd or just want a special Sunday night dinner with your family. It's bursting with the rustic and comforting flavours of rosemary and thyme, and it gets texture and umami from cremini mushrooms. A small amount of dry red wine gives it a sophisticated flavour (with the bonus of getting to enjoy the rest of the bottle with your meal!), but feel free to swap the wine for more broth if you are preparing this dish for children or those avoiding alcohol. Using a bag of frozen mixed veggies is my little secret here; it saves a ton of time and prep work! Look for a bag that contains small-diced carrots, peas, corn and green beans. If you'd like to change the mashed potato topping, feel free to swap it out for my garlic cauliflower mashed potatoes (see page 187). My Cosy Gravy (page 279) is also a delicious accompaniment for the pie, but admittedly, we enjoy it all on its own, too.

1. Preheat the oven to 400°F (200°C). Lightly oil a 3- or 4l casserole dish.

2. Put the potatoes in a large saucepan and add water to cover by 5cm. Bring to a boil, reduce the heat to medium, and simmer for 15 to 20 minutes, or until the potatoes are fork-tender. Drain and return to the pot. Add the minced garlic, garlic powder, salt and butter. Mash until smooth, adding almond milk as needed to achieve a spreadable consistency. Set aside.

3. While the potatoes are cooking, make the filling In an extra-large saucepan, heat the oil over medium heat. Add the leeks, garlic and a couple of pinches of salt. Stir to combine and sauté until the leeks are softened, 3 to 5 minutes.

4. Add the mushrooms, stir, and increase the heat to medium-high. Sauté until much of the liquid released by the mushrooms has cooked off, 10 to 13 minutes. (This is important, as it ensures the filling won't be too watery.)

5. Add the bag of frozen vegetables (no need to thaw beforehand) and sauté for a few minutes, until heated through. Stir in the potato flour until combined.

(recipe continues)

FOR THE POTATO TOPPING

1.125kg Yukon Gold, yellow, red or fingerling potatoes, peeled, if desired, and chopped

2 large cloves garlic, minced

1 teaspoon garlic powder, or to taste

1 to 1¼ teaspoons fine sea salt, to taste

55g dairy-free spread

4 to 6 tablespoons unsweetened unflavoured almond milk, as needed

FOR THE FILLING

2 tablespoons extra-virgin olive oil

2 medium leeks, or 1 large sweet onion, diced

6 medium cloves garlic, minced (heaping 2 tablespoons)

450g chestnut mushrooms, thinly sliced

1 450g bag frozen mixed vegetables (see headnote)

2 tablespoons potato flour

175ml low-sodium vegetable broth

60ml dry red wine (such as Merlot or Cabernet Sauvignon)

¼ teaspoon red pepper flakes (optional)

1½ teaspoons fine sea salt, or to taste

2½ teaspoons chopped fresh rosemary leaves, or 1 teaspoon dried

2½ teaspoons fresh thyme leaves, or 1 teaspoon dried, plus more for garnish

1 400g can lentils, drained and rinsed, or 300g cooked lentils

Paprika, for garnish

Fresh thyme leaves, for garnish

Cozy Gravy (page 279), for serving

6. Add the broth and wine and stir to combine. Simmer the mixture over medium to high heat until it thickens slightly. Add the red pepper flakes (if using), salt, rosemary, thyme and lentils. Sauté for a couple of minutes longer.

7. Spoon the filling into the prepared casserole dish and spread it out evenly.

8. Using a spoon (and a lightly oiled hand, if necessary), spread the potatoes out over the filling in an even layer. Sprinkle several dashes of paprika and some thyme leaves all over the top of the mashed potatoes.

9. Bake for about 25 minutes, then switch the oven to grill and grill for 4 to 7 minutes, until bubbling around the edges. Watch closely to avoid burning.

10. Serve with Cozy Gravy and (hopefully) any leftover wine! This will keep wrapped in the fridge for 4 to 5 days.

Make it soya-free Use soya-free vegan butter.

Make it grain-free Serve the Shepherd's Pie without the Cozy Gravy.

Chilli Cheese Nachos

VEGAN, GLUTEN-FREE, SOYA-FREE, ADVANCE PREP REQUIRED, KID-FRIENDLY, FREEZER-FRIENDLY

SERVES 4 OR 5

PREP TIME: **30 MINUTES (INCLUDING CHEESE SAUCE)**

COOK TIME: **25 MINUTES**

Growing up, I was a huge fan of Wendy's Chilli and Cheese Nachos (remember the 99 cent menu?). While it's been years since I've stepped foot inside, I still crave the idea of chilli and cheese nachos on occasion. I've finally created a wholesome version that's free of processed foods but that captures all the bold flavour of the original. You won't believe how decadent tasting—yet wholesome—the cheese sauce is, and how satisfying the smoky lentil and kidney bean chilli is. This dish makes a great appetizer (just serve the dip with a big spoon so guests can portion it into their own bowls) or you can serve it for dinner like we often do—it'll easily serve four. If you want to serve it to a crowd, try putting it in a warmed cast-iron pot or in a warmer to retain the heat. I like this dip spicy so I serve it with pickled sliced jalapeños on top—it adds a juicy kick of heat!

1. In a large saucepan, heat the oil over medium heat. Add the onion, garlic, and a pinch of salt, stir, and cook for 4 to 5 minutes, until the onion starts to soften.

2. Stir in the fresh jalapeño and three quarters of the bell pepper and cook for a few minutes more. Add the chilli powder, cumin, oregano, and paprika and stir to combine.

3. Pour in the diced tomatoes with their juices and stir. Increase the heat to medium-high and bring to a simmer.

4. Stir in the tomato paste, lentils and kidney beans. With a potato masher, roughly mash one-third of the mixture—don't try to mash it smooth, just until it's slightly thickened.

5. Add the vinegar, salt, black pepper and Sriracha. Cook over medium heat for 5 to 10 minutes, or longer if desired, until thickened to your liking.

6. Into individual bowls (or 2.5 to 3l cast-iron pot or glass dish), ladle a layer of chilli. Top with a layer of the cheese sauce. Keep layering until the chilli is used up and you've added as much cheese sauce as you prefer (I usually reserve 125ml of the sauce for another use). Top the dip with the remaining bell pepper, pickled jalapeño and a sprinkle of sea salt.

(recipe continues)

1 tablespoon extra-virgin olive oil

1 medium brown onion

3 large cloves garlic, minced (about 1 tablespoon)

½ to ¾ teaspoon fine sea salt, to taste, plus a pinch

1 medium/large jalapeño, seeded, if desired, and finely chopped

1 small red bell pepper, diced

1 tablespoon chilli powder

1 teaspoon ground cumin

1 teaspoon dried oregano

1 teaspoon smoked paprika

1 400g can chopped tomatoes, with juices

1 tablespoon tomato paste

1 400g can lentils, drained and rinsed, or cooked lentils

1 400g can red kidney beans, drained and rinsed

1½ teaspoons cider vinegar

Freshly ground black pepper

Sriracha or other hot sauce

2 batches All-Purpose Cheese Sauce (page 251)

Pickled sliced jalapeños, drained, for garnish

Corn tortilla chips, for serving

7. Serve immediately with corn tortilla chips. Let any leftovers cool completely (otherwise, the steam will create more water in the dip) before transferring to a container and refrigerating for up to 5 days. Reheat leftovers in a saucepan on the hob while stirring to combine with the 'cheese' sauce. Cooled leftovers can be frozen in freezer-safe zip-top bags with the air pressed out or in freezer-safe containers filled to the top (to prevent freezer burn) for up to 1 month.

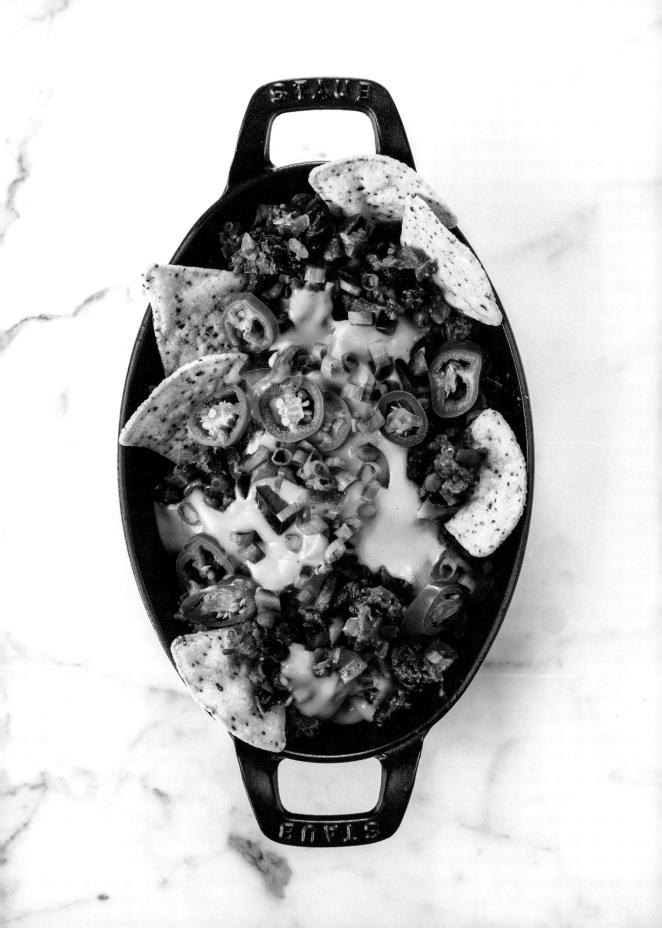

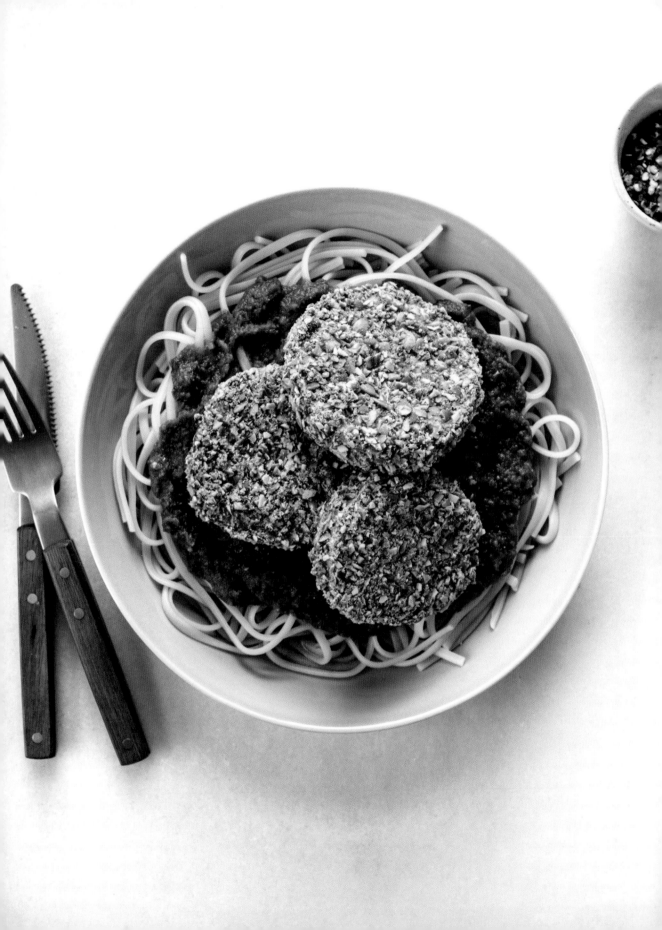

Aubergine Parmesan

VEGAN, GLUTEN-FREE OPTION, NUT-FREE, SOYA-FREE,
ADVANCE PREP REQUIRED, KID-FRIENDLY

MAKES 8 TO 12 CUTLETS (4 TO 6 SERVINGS)

PREP TIME: **25 TO 30 MINUTES**

COOK TIME: **16 TO 22 MINUTES**

This recipe has turned aubergine haters into lovers—just ask my husband, Eric. My nut-free Pumpkin Seed Vegan Parmesan Cheese coats the aubergine 'cutlets', which are then baked until crispy and golden. You'll want to eat them straight from the pan—I promise!—but it's also worth the wait to smother them in my Fail-Proof Tomato Sauce (page 175) or your favourite store-bought sauce and pair them with some freshly cooked pasta.

1. Sprinkle each aubergine cutlet liberally with salt (don't worry—we'll be washing it off later!). Place them in a large colander and let stand for 20 minutes in the sink while the salt draws out some water. The aubergines will 'sweat' during this time.

2. Preheat the oven to 450°F (230°C). Line a large baking sheet with parchment paper.

3. In a medium bowl, whisk together the milk, flour, vinegar, salt, pepper to taste, oregano, and basil. Place the parmesan in a large shallow dish.

4. Rinse the salt from the aubergine cutlets and pat dry with a dishcloth. Dip a cutlet into the milk and flour mixture and gently tap off any excess. Immediately dip it into the parmesan, pressing down gently to make sure the parmesan adheres. Flip the cutlet and press the other side into the parmesan until coated. Sprinkle any bare patches with additional parmesan. Place the cutlet on the prepared baking sheet and repeat with the remaining cutlets, setting them about 5cm apart. Wipe your hands clean after coating every one or two. You will likely have batter left over at the end, but this is normal. Simply discard any leftover batter.

5. Bake for 16 to 22 minutes, flipping once halfway through, until golden and crispy. Watch closely toward the end of the baking time to ensure the cutlets don't burn. Serve over cooked pasta topped with tomato sauce.

Tip To reheat leftover cutlets, bake for 5 minutes on each side at 450°F (230°C). Note that the cutlets will get soft in the fridge, so reheating in the oven is essential to crisp them up again!

Make it gluten-free Use plain gluten-free flour instead of spelt flour.

1 large aubergine (675 to 900g) peeled and sliced crosswise into 8 to 12 2cm thick cutlets

½ teaspoon fine sea salt, plus more as needed

250ml unsweetened unflavoured almond milk

86g white/light or whole grain spelt flour

1 teaspoon cider vinegar

Freshly ground black pepper

1 teaspoon dried oregano

1 teaspoon dried basil

Triple batch of Vegan Parmesan Cheese (page 267), made with pumpkin seeds

Cooked pasta, for serving

1 batch Fail-Proof Tomato Sauce (page 175) or store-bought

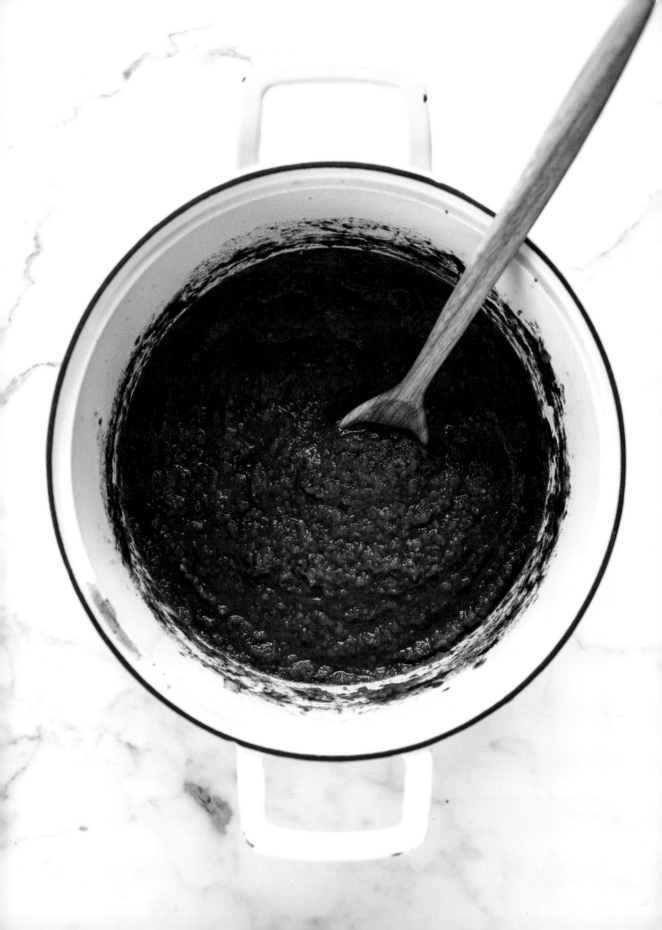

Fail-Proof Tomato Sauce

VEGAN, GLUTEN-FREE, NUT-FREE, SOYA-FREE, GRAIN-FREE,
FREEZER-FRIENDLY

MAKES 1.25L

PREP TIME: **10 MINUTES**

COOK TIME: **35 MINUTES**

Try this incredible garlic-basil tomato sauce on top of a bowl of pasta, courgette noodles, or spaghetti squash, or with my Aubergine Parmesan (page 173). You can use chopped, puréed, or crushed canned or jarred tomatoes—whatever you have in your pantry. You can purée the sauce with a stick blender or simply leave it chunky for added texture. To vary this sauce, try adding a splash of balsamic vinegar and some red pepper flakes for a flavourful twist.

1. In a large pot, heat the oil over medium heat. Add the onion, garlic, and a pinch of salt and stir to combine. Sauté over medium heat for 4 to 5 minutes, or until the onion is softened.

2. Stir in the tomatoes with their juices, bay leaves, oregano, salt and pepper to taste. Simmer for at least 30 minutes, until the sauce thickens. It should reduce in volume by one-third to one-half. Discard the bay leaves.

3. At this point, if you prefer a smooth sauce, you can purée it in a blender or directly in the pot using a stick blender. Otherwise, simply leave the sauce chunky. (I usually leave it chunky because I like the texture.)

4. Remove from the heat and stir in the basil. Taste and adjust the salt and pepper, if desired. Store the cooled sauce in an airtight container in the fridge for up to 1 week, or in the freezer in a freezer-safe zip-top bag or container for 1 to 2 months.

Tip I like to use Eden Organic Crushed Tomatoes (in a glass jar) for this recipe (I try to use glass if the option is available).

60ml extra-virgin olive oil

1 medium/large sweet onion, diced

5 or 6 medium cloves garlic, minced (about 2 tablespoons), to taste

1 teaspoon fine sea salt, or to taste, plus a pinch

2 794g cans or jars no-salt-added crushed, puréed, or chopped tomatoes, with juices

2 bay leaves

1 teaspoon dried oregano

Freshly ground black pepper

15g fresh basil leaves, finely chopped

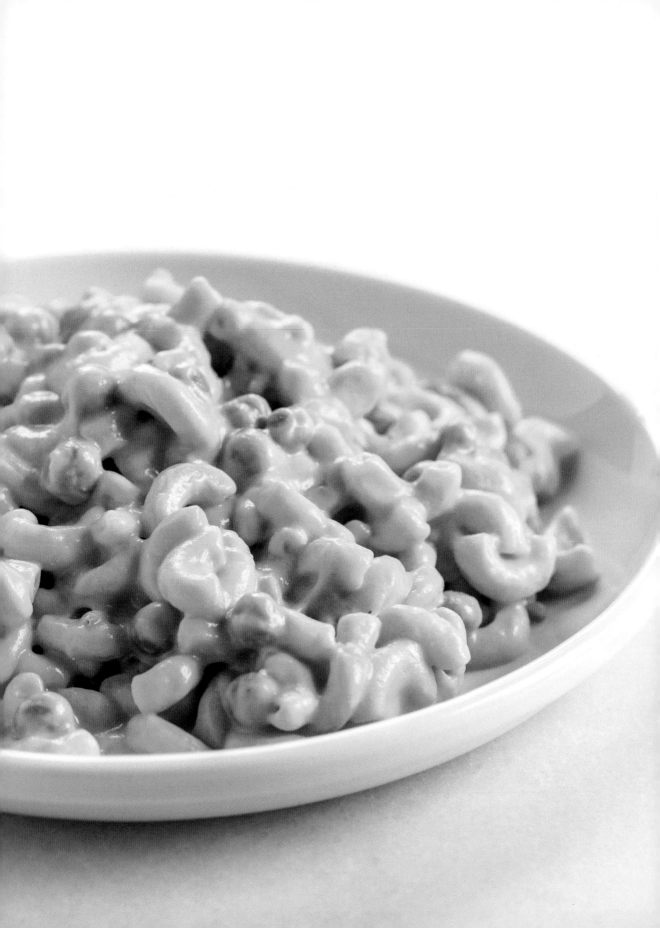

Mac and Peas

VEGAN, GLUTEN-FREE OPTION, SOYA-FREE, ADVANCE PREP REQUIRED, KID-FRIENDLY

SERVES 3 AS A MAIN OR 4 AS A SIDE

PREP TIME: **15 MINUTES**

COOK TIME: **20 MINUTES**

This mac and peas recipe uses my beloved All-Purpose Cheese Sauce. It's certainly different from traditional mac 'n' cheese, but if you can appreciate the more subtle flavours, as well as the creaminess that the vegetables add to the sauce, I promise you'll love it! We absolutely devour this in our house, because it's decadent-tasting and comforting yet still feels very light. Not surprisingly, this dish also earns rave reviews from kids! If serving this to children, you can omit the Sriracha and vinegar to keep the flavours more subtle. After mixing the cheese sauce into the pasta, be sure to taste and check for seasoning. Then, you can 'amp up the flavours' with a splash of white wine vinegar, Sriracha, Herbamare (or other sea salt), pepper, garlic powder and sweet paprika. These additions will take the dish to a whole other level, and I encourage you to have fun experimenting with it.

1. Bring a large pot of water to a boil for the pasta. Cook the pasta according to the package directions. Drain.

2. Return the pasta to the pot and add the peas and the cheese sauce. Stir and heat over low until heated throughout and slightly thickened.

3. Taste and season with vinegar, Sriracha, Herbamare, pepper, paprika and garlic powder to taste. Serve immediately with your desired toppings or simply enjoy it as it is.

Tip 1. Swap the peas for roasted or steamed broccoli to make Mac and *Trees*! 2. To quickly thaw the peas, add them to the pot of pasta during the last minute of cooking, then drain both at the same time. 3. To boost the protein, swap the peas for edamame.

Make it gluten-free Use gluten-free pasta of your choice.

225g dry pasta (such as macaroni or fusilli)

190g frozen peas, thawed (see Tip)

1 batch All-Purpose Cheese Sauce (page 251)

White wine vinegar (start with ½ teaspoon and add from there, if desired)

Sriracha or other hot sauce

Herbamare (see page 307) or fine sea salt

Freshly ground black pepper

Sweet paprika

Garlic powder

TOPPING SUGGESTIONS

Chopped avocado

Sun-dried tomatoes, rehydrated (if necessary) and chopped

Sriracha (or other hot sauce)

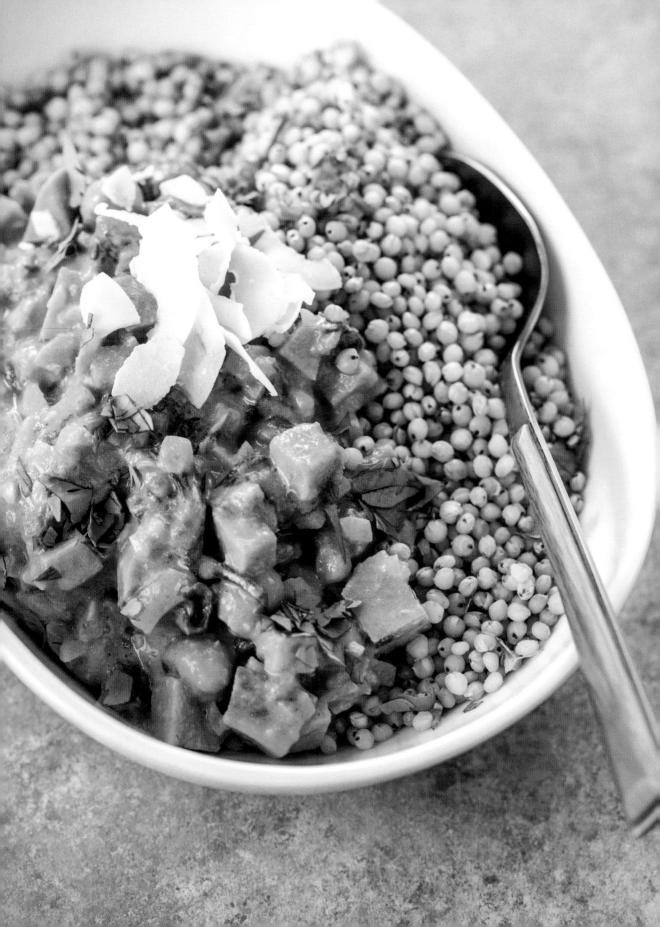

Sweet Potato, Chickpea and Spinach Coconut Curry

VEGAN, GLUTEN-FREE, SOYA-FREE, GRAIN-FREE OPTION, FREEZER-FRIENDLY

SERVES 6

PREP TIME: **25 MINUTES**

COOK TIME: **25 MINUTES**

This curry is just divine! The coconut milk brings it all together, mellowing and integrating the spices while adding a light sweetness that pairs wonderfully with the sweet potato. It's the perfect comfort food! This is a thick, stew-like curry—not runny or soupy. It's the kind you'll love to scoop up with a hunk of bread. Because the recipe moves quickly once you've started, be sure to have the ingredients prepped and ready to toss into the pot as soon as they're called for. (Keep them separate after prepping, as they are added at different stages.) This helps you avoid burning the spices. I also recommend chopping the sweet potatoes very small (5mm to 1cm pieces); they will cook much faster this way. I'm all about getting food into our bellies as fast as humanly possible.

1. In a large saucepan, heat the oil over medium heat. The oil is hot enough when a cumin seed sizzles when tossed into the pan. Add the cumin seeds and toast for about a minute, until fragrant and lightly darkened in color (be careful not to burn them). Immediately stir in the onion, season with a pinch of salt, and cook for 3 to 5 minutes, or until the onion is soft and translucent.

2. Add the garlic, ginger, turmeric, coriander and red pepper flakes. Stir to combine and sauté for a couple of minutes, until the garlic softens.

3. Add the sweet potato, chickpeas, tomatoes with their juices and coconut milk. Stir to combine, cover, and simmer over medium heat for 20 to 30 minutes, until the potatoes are fork-tender. At this point, I always mash one-third of the mixture to thicken the sauce (using a potato masher), but this step is optional.

4. Stir in the spinach and cook until wilted. Season with the salt and black pepper to taste.

5. Serve on a bed of cooked grains, garnished with coriander and coconut. If desired, offer lime wedges for squeezing over the curry. Store the cooled curry in an airtight container in the fridge for 4 to 5 days, or in the freezer for up to 1 month.

Make it grain-free Serve this curry without cooked grains.

4 teaspoons virgin coconut oil

1 tablespoon cumin seeds

1 medium onion, finely chopped

¾ to 1 teaspoon fine sea salt, to taste, plus a pinch

3 large cloves garlic, minced

4 teaspoons grated fresh ginger

1 teaspoon ground turmeric

1 teaspoon ground coriander

¼ teaspoon red pepper flakes, or to taste

1 medium/large sweet potato, peeled and cut into 5mm to 1cm dice (600g)

1 400g can chickpeas, drained and rinsed, or 250g cooked chickpeas

1 400g can chopped tomatoes, with juices

1 400ml can light coconut milk

1 142g pack baby spinach

Freshly ground black pepper

FOR SERVING

Cooked basmati rice, quinoa, millet or sorghum

Chopped fresh coriander leaves

Unsweetened shredded or large-flake coconut

Lime wedges (optional)

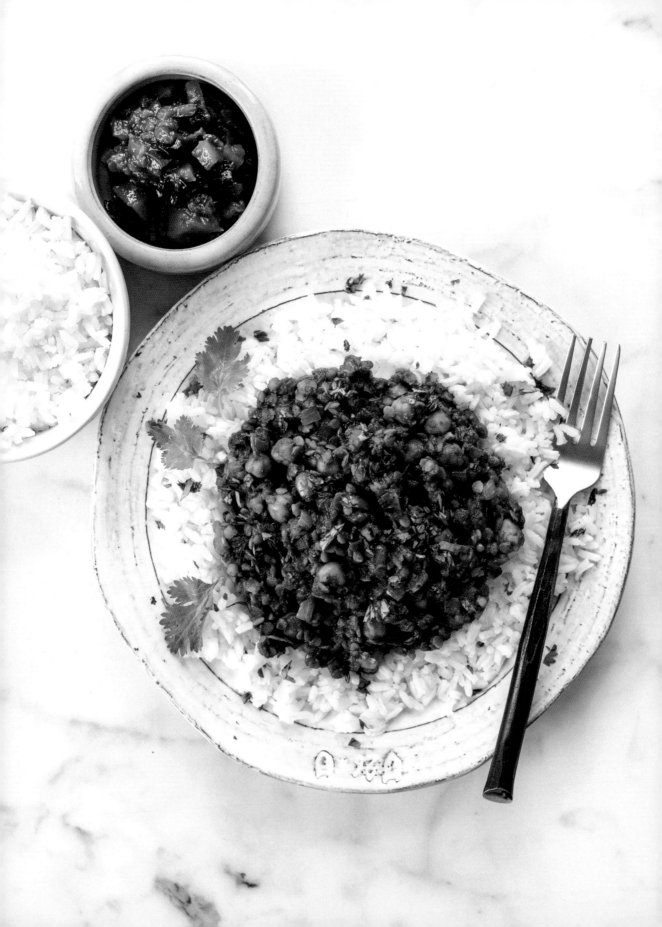

Comforting Red Lentil and Chickpea Curry

VEGAN, GLUTEN-FREE, NUT-FREE, SOYA-FREE, GRAIN-FREE OPTION,
KID-FRIENDLY, FREEZER-FRIENDLY

SERVES 6, WITH ACCOMPANIMENTS

PREP TIME: 20 MINUTES

COOK TIME: 20 MINUTES

Packed with protein and anti-inflammatory spices, this dish will energize you and keep you full for hours. It's such a quick-and-easy recipe, not to mention comforting, satisfying and delicious! It makes for a fast week-night dinner, and it ought to give you leftovers for lunch the next day, which we always encourage. If you have some baby spinach on hand, stir it in at the end of cooking for a healthful and colourful addition. Serve this curry on a bed of basmati rice and finish it with a lightly sweet scoop of Apple-Mango Chutney (page 277) for a meal you won't soon forget.

1. Rinse the lentils in a fine-mesh sieve, then put them in a medium pot and add 625 to 750ml water. Bring to a boil over medium-high heat, then reduce the heat to medium-low, cover, and simmer for 8 to 15 minutes, until just tender, adding more water if necessary. Drain. The lentils will look a bit paste-like, but this is normal.

2. In a large skillet, heat the oil over medium heat. Add the onion and garlic and cook until the onion is soft and translucent, 4 to 5 minutes. Stir in the ginger and cook for 1 to 2 minutes more.

3. Stir in the curry paste, curry powder, turmeric, cumin, salt and sugar. Increase the heat to medium-high and cook, stirring frequently, until fragrant, 1 to 2 minutes.

4. Stir in the tomatoes, chickpeas and cooked red lentils. Cook until heated through, reducing the heat, if necessary, or simmer longer, if you wish.

5. Serve over a bed of hot rice with a scoop of warm chutney and a sprinkle of coriander, if desired. Store the cooled curry in an airtight container in the fridge for 4 to 5 days, or freeze for up to 1 month. I like to freeze leftovers flat in freezer-safe zip-top bags.

Tip This curry is moderately spicy, but if you aren't a fan of spicy food, I recommend starting with 1 tablespoon curry paste and increasing from there, if desired.

Make it grain-free Serve without the rice.

210g uncooked red lentils, or 350g cooked red lentils

4 teaspoons virgin or refined coconut oil or extra-virgin olive oil

1 medium sweet onion, diced (about 300g)

3 medium cloves garlic, minced

2 teaspoons minced fresh ginger

2 tablespoons red curry paste, or to taste (see Tip)

1 tablespoon good-quality curry powder

½ teaspoon ground turmeric

1 teaspoon ground cumin

½ to ¾ teaspoon fine sea salt, to taste

1 teaspoon natural cane sugar

300g chopped tomatoes or passata (I use one 396g jar Eden Organic no-salt-added crushed tomatoes)

1 400g can chickpeas, drained and rinsed, or 250g cooked chickpeas

490g to 730g cooked basmati rice or rice of your choice, for serving

Apple-Mango Chutney (page 277), for serving

Chopped fresh coriander, for garnish (optional)

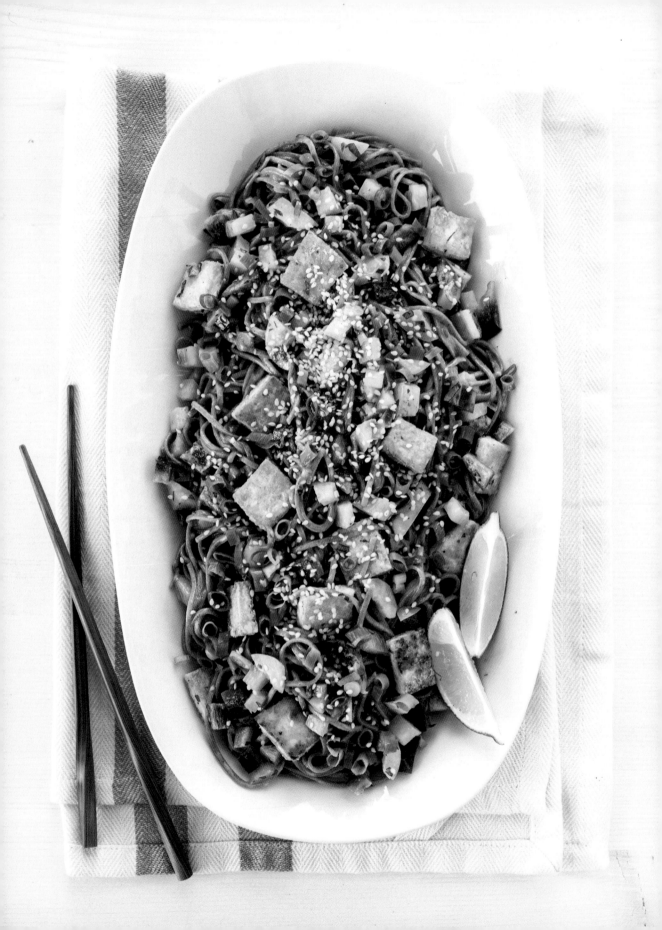

Soba Noodle Salad

VEGAN, GLUTEN-FREE OPTION, NUT-FREE, ADVANCE PREP REQUIRED,
KID-FRIENDLY

SERVES 6

PREP TIME: **20 MINUTES**

COOK TIME: **30 MINUTES**

Once I start eating this beautiful soba noodle salad, it's hard to stop! It's light and energizing, but the fibre-rich soba noodles and crispy tofu give it plenty of protein and staying power. The simple sesame-tahini dressing is both sweet and tangy, thanks to the combo of rice vinegar and maple syrup, and sometimes I like to add it to stir-fries and other grain bowls as well as this dish. The soba salad can be served warm or cold, making it a great option for any season. If you'd like to experiment with different textures, you can use spiral or bow-tie pasta or even spiralized carrot or courgette 'pasta' in lieu of the soba noodles.

1. Prepare the Cast-Iron Tofu (page 137).

2. Make the dressing In a small bowl, whisk together the dressing ingredients until smooth. Cover and refrigerate to thicken slightly.

3. Make the salad Bring a pot of water to a boil. Cook the noodles according to the package directions. Drain and place in a large bowl.

4. Add the bell peppers, spring onions and coriander to the bowl with the noodles. Add the dressing and toss to coat. Add half the tofu cubes and toss again. Taste and season with sea salt if necessary.

5. Top the salad with the remaining tofu, sesame seeds, and coriander scattered on top. You can also add a squeeze of lime juice on top of each bowl just before serving or simply serve with a lime wedge. The salad can be stored in an airtight container in the fridge for up to 3 days. The tofu will soften as it sits, but it's still very tasty!

Tip 1. You can use untoasted or toasted sesame oil; it's totally up to you! Toasted sesame oil has a much more robust flavour, while untoasted is more mellow, so feel free to use whichever you prefer. 2. The veggies have a tendency to fall to the bottom of the bowl, so I like to scoop them up and add them back on top just before serving.

Make it gluten-free Use 100% buckwheat soba noodles. Traditional soba noodles are made with buckwheat flour; however, some contemporary brands incorporate wheat flour. Be sure to check the label carefully and use a brand made with just buckwheat flour.

FOR THE DRESSING

60ml toasted or untoasted sesame oil (see Tip)

3 to 4 tablespoons rice vinegar, to taste (I like it tangy, so I use 4)

25ml tahini

1 tablespoon pure maple syrup, or to taste

1 tablespoon low-sodium tamari

2 cloves garlic, grated on a Microplane

FOR THE SALAD

1 225g pack soba noodles

1 medium red bell pepper, seeded and diced (about 220g)

1 medium yellow bell pepper, seeded and diced 220g

3 to 4 onions, finely chopped (80g)

50g coriander leaves, minced

1 batch Cast-Iron Tofu (page 137)

Fine sea salt

1 tablespoon sesame seeds, for garnish

Fresh lime juice, for serving (optional)

Sriracha, for serving

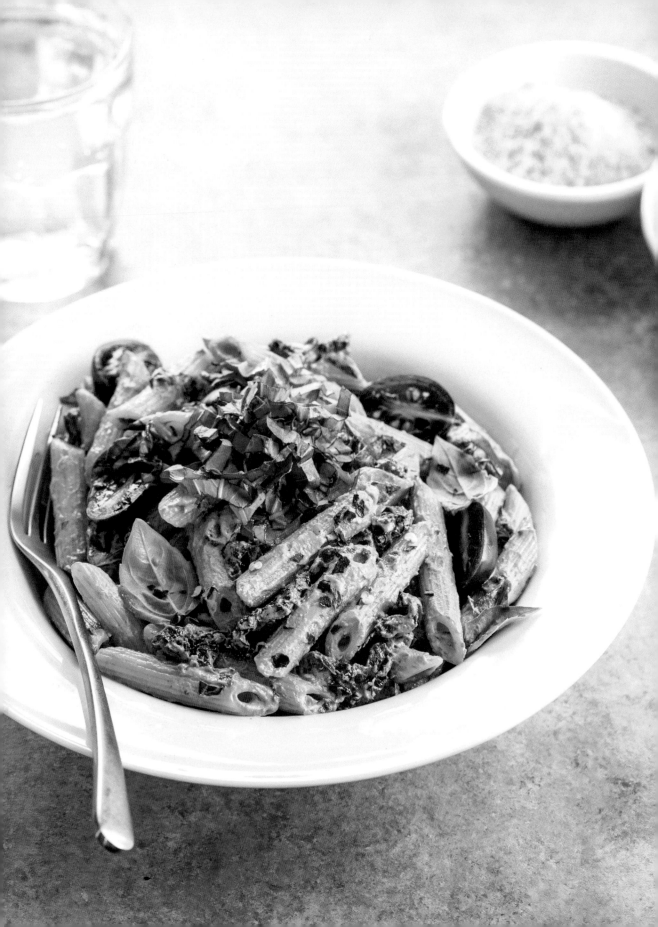

Sun-Dried Tomato Pasta

VEGAN, GLUTEN-FREE OPTION, SOYA-FREE, ADVANCE PREP REQUIRED,
KID-FRIENDLY OPTION

SERVES 4

SOAK TIME: **1 TO 2 HOURS, OR OVERNIGHT**

PREP TIME: **15 TO 20 MINUTES**

COOK TIME: **10 MINUTES**

This is a new spin on our favourite creamy tomato pasta dish from my first cookbook. It's on heavy rotation around here and I think you are going to love it. If you are a fan of salty and sweet flavours, like umami-rich sun-dried tomatoes, then you will love this simple yet elegant dinner dish. It's bursting with intense tomato flavour, basil, and lemon, and it'll be on the table in under thirty minutes, which makes it an ideal week-night dish. You can definitely save leftovers (or double the recipe and enjoy it two nights in a row), but keep in mind that once the sauce has been mixed into the pasta, the texture won't reheat well. Don't despair, though! I recommend chilling any leftover sauce separately from the pasta. The next day, simply mix the sauce and pasta together and reheat, or make fresh pasta to go with leftover sauce.

1. **Make the sun-dried cashew cream** Put the cashews in a bowl and add water to cover by a couple of inches. Soak for 8 to 12 hours or overnight. (For a quick-soak method, cover with boiling water and soak for 30 to 60 minutes.) Drain and rinse.

2. In a high-speed blender, combine the cashews, water, garlic, sun-dried tomatoes, lemon juice and salt. Blend on high until super smooth. If you have a Vitamix, use the tamper to help the mixture blend. If your blender is having a hard time getting the mixture smooth, add a splash or two of olive oil and blend again. Set aside.

3. **Make the pasta** Bring a large pot of water to a boil. Cook the pasta according to the pack directions.

4. Place the spinach in a large colander in the sink. When the pasta is cooked, carefully and slowly empty the pot over the spinach in the colander to drain. (This is a quick way to wilt the spinach.) Return the pasta and spinach to the pot and set over low-medium heat.

5. Stir in the sun-dried tomatoes, basil, and sun-dried cashew cream until combined. Add a splash of olive oil if the sauce seems too thick.

(recipe continues)

FOR THE SUN-DRIED CASHEW CREAM

65g raw cashews

140ml water

2 or 3 medium cloves garlic, to taste

20g oil-packed sun-dried tomatoes, drained

2 tablespoons fresh lemon juice

1/2 teaspoon fine sea salt

Splash of olive oil, if needed

FOR THE PASTA

450g dry pasta of your choice (such as fusilli, penne, macaroni, etc.)

1 142g pack baby spinach

40g oil-packed sun-dried tomatoes, drained and chopped

20g fresh basil leaves, chopped

Splash of olive oil, if needed

Zest of 1 lemon (about 1 tablespoon)

1 to 2 teaspoons white wine vinegar, to taste (optional)

Red pepper flakes

Herbamare (see page 307) or fine sea salt

Freshly ground black pepper

Vegan Parmesan Cheese (page 267), made with cashews (optional)

Sliced cherry or grape tomatoes (optional)

Fresh basil leaves, for garnish (optional)

6. Stir in the lemon zest and vinegar (use only if you like a tangy kick!) and season with red pepper flakes, salt and black pepper. Serve immediately, garnished with parmesan, sliced tomatoes and basil, if desired. The sauce will thicken and dry out fairly quickly, so I recommend serving the pasta immediately and not letting it sit in the pot for long.

Make it gluten-free Use gluten-free pasta of your choice.

Make it kid-friendly Mince the spinach and basil in a food processor so it blends into the pasta without being detected. Also, try serving the dish with fun pasta shapes like fusilli or ditalini.

Marinated Portobello Mushroom Bowl

VEGAN, GLUTEN-FREE, SOYA-FREE OPTION, GRAIN-FREE,
ADVANCE PREP REQUIRED, KID-FRIENDLY

SERVES 4

MARINATE TIME: **1 HOUR MINIMUM OR OVERNIGHT**

PREP TIME: **20 MINUTES**

COOK TIME: **25 TO 35 MINUTES**

Portobello mushrooms are marinated in a delicious garlic-balsamic dressing and then grilled for unbeatable flavour and texture. My favourite way to serve them is with garlic cauliflower mashed potatoes and grilled seasonal vegetables alongside. This recipe calls for eight mushroom caps, which might seem like a lot, but keep in mind that they shrink down considerably as they cook. I can easily enjoy a few all on my own, but then again, I've never been one to turn away a mushroom! If you have any leftovers, the caps are great sliced up and served in a wrap the following day.

1. Make the mushrooms Rub the outside of the mushroom caps with a damp towel to remove any debris. With a small spoon, scrape the black 'gills' out and discard.

2. In a large zip-top freezer bag or an extra-large container with a lid, combine the oil, vinegar, coconut aminos, garlic, salt and pepper to taste. Seal the bag (or secure the container lid) and shake vigorously to combine. Add the mushroom caps, seal the bag and gently shake until the caps are coated with the marinade. Marinate the mushrooms in the fridge for a minimum of 1 hour or up to 8 to 9 hours, shaking the bag (or container) a few times during this time to redistribute the marinade.

3. Make the garlic cauliflower mashed potatoes Steam or boil the cauliflower and potatoes together until fork-tender, 15 to 25 minutes. Drain.

4. In a 3- or 4l pot, melt the spread over medium heat. Add the garlic and lightly sauté for a couple of minutes. Add the cauliflower and potatoes and mash until mostly smooth. Season with the salt and pepper to taste.

(recipe continues)

FOR THE MUSHROOMS

8 small/medium portobello mushroom caps (about 675g)

75ml extra-virgin olive oil

75ml balsamic vinegar

75ml coconut aminos

3 cloves garlic, minced

Fine sea salt and freshly ground black pepper

FOR THE GARLIC CAULIFLOWER MASHED POTATOES

1 medium/large head cauliflower (900g), cut into 1cm pieces

2 medium/large Yukon Gold or new potatoes (340g), unpeeled, cut into 1cm dice

3 tablespoons dairy-free spread

2 or 3 large cloves garlic, minced, to taste

½ to 1 teaspoon fine sea salt, to taste

Freshly ground black pepper

Grilled or roasted vegetables of choice (such as asparagus or green beans), for serving

Herbamare (see page 307) or fine sea salt

Freshly ground black pepper

5. Heat a grill to medium-high. If using a grill with two racks, I recommend using the top rack to avoid burning. Remove the mushrooms from the marinade (reserve the marinade) and set on the grill gill-side down. Grill for 3 to 5 minutes, then flip the caps and spoon a teaspoon of the marinade into each cap. Grill for 3 to 5 minutes more, or until the caps have reduced in size and are tender. They should have grill marks and be slightly shrivelled in appearance. Discard any water in the caps after cooking. Grill any vegetables you'd like to serve with the mushrooms, brushing them with the marinade as they cook.

6. Reheat the cauliflower mashed potatoes, if necessary, then scoop some onto each plate and top with a couple of the grilled mushroom caps. Serve the grilled or roasted vegetables on the side. Shake up the marinade and add a tablespoon of marinade on top before serving. Season with Herbamare and additional pepper.

Tip 1. The cauliflower mashed potatoes have a bit of texture to them when you mash them by hand (thanks to little cauliflower bits that never fully mash smooth). If you want a smoother texture you can purée the cooked cauliflower in a food processor and then stir it into the mashed potatoes (I don't recommend puréeing the potatoes with the cauliflower because potatoes become 'gluey' when processed). If going this route, you'll have to cook the potatoes and cauliflower in two separate pots.
2. If you have any leftover mushroom caps, you can simply toss them back into the marinade bag and place them in the fridge. The next day, heat them up in a skillet before serving. The leftover marinade can be used as salad dressing, as well. 3. If you don't want to use an outdoor barbecue to grill the vegetables, feel free to use a grill pan on the stovetop.

Make it soya-free Use soya-free dairy-free spread.

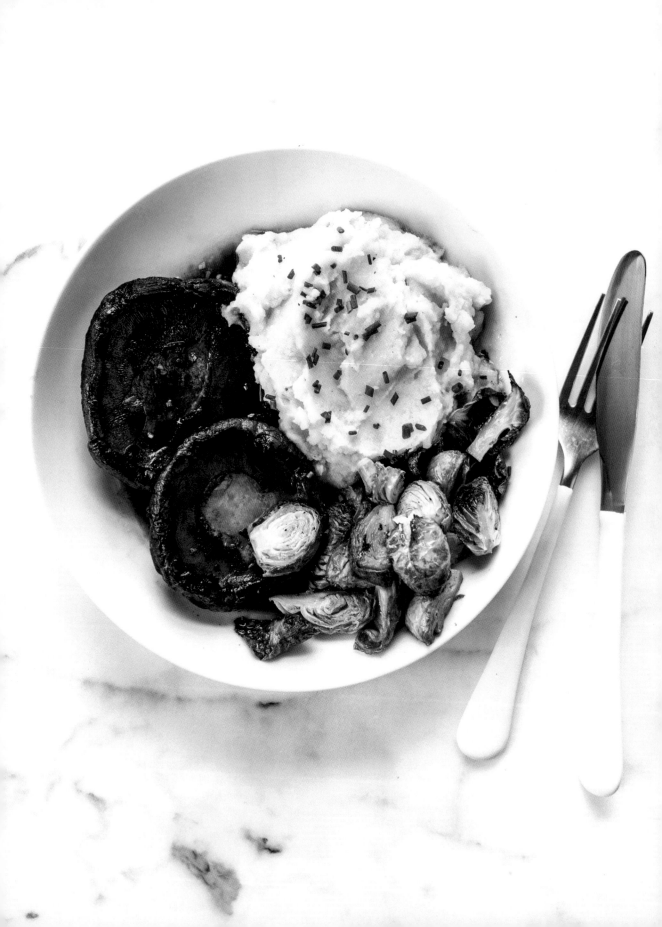

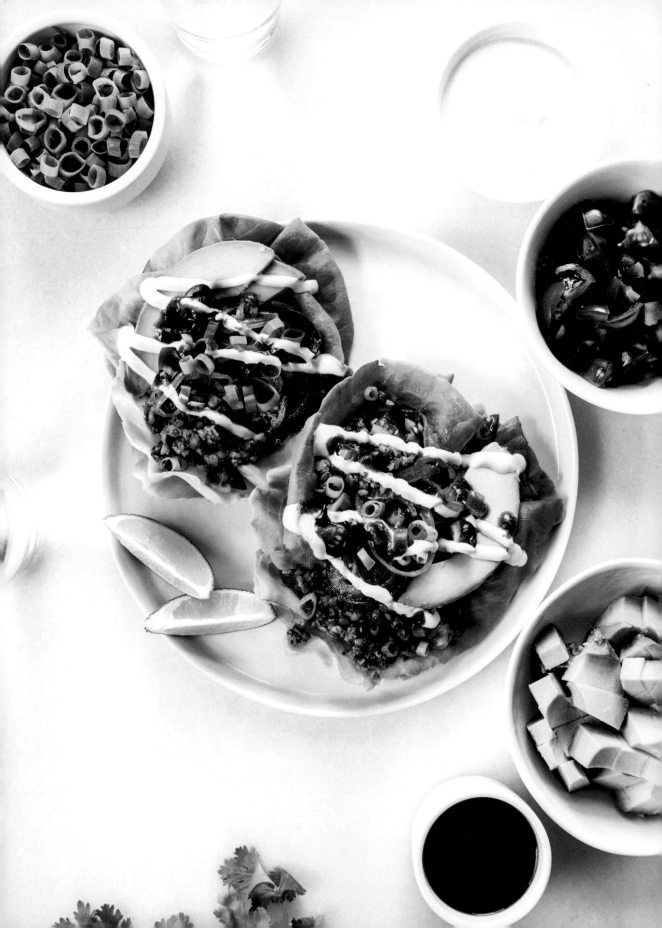

Ultimate Green Taco Wraps

VEGAN, GLUTEN-FREE, NUT-FREE OPTION, SOYA-FREE, GRAIN-FREE,
KID-FRIENDLY OPTION

MAKES 8 TO 10 WRAPS (4 OR 5 SERVINGS)

PREP TIME: **30 MINUTES**

COOK TIME: **30 MINUTES**

Don't let the long ingredient list for these taco wraps deter you; you can prepare the recipe with as few or as many toppings as you wish! On nights when we're crunched for time, we make the tacos very simple, using only the lentil 'meat', chopped tomato, and sliced avocado, all wrapped up in soft tortillas or lettuce leaves. You can also swap in vegan mayo in lieu of the cashew cream; it works great at a pinch, and I like to add a dollop of it on top whenever we don't have cashew cream on hand. It comes together fast. You can also save loads of time by preparing the 'meat' and cashew cream the day before.

If you haven't tried my chewy, crumbly lentil-walnut taco meat yet, this recipe is a perfect introduction. It's high protein, and the taco seasonings give it plenty of flavour. The nut-free version, which uses roasted pumpkin seeds, is just as tasty, so it's a great option if you can't have nuts, or simply want to change it up. Feel free to use soft tortilla wraps instead of lettuce wraps, or you can even make this recipe into a big salad. The sky is the limit!

1. Make the lentil-walnut taco meat Cook the lentils according to the instructions on page 287. Drain off excess water.

2. In a food processor, mince the garlic. Add the lentils and walnuts and pulse until chopped (make sure not to purée it, as you want some texture). Transfer the mixture to a large bowl. Stir in the oregano, cumin, chilli powder and salt. Finally, stir in the oil (start with 4 teaspoons and 1 tablespoon of the water until combined. The taco 'meat' should be nice and moist and not dry—if it's too dry, add more oil or water and stir again. Taste and adjust the seasonings, if desired. I love to add a splash of vegan Worcestershire sauce! Keep in mind that some brands contain soya, however.

3. Make the filling In a very large skillet or wok, heat the oil over medium heat. Add the bell peppers, onion, and a pinch each of salt and black pepper. Cook, uncovered, reducing the heat if necessary and stirring frequently for 15 to 20 minutes, until the onion is translucent and the bell peppers are soft.

(recipe continues)

FOR THE LENTIL-WALNUT TACO MEAT

150g uncooked French green lentils, or 1 400g can lentils, drained and rinsed

1 medium clove garlic

120g walnut pieces or pumpkin seeds, toasted (see Tip)

1½ teaspoons dried oregano

1½ teaspoons ground cumin

1½ teaspoons chilli powder

½ teaspoon fine sea salt, or to taste

4 teaspoons to 3 tablespoons extra-virgin olive oil, as needed

1 to 2 tablespoons water, as needed

Vegan Worcestershire sauce (optional)

FOR THE FILLING

2 tablespoons extra-virgin olive oil

2 medium/large bell peppers, sliced into thin strips (I prefer red and orange, but any will work)

1 medium/large onion, sliced into thin strips

Fine sea salt and freshly ground black pepper

Green wraps (butter, romaine or iceberg lettuce, or chard leaves) or tortillas

Cashew Sour Cream (page 261) or Homemade Vegan Mayo (page 269) or Vegenaise

Fresh Cherry Tomato Salsa (page 63)

Sliced spring onion

Fresh lime juice

Sliced avocado

Sriracha or other hot sauce

Chopped fresh coriander

4. On a plate, place two large lettuce leaves stacked on top of one another. Top with taco meat, filling and any other desired toppings. If the wraps are too delicate to eat with your hands, feel free to eat them with a knife and fork, salad style. Leftovers can be stored in the fridge in separate airtight containers and enjoyed over the next couple of days.

Tip To toast the walnuts or pumpkin seeds: Preheat the oven to 300°F (150°C). Spread the walnuts over a rimmed baking sheet and toast in the oven for 10 to 13 minutes, watching closely, until lightly golden and fragrant. Set aside to cool for a few minutes.

Make it nut-free Swap the walnuts for toasted pumpkin seeds. Leave out the cashew cream, or swap it for Sunflower Seed Cream (see page 145).

Make it kid-friendly Wrap an assembled taco (lettuce 'shell' and all) in a soft wholegrain tortilla and secure it with a cocktail toothpick (if your child is old enough to know to remove the toothpick, that is). For even more fun, you can tie a spring onion 'ribbon' around the centre to hold it all together.

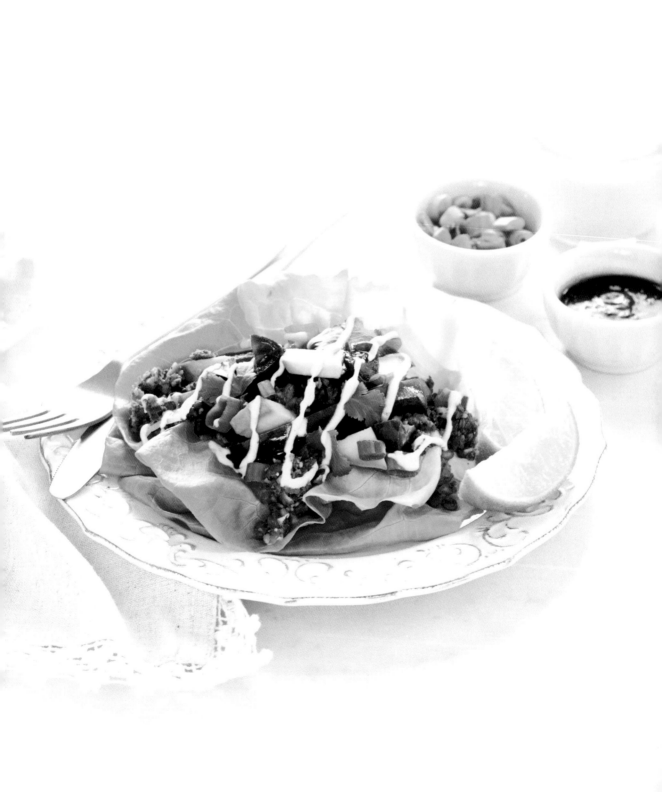

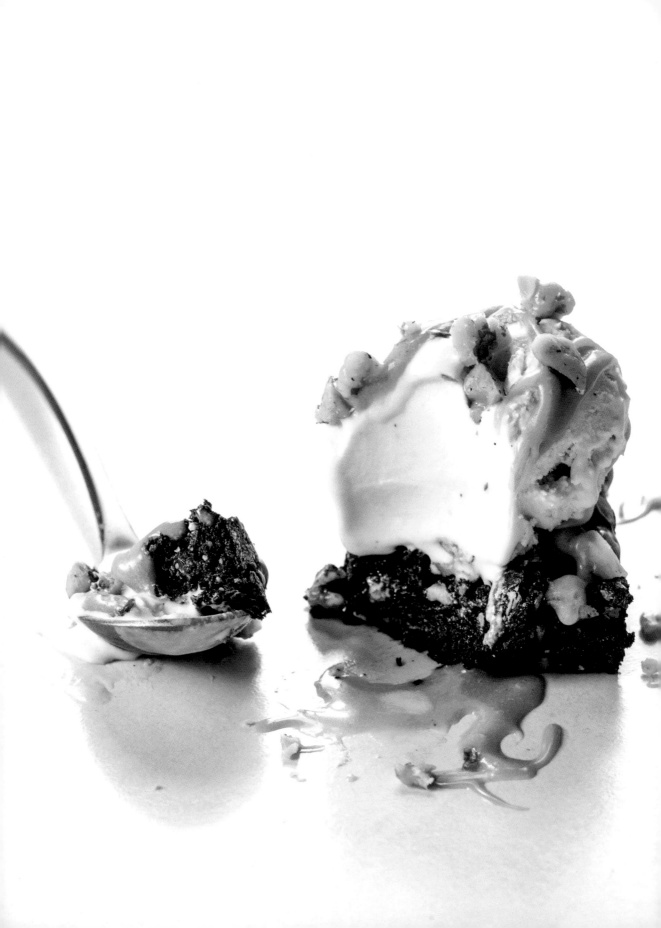

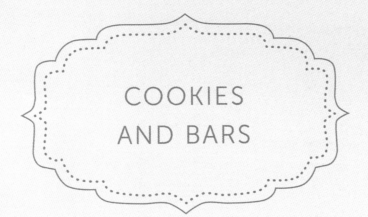

COOKIES AND BARS

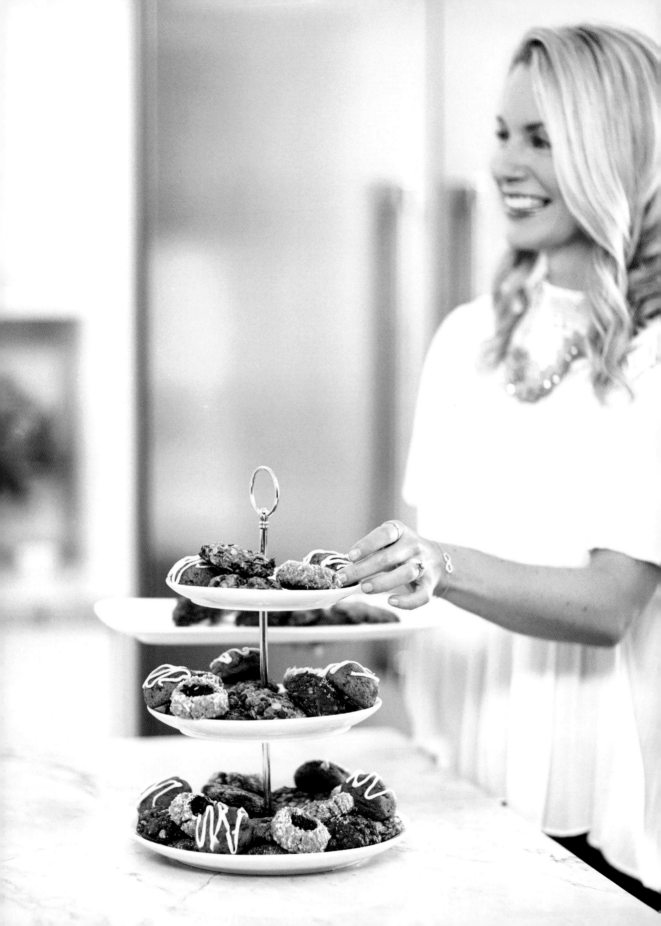

IN MY FIRST COOKBOOK, I included one cookie recipe: Crispy Almond Butter Chocolate Chip Cookies, which were my most beloved cookies at the time. The feedback I've received from readers since the first book came out is that first, you really love this cookie recipe, and second, you want even more cookies! A whole chapter of cookies! Well, I like the way you think. Here's your chapter devoted to cookies. You'll find my go-to recipes for holidays, special occasions, and everyday baking, too. Bring on the cookies!

To be honest, this chapter caused me a few grey hairs (vegan cookie recipes are notoriously temperamental and sensitive to even small changes), but after hundreds of recipe trials (and a whole lot of cookie eating), it was so worth it! The award for Most Recipe Trials Ever goes to my Ultimate Flourless Brownies—they are totally flourless, vegan, gluten-free, grain-free, and incredibly dense and fudgy, and, unlike a lot of flourless vegan brownies, they don't contain beans, avocado or tofu. They took some time to perfect, but I promise, this recipe will blow you away. There's even a nut-free option, too! My Nut-Free Dream Bars were created especially for those of you with nut allergies, but to my delight everyone adores these easy, no-bake 'candy' bars, and they are a hit with kids and adults alike. If you have some holiday baking in mind, my Chocolate-Almond Espresso Cookies, Pillowy Pumpkin Snacking Cookies, Flourless Peanut Butter Cookies, Chewy Molasses Spelt Cookies and Triple Almond Thumbprint Cookies are definitely ones to include on your baking list. And don't forget about my favourite Chocolate-Dipped Vanilla Bean Macaroons—pop a batch into the oven before your guests arrive, and your entire house will be filled with the delightful aromas of vanilla, cinnamon and almond! Just don't forget to invite the Liddons.

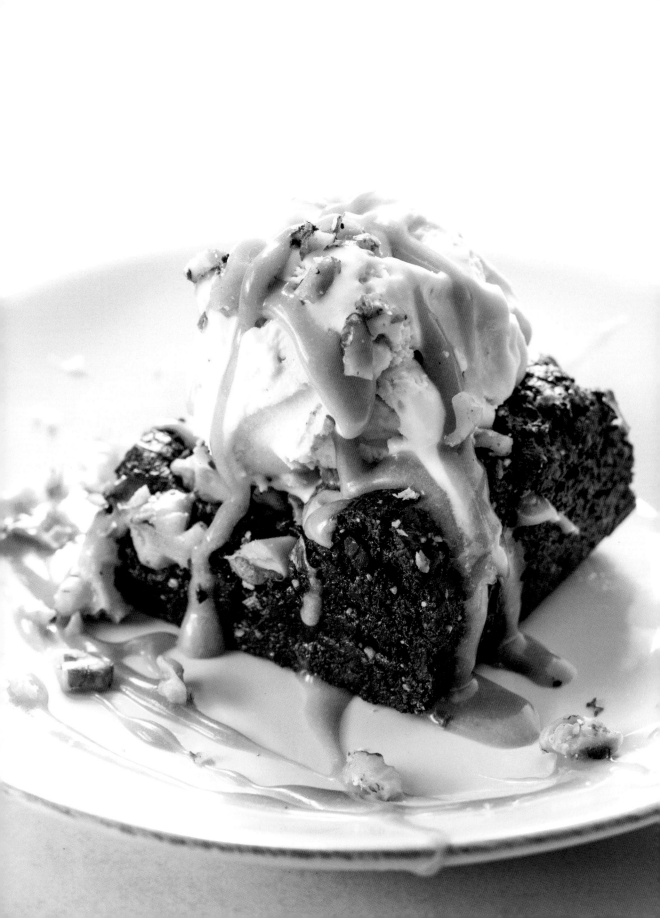

The Ultimate Flourless Brownies

VEGAN, GLUTEN-FREE, NUT-FREE OPTION, SOYA-FREE, GRAIN-FREE, OIL-FREE,
KID-FRIENDLY, FREEZER-FRIENDLY

MAKES 8 (6CM SQUARE) BROWNIES

PREP TIME: **15 MINUTES**

BAKE TIME: **24 TO 28 MINUTES**

I'm pretty serious about my brownies, as you may recall from my first book. This time, my goal was to create brownies that were flourless and grain-free, in addition to being vegan and gluten-free. I even have a nut-free option for you below! Am I crazy, or was it just an excuse to eat a ton of brownies? I guess we'll never know. In the end, I created super-fudgy and dense brownies with crisp edges (aka my brownie nirvana) by using nut or seed butter as the base—nope, not a stitch of flour required! A few tips: Be sure to use 100% natural almond butter (you only want to see almonds on the label—whether you use roasted or raw is up to you). My Homemade Almond Butter (page 75) works perfectly in this recipe, but if you'd like to use store-bought almond butter, you can do that, too. I just recommend pouring off and discarding any oil at the top of the jar, and then stirring the almond butter well before measuring. Also, avoid using the super-dry almond butter at the bottom of the jar—it's simply too firm to mix into this extra-thick brownie batter. (These tips apply to all my recipes that call for nut butter, so they're good to keep in mind.) As for the taste, these brownies have a rich chocolate flavour that becomes even more complex thanks to the nuttiness of the almonds. The addition of chopped dark chocolate is key, and makes the brownies even more decadent. Prepare for an obsession . . .

1. Preheat the oven to 350°F (180°C). Line a 23cm × 13cm (2l) loaf pan with parchment paper cut to fit the length of the pan, with overhang so you can lift out the slab after cooling.

2. In a large bowl, whisk together the ground flax and water. Let the mixture sit for a few minutes, then stir in the salt, baking soda, maple syrup, vanilla, arrowroot, cocoa powder and sugar—in the order listed—until thoroughly combined. The batter will be very thick!

3. Stir in the almond butter until thoroughly combined. You want to mix the dough for a while to make sure the almond butter is fully and evenly distributed. Don't worry about overmixing, since there's no flour in this recipe. You will be left with a very thick and very sticky dough. I repeat, this is normal! Stir in the chopped chocolate until combined.

4. Scoop the thick dough into the prepared pan. Place a piece of parchment paper on top of the dough and press down, starting in the centre and pushing outwards until even. You can remove the paper and lightly dampen your hands with water to help smooth it out evenly.

(recipe continues)

FOR THE BROWNIES

1 tablespoon plus 1½ teaspoons milled linseed

3 tablespoons water

¾ teaspoon fine sea salt

¼ teaspoon baking soda

60ml pure maple syrup

1 teaspoon pure vanilla extract

2 tablespoons arrowroot powder

60g unsweetened cocoa powder, sifted if necessary

90g natural cane sugar

175ml Homemade Almond Butter (page 75) or store-bought (see headnote)

100g non-dairy dark chocolate (55 to 70% cocoa), finely chopped

60g walnuts, toasted and chopped (optional)

FOR SERVING

Magic No-Cook Caramel Sauce (page 253)

Non-dairy vanilla ice cream

Flaky sea salt (such as Maldon), for garnish

5. If desired, scatter the walnuts on top and press them gently into the dough to adhere.

6. Bake for 24 to 28 minutes, until the edges are starting to firm up. The middle will still look underdone and will be soft to the touch. If you insert a toothpick into the middle, it *won't* come out clean. But don't worry. The edges will be higher and the middle will look sunken down a bit—this is all normal! Let the brownies cool in the pan on a cooling rack for 20 to 30 minutes.

7. After cooling, you can either slice the brownies while still warm (note that they might break apart a bit if sliced warm) or you can pop the pan into the freezer, uncovered, for 20 to 30 additional minutes before slicing (they will slice cleaner when chilled). To remove the brownie slab, slide a knife around the ends and carefully lift it out. The brownies might be a bit greasy on the bottom because of the oils in the almond butter; if so, place the brownies on two or three layers of paper towel for about 5 minutes (this absorbs most of the oil), or simply enjoy right away.

8. Serve each brownie with a scoop of ice cream, a drizzle of Magic No-Cook Caramel Sauce, and a pinch of flaky sea salt, if desired. Store leftovers in an airtight container in the fridge for up to a few days. You can also wrap the cooled brownies individually in aluminium foil and place them into an airtight container in the freezer for 4 to 6 weeks. Thaw in the fridge or at room temperature before enjoying.

Tip To thaw a frozen brownie quickly, bake it in the oven for about 7 minutes at 350°F (180°C) for a warm, gooey brownie that's amazing served à la mode!

Make it nut-free Swap the almond butter for natural sunflower seed butter and replace the walnuts with 1 tablespoon hulled sunflower seeds.

Chocolate-Dipped Vanilla Macaroons

VEGAN, GLUTEN-FREE, SOYA-FREE OPTION, GRAIN-FREE, FREEZER-FRIENDLY

MAKES 13 LARGE MACAROONS

PREP TIME: **15 MINUTES**

BAKE TIME: **25 TO 30 MINUTES**

FREEZE TIME: **20 MINUTES**

This is what I like to call macaroon *perfection*! It's the go-to quick-and-easy dessert that I pop in the oven before company comes over. Not only does everyone go nuts over the macaroons, but they fill the house with a delicious vanilla, cinnamon, and almond scent as they bake. The macaroons have achieved *vault status* in our household. My secret is slow baking the macaroons at a very low oven temperature to ensure that the delicate coconut and almonds don't burn before the interior is baked. Drizzle them in melted dark chocolate for the ultimate treat. Be sure to use melted coconut butter (see page 281 for a homemade version) and not coconut oil in this recipe. The coconut butter is necessary for proper binding, and coconut oil will not work in this recipe.

140g raw almonds, ground into a fine meal (see page 290)

90g unsweetened shredded coconut

½ teaspoon plus ⅛ teaspoon fine sea salt

½ teaspoon ground cinnamon

125ml pure maple syrup

60g Homemade Coconut Butter (page 281) or store-bought, melted

1 teaspoon pure vanilla extract

1 vanilla pod, seeds scraped, or ¼ teaspoon pure vanilla powder

100g non-dairy dark chocolate

1 teaspoon virgin coconut oil

1. Preheat the oven to 275°F (140°C). Line a baking sheet with parchment paper. Line a large plate with parchment paper.

2. In a large bowl, stir together the almond meal, shredded coconut, salt, cinnamon, maple syrup, melted coconut butter, vanilla extract and vanilla pod seeds until thoroughly combined. The dough will be thick and sticky.

3. With a 2-tablespoon retractable cookie scoop, scoop a ball of dough and pack it in so the top is flat. Release the dough onto the prepared baking sheet. Repeat with the rest of the dough, setting the macaroons about 5cm apart on the baking sheet.

4. Bake for 15 minutes, then rotate the pan and bake for 10 to 15 minutes more, until the macaroons are a bit golden around the edges. Watch them closely during the last 5 to 10 minutes.

5. Let cool on the baking sheet for 10 minutes, then carefully transfer to a cooling rack to cool completely.

6. In the top of a double boiler, melt the chocolate and coconut oil together over low-medium heat, stirring frequently until smooth. (Alternatively, melt them together in a small pot over low heat, stirring frequently.) Turn off the heat.

7. Dip the flat base of each cooled macaroon into the chocolate and twirl the macaroon until the base is coated in chocolate. As you dip them, place each macaroon onto the parchment paper-lined plate, upside down, so the chocolate coating is facing upwards. Freeze the macaroons for 10 to 15 minutes, or until the chocolate has hardened.

(recipe continues)

8. Flip each macaroon chocolate-side down and drizzle the remaining chocolate on top (reheat the chocolate until liquid, if necessary). Freeze for 5 to 10 minutes, until the chocolate drizzle is firm.

9. Store leftover macaroons in an airtight container in the fridge for up to 1 week. You can also wrap the macaroons in foil, place them in an airtight container or freezer-safe zip-top bag, and freeze for up to 1 month.

Make it soya-free Use a soya-free non-dairy chocolate, such as Enjoy Life brand.

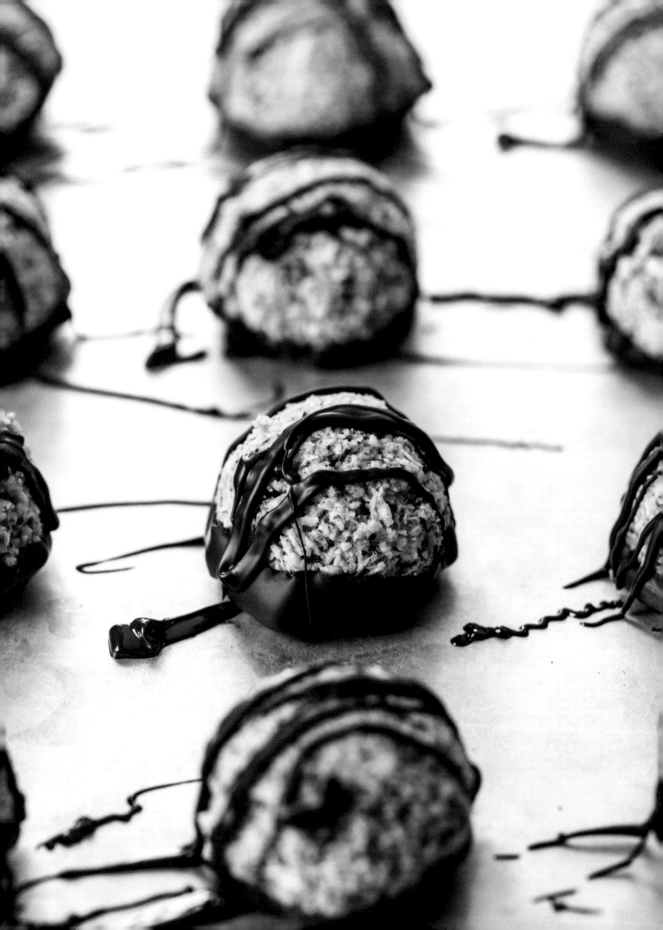

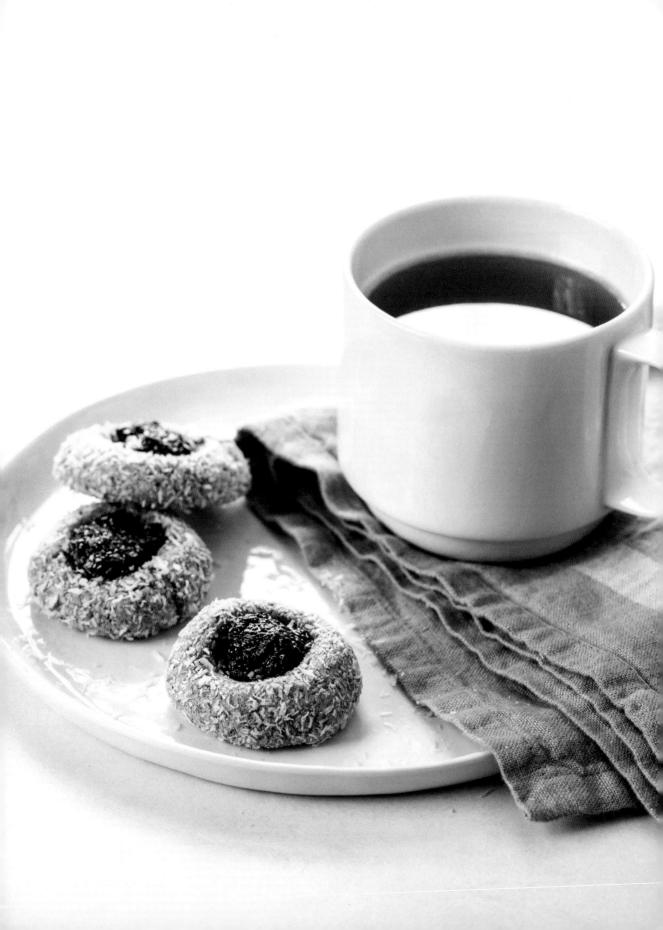

Triple Almond Thumbprint Cookies

VEGAN, GLUTEN-FREE, SOYA-FREE, OIL-FREE, ADVANCE PREP OPTION,
KID-FRIENDLY, FREEZER-FRIENDLY

MAKES 16 COOKIES

PREP TIME: **20 MINUTES**

BAKE TIME: **10 TO 12 MINUTES**

A while ago, I set my heart on making a thumbprint cookie that would capture traditional flavours of raspberry and almond. This cookie, which has almonds, almond butter, almond extract, and my Raspberry Almond Chia Seed Jam, far exceeded my expectations! The cookies are fantastic—lightly sweet and very dense, with a buttery almond flavour and aroma plus a pop of tart raspberry. If you are a fan of peanut butter and jam, you will love this bite-size, 'grown-up' version! And no matter how grown up you are, the cookie dough is so delicious that it will be hard to convince yourself not to polish it off before it reaches the oven!

1. Preheat the oven to 350°F (180°C). Line a large baking sheet with parchment paper.

2. In a food processor, combine the almond meal, brown rice flour, milled linseed, salt, and baking powder. Process just to combine.

3. Add the almond butter, maple syrup and almond extract and process for only 4 or 5 seconds, just until a dough forms. Do not overmix. The dough will be very wet and sticky, but this is normal.

4. Remove the blade from the processor bowl. Lightly wet your hands and roll the dough into balls just smaller than golf balls. You should have about 16 balls. Place the balls on the prepared baking sheet for now.

5. Put the shredded coconut in a small bowl. Roll each ball of dough in the coconut until completely coated.

6. Place the balls at least 5cm apart on the baking sheet. With your thumb, press into the middle of each ball, creating a round well. Make sure the cookie stays in a uniform round shape, and readjust its shape with your fingers if necessary. Add about 1 teaspoon of the jam into each well.

(recipe continues)

185g raw almonds, ground (see page 290) or 185g ground almonds

40g brown rice flour (see Tip)

2 tablespoons milled linseed

½ teaspoon fine sea salt

1 teaspoon baking powder

125g natural smooth raw or roasted almond butter

105ml pure maple syrup

½ teaspoon pure almond extract

30g unsweetened shredded coconut, for rolling

5 to 6 tablespoons Raspberry-Almond Chia Seed Jam (see page 44) or jam of your choice

7. Bake for 10 to 12 minutes, until the cookies have expanded, cracked a bit in some places, and are lightly golden on the bottom. The cookies will be very soft and delicate when coming out of the oven, but trust me, this is totally fine. Let the cookies cool on the baking sheet for 5 to 10 minutes and then carefully transfer them with a spatula onto a cooling rack until completely cool. Again, the cookies will still seem very delicate, but they will firm up a lot once they cool. Store leftover cookies in an airtight container in the fridge for up to 1 week, or in the freezer for up to 1 month.

Tip 1. I love to eat these cookies semi-frozen—try it! 2. If you don't have any brown rice flour on hand, you can use oat flour. I prefer to use brown rice flour because the cookies come out less dense than when you use oat flour, but it'll work at a pinch.

Chocolate-Almond Espresso Cookies

VEGAN, GLUTEN-FREE, SOYA-FREE OPTION, OIL-FREE, FREEZER-FRIENDLY

MAKES 13 OR 14 COOKIES

PREP TIME: **10 MINUTES**

BAKE TIME: **10 TO 12 MINUTES**

If my Flourless Peanut Butter Cookies (page 213) and Ultimate Flourless Brownies (page 199) had a love child, it would resemble these decadent cookies. They do without flour entirely, and instead use ground almonds, rolled oats and a touch of shredded coconut to achieve an irresistible, chewy texture. The cocoa powder and chocolate chips give a powerful dose of chocolatey flavour, and the hint of espresso brings out the chocolate flavour even more. Don't worry if you aren't an espresso fan, though: The cookies don't have a strong coffee flavour if you use the smaller amount of espresso powder I recommend (¼ teaspoon). If you'd like a slightly stronger espresso flavor, feel free to use ½ teaspoon. Of course, if you can't find any you can leave it out and the cookies will still taste lovely, just not quite as rich and chocolatey.

1. Preheat the oven to 350°F (180°C). Line a large baking sheet with parchment paper.

2. In a medium bowl, whisk together the milled linseed and the water. Set aside to thicken.

3. In a large bowl, whisk together the almond meal, coconut, oats, brown sugar, chocolate, cocoa powder, baking powder, salt, and espresso powder.

4. Add the almond butter, maple syrup and vanilla to the bowl with the linseed mixture. Stir until thoroughly combined. The mixture will be very thick.

5. Spoon the wet ingredients into the dry ingredients and stir until thoroughly combined. The batter will likely appear very dry at first, but this is normal. Knead the dough with your hands to make it all come together. (You can also use electric beaters, but I prefer to just get right in there with my hands!) If for some reason your dough is still too dry to shape into balls, add 1 teaspoon water and mix again. The dough will be sticky and dense.

6. Lightly wet your hands and form the dough into 13 or 14 balls, about 2 tablespoons of dough each. If the chocolate chips fall out of the dough, simply push the dough balls into the chips in the bottom of the bowl so they adhere. Place the dough balls on the prepared baking sheet 5 to 8cm apart. Do not press down to flatten the balls, or they will not be as fluffy.

(recipe continues)

1 tablespoon milled linseed

2 tablespoons water

45g ground almonds (see page 290)

3 tablespoons unsweetened shredded coconut

43g gluten-free rolled oats

100g brown sugar

40g non-dairy mini chocolate chips

2 tablespoons unsweetened cocoa powder

1 teaspoon baking powder

½ teaspoon fine sea salt

¼ to ½ teaspoon instant espresso powder, to taste

125ml natural smooth almond butter (see Tip)

2 tablespoons plus 2 teaspoons pure maple syrup

1 teaspoon pure vanilla extract

Flaky sea salt (such as Maldon), for garnish

7. Bake for 10 to 12 minutes, until they spread out slightly but are still a bit puffy. The cookies will be very soft and delicate coming out of the oven, but they will firm up as they cool. Let the cookies cool on the baking sheet for 7 to 8 minutes before carefully transferring to a cooling rack to cool completely. Garnish with flaky sea salt, if desired. Store the cooled cookies in an airtight container in the fridge for 3 to 4 days or freeze them for up to 1 month. I like to wrap them individually in foil and then place them in a freezer-safe zip-top bag or airtight container.

Tip The thickness of your cookies will depend on the thickness of the almond butter you use. I don't recommend using dry almond butter (stay away from almond butter that collects at the bottom of the jar). However, before you measure the almond butter, be sure to pour off any oil at the top of the jar and mix it well so that you don't end up with greasy cookies.

Make it soya-free Use soya-free non-dairy chocolate chips, such as Enjoy Life brand.

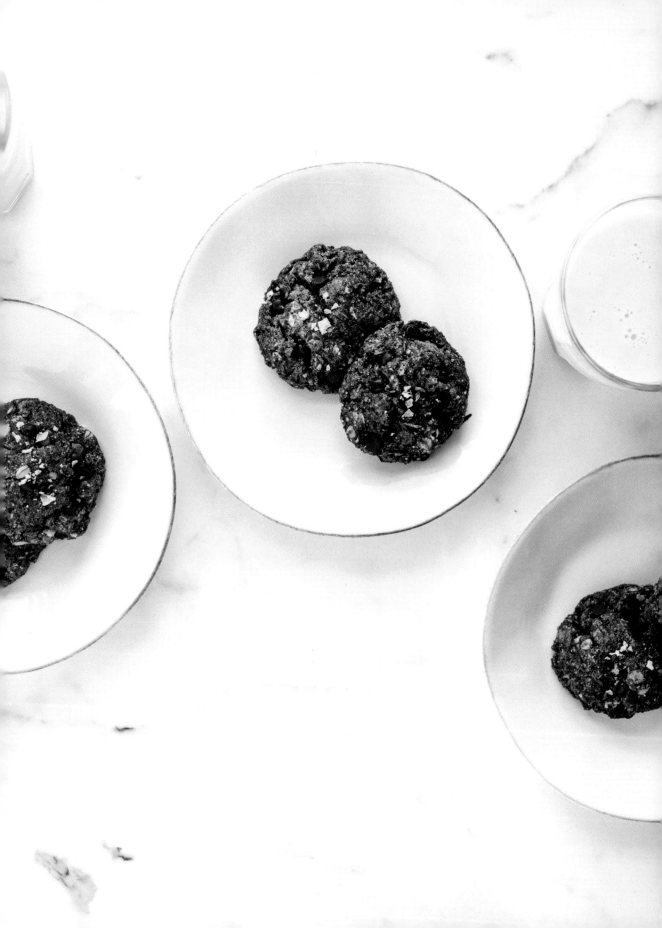

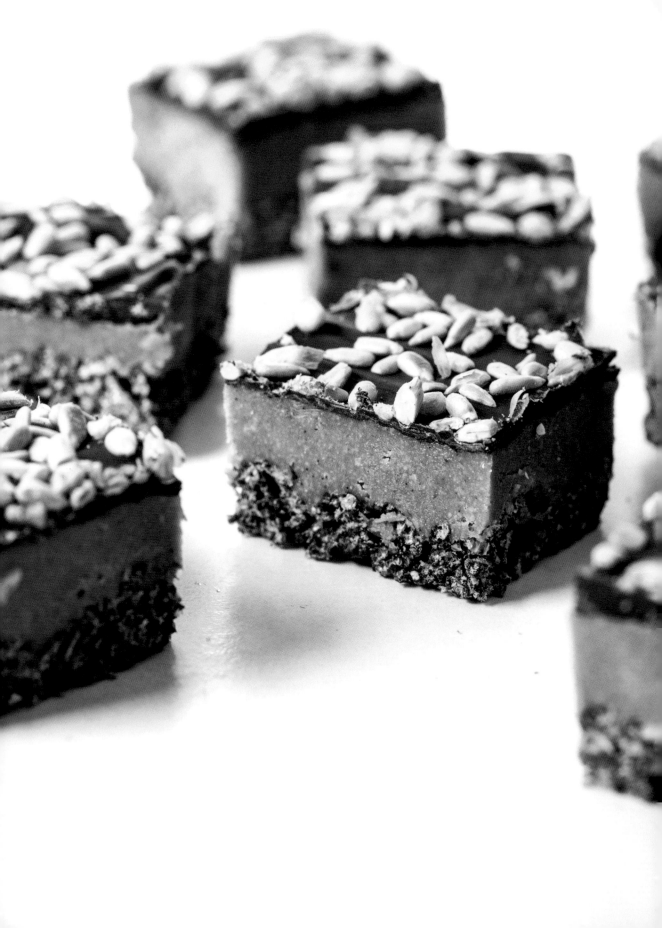

Nut-Free Dream Bars

VEGAN, GLUTEN-FREE, NUT-FREE, SOYA-FREE OPTION, KID-FRIENDLY, FREEZER-FRIENDLY

MAKES 20 SMALL SQUARES

PREP TIME: **25 MINUTES**

FREEZE TIME: **90 MINUTES**

You'll think you're dreaming when you sink your teeth into these delightful nut-free bars! I know I did. These are a healthier version of a no-bake candy bar. I formulated the recipe to be friendly for kids and adults with nut allergies, but whether you need a nut-free treat or not, I promise you'll fall in love with these sweet, crispy bars. They have a lot of different textures in the layers, from crispy rice cereal to creamy sunflower butter, and they are best to eat cold—straight from the fridge or freezer. If you don't want to use sunflower seed butter, you can easily replace it with almond or peanut butter (and you can do the same for the topping, replacing the seeds with toasted sliced almonds or peanuts) and create totally new flavours!

1. **Make the crust** Oil a large loaf pan (about 25cm x 15cm(3l)) and then line it with a piece of parchment paper cut to fit the length of the pan.

2. In a medium bowl, mix together the crust ingredients until the cereal is fully coated. Spoon the mixture into the prepared loaf pan and spread it out evenly with the back of a spoon. It'll be very sticky, but this is normal. With lightly wet hands, press the mixture down firmly and evenly into the pan. The crust mixture will seem very loose at this stage. Place in the freezer.

3. **Make the filling** Rinse and dry the bowl you used to make the crust. In the bowl, combine all the filling ingredients and stir until combined and smooth.

4. Remove the pan from the freezer (the crust should be firm) and spoon the filling on top of the crust. Spread it out evenly with a spatula. Return the pan to a flat surface in the freezer for about 1 hour, or until the filling is firm.

5. **Make the chocolate coating** In a small skillet, toast the sunflower seeds over medium heat, stirring often, for 3 to 5 minutes, until the seeds are lightly golden.

(recipe continues)

FOR THE CRUST

1 tablespoon virgin coconut oil, melted, plus more for the pan

38g crispy rice cereal

2 tablespoons unsweetened cocoa powder

2 tablespoons plus 1½ teaspoons brown rice syrup

Pinch of fine sea salt

FOR THE SUNFLOWER SEED BUTTER FILLING

250ml Homemade Sunflower Seed Butter (page 79) or store-bought

67ml pure maple syrup

60ml virgin coconut oil, melted

1 teaspoon pure vanilla extract

2 pinches of fine sea salt

FOR THE CHOCOLATE COATING

35g hulled sunflower seeds

40g non-dairy chocolate chips or chopped chocolate

1 teaspoon virgin coconut oil

6. Once the filling is firm, in the top of a double boiler melt the chocolate and coconut oil over low-medium heat, stirring frequently, until smooth. (Alternatively, melt them in a small pot over low heat, stirring frequently.) Turn off the heat. Spread the chocolate quickly on top of the filling (working fast ensures it doesn't harden up before you've finished spreading the chocolate). Immediately sprinkle on the toasted sunflower seeds before the chocolate sets. Return the pan to the freezer until the chocolate coating is solid, about 30 minutes.

7. Run a knife around the edges of the pan to loosen. Lift out the slab by holding the parchment paper and lifting up. Run very hot water over a sharp knife for a couple of minutes (this helps the knife cut through the frozen chocolate). Slice the bar into small squares and serve immediately, as they will begin to melt at room temperature. Store any leftovers in an airtight container in the freezer for up to 1 month.

Tip These squares soften at room temperature, so I don't recommend letting them sit out on the counter very long. They are best served chilled.

Make it soya-free Use soya-free non-dairy chocolate, such as Enjoy Life brand.

Flourless Peanut Butter Cookies

VEGAN, GLUTEN-FREE, NUT-FREE OPTION, SOYA-FREE OPTION, OIL-FREE,
KID-FRIENDLY, FREEZER-FRIENDLY

MAKES 12 COOKIES

PREP TIME: **15 MINUTES**

BAKE TIME: **12 TO 14 MINUTES**

These chewy cookies are completely flourless, in addition to being vegan and gluten-free, but no one will be any the wiser! I actually created this cookie recipe for my first cookbook, but I didn't have room to include it. My sister, Kristi, was shocked it didn't make the cut, so I was firmly told I simply *must* include it in this book. Who am I to deny my sister her favourite cookie recipe? The thickness of the cookies will depend on the consistency of the peanut butter—if your peanut butter is super dry, you will get very thick cookies (I don't recommend using overly dry peanut butter!), and if it's oily and runny, you will get thinner cookies. For best results, use all-natural peanut butter and stir well before measuring. Keep in mind that conventional peanut butter (the kind with added oils and sugars) will not work in this recipe—stick to the all-natural stuff (just roasted peanuts on the ingredients list) for best results! If you prefer homemade, you can easily make your own peanut butter if you have a heavy-duty food processor (see page xv).

1. Preheat the oven to 350°F (180°C). Line a large baking sheet with parchment paper.

2. In a medium bowl, whisk together the milled linseed and water, and set aside for a few minutes.

3. In a large bowl, whisk together the coconut, rolled oats, brown sugar, baking powder, salt and chocolate.

4. Add the peanut butter, vanilla and maple syrup to the bowl with the flax mixture and stir until thoroughly combined. The mixture will be very thick.

5. Spoon the wet ingredients into the dry ingredients and stir until thoroughly combined. The batter will likely appear very dry at first, but this is normal. Knead the dough with your hands to make it all come together. (You can also use an electric mixer, but I prefer to just get right in there with my hands!) If for some reason your dough is still too dry to shape into balls, add 1 teaspoon of water and mix again. The dough will be sticky.

6. Lightly wet your hands (shaking off excess water) and form the dough into 12 balls about the size of golf balls. If any chocolate chips fall out of the dough, simply push the dough balls into the chips at the bottom of the bowl. Place the balls on the prepared baking sheet 5 to 8cm apart. Gently press down on each ball to flatten slightly.

1 tablespoon milled linseed

3 tablespoons water

30g unsweetened shredded coconut

85g gluten-free rolled oats

100g brown sugar

1 teaspoon baking powder

½ teaspoon fine sea salt (see Tip)

40g non-dairy mini chocolate chips (such as Enjoy Life brand)

125g natural smooth peanut butter

1 teaspoon pure vanilla extract

2 tablespoons pure maple syrup

(recipe continues)

7. Bake for 12 to 14 minutes. The cookies will be very soft and delicate coming out of the oven, but they will firm up as they cool. The bottoms will be golden brown. Let the cookies cool on the baking sheet for 5 to 8 minutes before carefully transferring to a cooling rack to cool completely. Store the cookies in an airtight container in the fridge for 3 to 4 days or freeze them for up to 1 month. I like to wrap them individually in foil and then place them in a freezer-safe zip-top bag or airtight container.

Tip Reduce the salt quantity if using salted peanut butter.

Make it nut-free Replace the peanut butter with natural sunflower seed butter.

Make it soya-free Use soya-free mini chocolate chips, such as Enjoy Life brand.

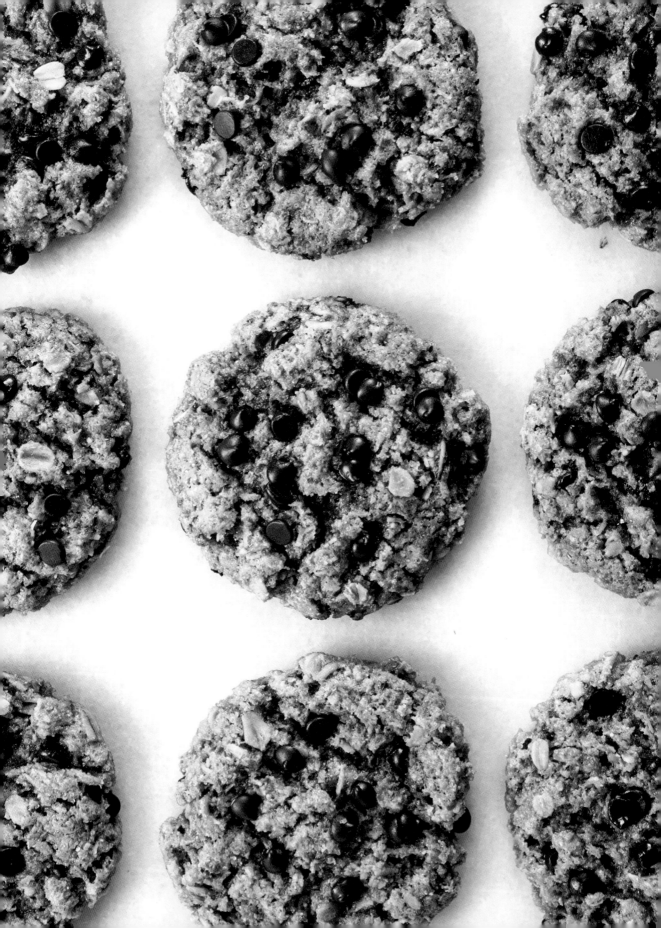

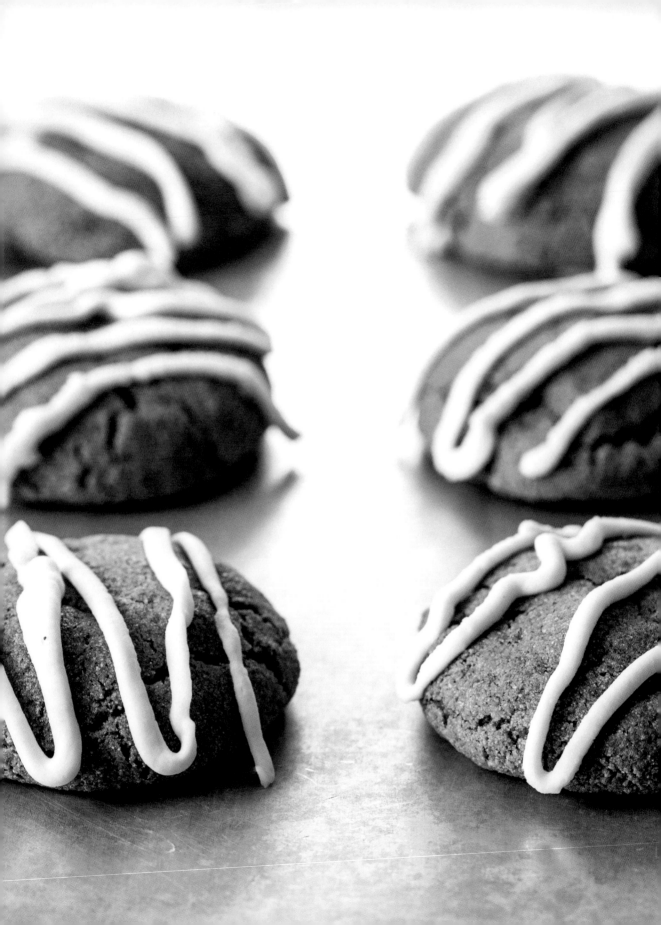

Pillowy Pumpkin Snacking Cookies

VEGAN, NUT-FREE, SOYA-FREE, KID-FRIENDLY, FREEZER-FRIENDLY

MAKES 11 COOKIES

PREP TIME: **10 TO 15 MINUTES**

BAKE TIME: **12 TO 14 MINUTES**

I love crispy cookies, but sometimes I want a soft, thick, pillowy cookie, and these spicy treats are my favourite way to satisfy the craving! In this recipe, pumpkin purée is spiced with cinnamon, ginger, vanilla, nutmeg, cloves and cardamom—you'll be dreaming of fall leaves and cosy sweaters as the cookies bake. I top these with Coconut Whipped Cream (page 275) for a truly irresistible, 'pumpkin-pie' flavoured cookie. My Magic No-Cook Caramel Sauce (page 253) is also a lovely topping. Or skip the topping for a more portable option; the cookies taste great either way!

1. Preheat the oven to 350°F (180°C). Line a large baking sheet with parchment paper.

2. In a large bowl using an electric mixer, beat together the coconut oil, sugar, pumpkin and vanilla until smooth.

3. Add the cinnamon, linseed, ginger, baking soda, nutmeg, cloves, cardamom and salt. Beat until combined. Add the flour and beat again until combined. The dough should be moist and easy to roll into balls.

4. Shape the dough into large balls, about 2 packed tablespoons each. Place the balls 5 to 8cm apart on the prepared baking sheet. Do not flatten the balls, or the cookies will not be as fluffy.

5. Bake for 12 to 14 minutes, until the cookies have puffed up. Some might be lightly cracked on the surface.

6. Let cool on the pan for 5 minutes before transferring to a cooling rack to cool completely.

7. Pipe Coconut Whipped Cream onto the cookies, if desired (make sure they are completely cool or the cream will melt). Store the cooled cookies in an airtight container in the fridge for 2 to 3 days or freeze them for up to 2 weeks. I like to wrap them individually in foil and then place them in a freezer-safe zip-top bag or airtight container.

3 tablespoons virgin coconut oil, softened

50g brown sugar

75g unsweetened pumpkin purée

½ teaspoon pure vanilla extract

2 teaspoons ground cinnamon

2 teaspoons milled linseed

¾ teaspoon ground ginger

½ teaspoon baking soda

½ teaspoon freshly grated nutmeg

⅛ teaspoon ground cloves

Dash of ground cardamom

¼ teaspoon fine sea salt

115g white/light spelt flour

Coconut Whipped Cream (page 275), for topping (optional)

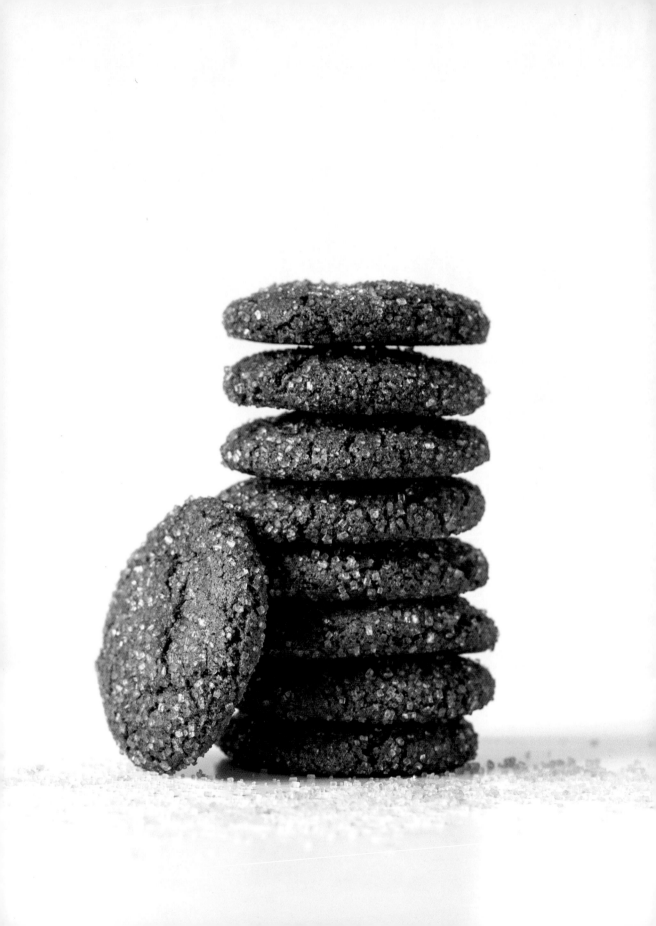

Chewy Molasses Spelt Cookies

VEGAN, NUT-FREE, SOYA-FREE OPTION, KID-FRIENDLY, FREEZER-FRIENDLY

MAKES 12 COOKIES

PREP TIME: 15 MINUTES

BAKE TIME: 8 TO 13 MINUTES

With crispy edges and chewy centres, these richly spiced cookies are hard to resist! I use moderate amounts of sweetener here, so the molasses cookies are sweet but not too sweet. The combination of molasses, ginger, cinnamon and cloves will make your home smell heavenly as the cookies bake—you'll be tempted to have a batch in the oven throughout the Christmas season. The texture of these cookies is variable; the longer you leave them in the oven, the crispier they become. Extend the baking time a bit for a traditional ginger snap texture or bake for the shorter time if you prefer a softer cookie.

1. Preheat the oven to 350°F (180°C). Line a large baking sheet with parchment paper.

2. In a mug, stir together the ground flax and water and set aside for a few minutes to thicken.

3. In a large bowl using an electric mixer, beat together the butter, cane sugar, maple syrup, molasses, vanilla and linseed mixture until smooth and combined.

4. One by one, beat in the ginger, baking soda, cinnamon, salt, cloves and flour until just combined. Be sure not to overmix the batter.

5. Put the turbinado sugar in a bowl. Shape the dough into small 2.5cm balls and roll in the sugar. Place the balls 5cm apart on the prepared baking sheet. Do not press down.

6. Bake for 8 to 10 minutes for a softer cookie and 12 to 13 minutes for a crispier cookie.

7. Let cool on the pan for 5 minutes before transferring to a cooling rack for 10 to 15 minutes. Store the cookies in an airtight container in the fridge for 3 to 4 days or freeze for up to 1 month.

Make it soya-free Use soya-free vegan butter or coconut oil.

1½ teaspoons ground flax

2 tablespoons water

55g dairy-free spread or virgin coconut oil, softened

65g natural cane sugar

2 tablespoons pure maple syrup

2 tablespoons blackstrap molasses

½ teaspoon pure vanilla extract

1 teaspoon ground ginger

½ teaspoon baking soda

½ teaspoon ground cinnamon

¼ teaspoon fine sea salt

¼ teaspoon ground cloves

130g white spelt flour or wholegrain spelt flour

2 tablespoons turbinado sugar or natural cane sugar, for rolling

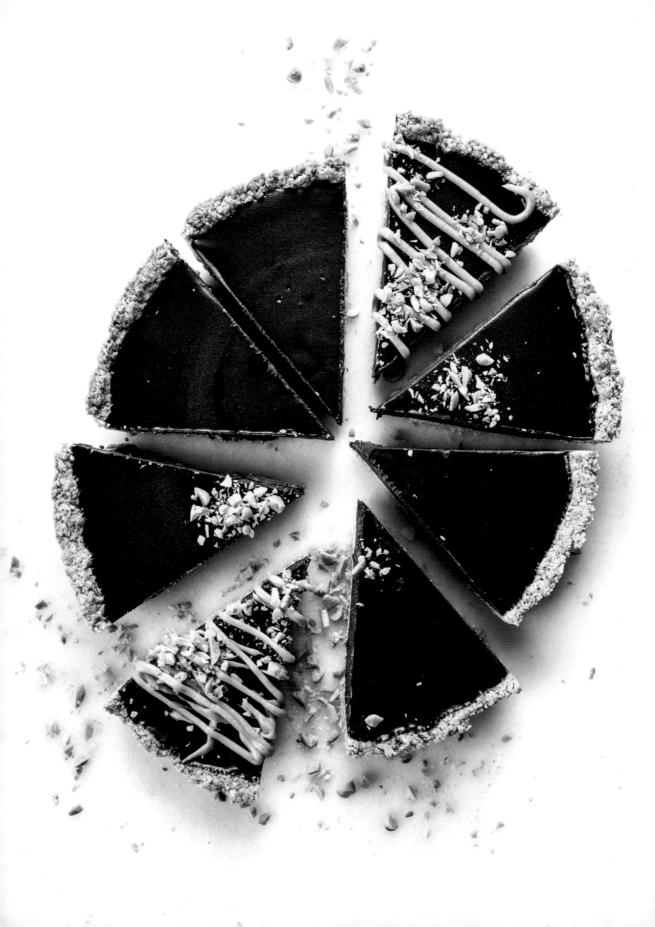

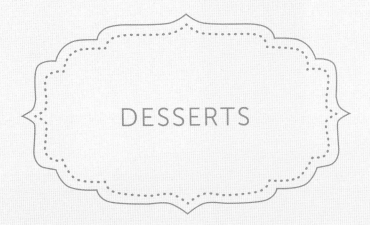

DESSERTS

ANYONE WHO READS my blog regularly knows that I love desserts, and while I try my best to enjoy them in moderation, I'll never shun them entirely. I like to create desserts that use as many whole ingredients as possible, without sacrificing flavour or texture. Some of my favourite desserts are quite simple—a couple of squares of dark chocolate at the end of the day, my Secret Ingredient Chocolate Pudding, or even a banana spread with almond butter. But when there's a special occasion, I love to spoil my friends and family with a homemade dessert made with as many wholesome ingredients as I can pack in.

During the cooler months, I love to make my High-Rise Pumpkin Cupcakes with Spiced Buttercream Frosting. For special and 'anytime' occasions, my Peanut Better Balls, Mile-High Black-and-White Freezer Fudge, and Peanut Butter Lover's Chocolate Tart are always a hit. When it's warmer outside, try my Lemon Cheesecake—it's a no-bake dessert that's delicious chilled, and even people who claim they aren't fans of lemon go absolutely crazy over this one! For a warm-weather dessert that's ready in minutes, be sure to make my vibrant Mango-Coconut-Lime and Raspberry-Banana Sorbet. I make it time and time again for our family (even during winter if the craving strikes!). It's a refreshing treat, and I think you'll love it, too.

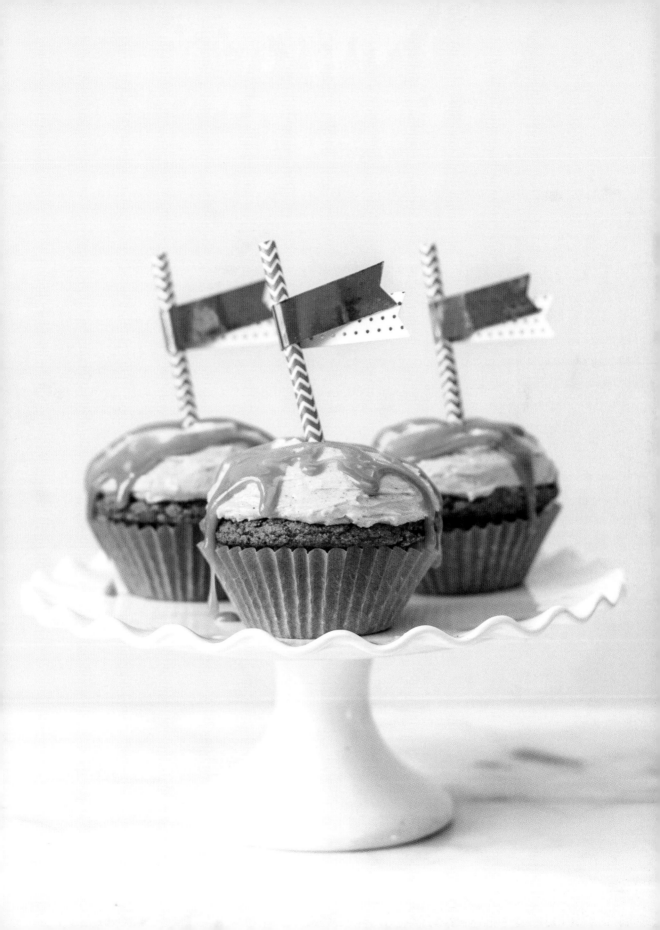

High-Rise Pumpkin Cupcakes

PREP TIME: **20 MINUTES**

BAKE TIME: **24 TO 30 MINUTES**

VEGAN, NUT-FREE OPTION, SOYA-FREE OPTION, ADVANCE PREP REQUIRED, KID-FRIENDLY, FREEZER-FRIENDLY

MAKES 12 CUPCAKES

300g white/light spelt flour (see Tip)

125g natural cane sugar

2 teaspoons baking powder

2 teaspoons ground cinnamon

1½ teaspoons freshly grated nutmeg

½ teaspoon baking soda

½ teaspoon fine sea salt

¼ teaspoon ground allspice

⅛ teaspoon ground cloves

185g unsweetened pumpkin purée

250ml unsweetened almond milk

60ml pure maple syrup

60ml grapeseed oil or refined coconut oil, melted (see Tip)

1 tablespoon fresh lemon juice

2 teaspoons pure vanilla extract

Spiced Buttercream Frosting (page 227) or Orange-Maple Coconut Whipped Cream (see page 275)

These irresistible pumpkin spice cupcakes (photo on previous page) are amazing in the fall or winter months—but I certainly don't hesitate to make them in the summer, too! The cupcakes are surprisingly light and fluffy, and if you're anything like me you might scream with delight when you see how much they rise while they bake. I use white (or light) spelt flour to give these a wonderful, moist and light texture. If you can't find any, you can use whole spelt flour in the recipe, but be aware that the cupcakes will be more dense (yet still tasty!). A big thanks to Dreena Burton, talented cookbook author and blogger at plantpoweredkitchen. com, for inspiring this recipe!

1. Preheat the oven to 350°F (180°C). Lightly grease a 12-cup muffin tin with oil or line it with non-stick paper liners (I prefer If You Care brand Large Baking Cups, as I've found other brands, such as Reynolds, can stick).

2. In a large bowl, whisk together the flour, sugar, baking powder, cinnamon, nutmeg, baking soda, salt, allspice and cloves until combined.

3. In a medium bowl, whisk together the pumpkin purée, milk, maple syrup, oil, lemon juice and vanilla until smooth.

4. Add the wet mixture to the dry mixture and stir until combined. Stop mixing as soon as there are no dry patches of flour on the bottom of the bowl; it's important not to overmix spelt flour as it can result in a dense cupcake. The batter will be quite thick (like a muffin batter), but this is normal.

5. Scoop the batter (I like to use a retractable ice-cream scoop) into each well of the prepared muffin tin, filling them two-thirds to three-quarters full. Smooth out the tops a bit. Bake for 24 to 30 minutes, or until a toothpick inserted into the centre of each cupcake comes out clean and the cake springs back—very slowly—when touched. The cupcakes rise beautifully—you might actually scream with joy when you see the beautiful rounded tops!

6. Let cool in the pan on a cooling rack for about 10 minutes. Gently transfer the cupcakes to the rack and let cool completely. (Be sure the cupcakes are not warm when you frost them, or the frosting will melt.)

7. Frost the cooled cupcakes with Spiced Buttercream Frosting or Orange-Maple Coconut Whipped Cream. Store any leftovers in an airtight container in the fridge for up to 5 days. You can also freeze the cupcakes: Place the frosted cupcakes on a plate and freeze, uncovered. Once the frosting has hardened, remove the cupcakes from the freezer and wrap them individually in clingfilm. Transfer them to an airtight container and freeze for up to 1 month. To thaw, unwrap the cupcake and place it in the fridge or on the counter until thawed throughout.

Tip 1. Feel free to substitute all-purpose white flour instead of spelt flour. 2. I use grapeseed oil in this cake because it's neutral, with virtually no flavour. I don't recommend using a strong-tasting oil like extra-virgin olive oil. If you don't have grapeseed oil or refined coconut oil (which is also flavourless), you can use melted virgin coconut oil. Just note that the cake will have a light coconut flavour. When using melted coconut oil, make sure the rest of your ingredients are at room temperature to prevent the coconut oil from solidifying.

Make it nut-free Swap the almond milk for coconut milk or another nut-free milk of your choice.

Make it soya-free Use soya-free dairy-free spread for the Spiced Buttercream. Or simply prepare the Orange-Maple Coconut Whipped Cream as an alternative.

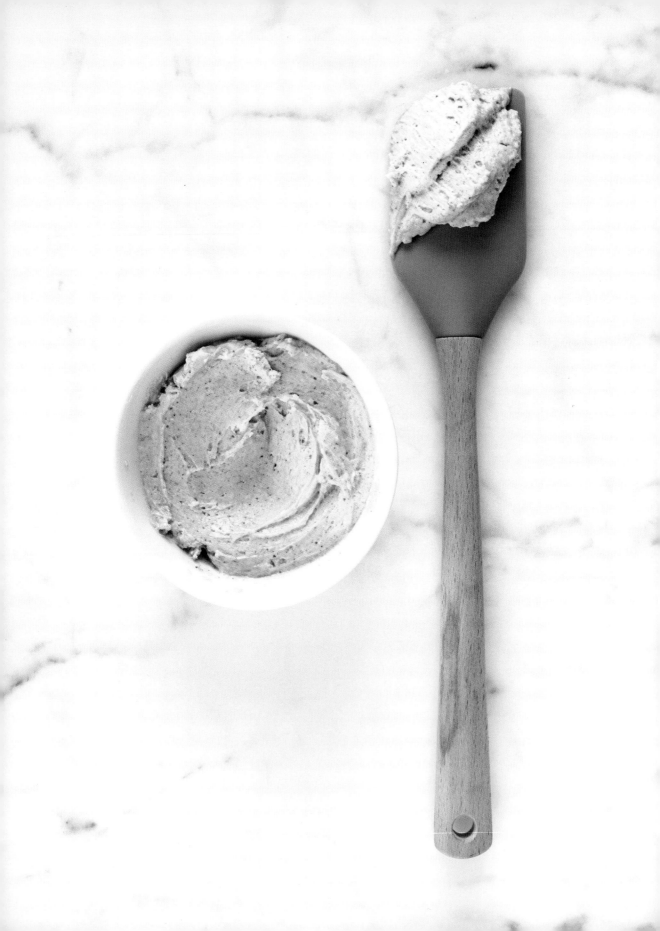

Spiced Buttercream Frosting

VEGAN, GLUTEN-FREE, NUT-FREE OPTION, SOYA-FREE OPTION, GRAIN-FREE, KID-FRIENDLY

MAKES 300ML

PREP TIME: **10 MINUTES**

Buttery, sweet and lightly spiced with nutmeg, cinnamon and vanilla, this dairy-free 'buttercream' is a perfect complement to the High-Rise Pumpkin Cupcakes (page 224). You can use the spiced buttercream version or the double vanilla variation (see below) depending on your mood.

1. In a large bowl using an electric mixer or in the bowl of a stand mixer fitted with the whisk attachment, beat the butter for about 30 seconds until fluffy and smooth.

2. Add the sugar, 1 teaspoon of milk, vanilla, cinnamon, nutmeg and salt. Beat again, starting on low speed and covering the bowl or stand mixer with a tea towel, until smooth and fluffy, stopping to scrape down the bowl as necessary. If your buttercream is still too thick, you can thin it with a touch more milk. If it becomes too thin, you can thicken it by beating in more sugar.

Tip For the dairy-free spread, I use soya-free Earth Balance buttery spread. You can use whichever dairy-free spread you prefer, though.

Make it nut-free Swap the almond milk for a nut-free milk of your choice, such as coconut milk.

Make it soya-free Use soya-free dairy-free spread.

For Double Vanilla Buttercream Add ½ teaspoon pure vanilla powder or the seeds from vanilla pods and omit the cinnamon and nutmeg.

170g dairy-free spread (see Tip)

190g icing sugar, plus more if needed

1 to 3 teaspoons almond milk, as needed

½ teaspoon pure vanilla extract

½ teaspoon ground cinnamon, or to taste

¼ teaspoon freshly grated nutmeg, or to taste

Pinch of fine sea salt

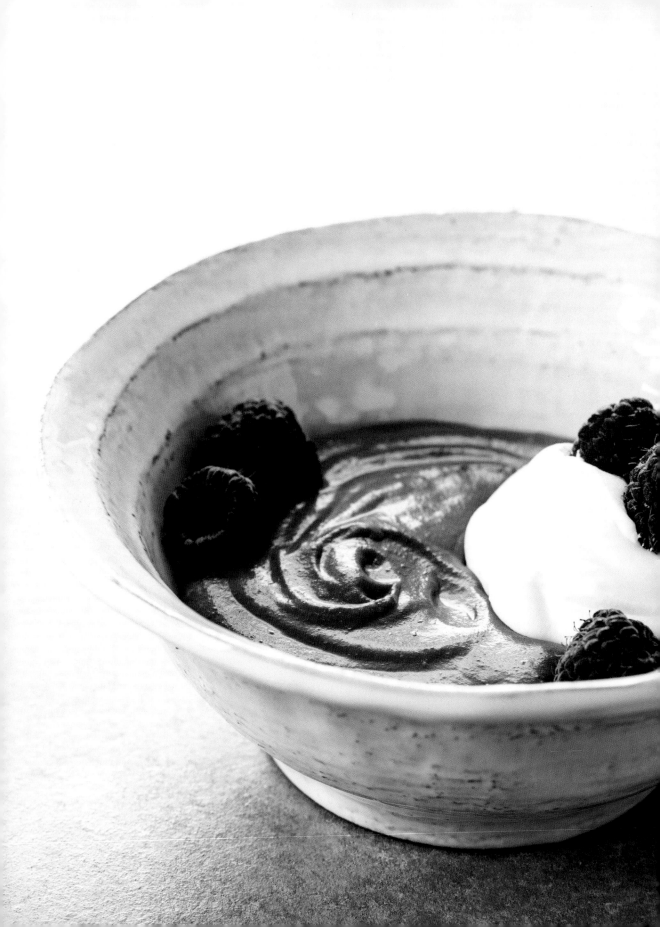

Secret Ingredient Chocolate Pudding

VEGAN, GLUTEN-FREE, SOYA-FREE, GRAIN-FREE, KID-FRIENDLY

MAKES 325ML (3 SERVINGS)

PREP TIME: **10 MINUTES**

COOK TIME: **10 TO 15 MINUTES**

You can use many ingredients as a creative non-dairy base for vegan puddings. Most recipes call for avocado, tofu or even black beans, but I developed a personal favourite version using sweet potato. The sweet potato flavour is virtually undetectable, and no one ever guesses it's the hidden ingredient, but it provides thickness and body, as well as a light sweetness. This pudding is rich, smooth and chocolatey, just like choco-late pudding should be! If you'd like to enhance the chocolate flavour even more, try adding ¼ teaspoon espresso powder for a fun twist. One of my recipe testers calls this pudding 'brownie batter', which makes it all the more remarkable that it's free of dairy and refined sugars. The serving size is fairly small for this pudding because it's quite rich and a little bit goes a long way, but feel free to double the batch if you want a generous portion. After chilling, this pudding will thicken a great deal, almost taking on a thick mousse texture. You can decide for yourself which way you prefer it!

1. Bring a medium pot of water to a boil and set a steamer basket on top. Steam the sweet potato in the basket, covered, for 10 to 15 minutes, until fork-tender. You may also use a steamer appliance. Turn off the heat and let sit for 5 minutes.

2. Transfer the sweet potato to a food processor and add the maple syrup. Process until smooth. Add the rest of the ingredients and process until smooth, stopping to scrape down the bowl as necessary. Taste and adjust the sweetness, if desired. I find this pudding tastes a bit sweeter after chilling, so keep that in mind. You can always adjust the sweetness after it chills.

3. Transfer to an airtight container and refrigerate for at least a few hours or up to overnight to thicken. If the pudding is too thick for your liking, you can thin it out with a splash of almond milk.

4. Serve the pudding with Coconut Whipped Cream, fresh berries and toasted sliced almonds, if desired. You can also enjoy it on its own, or with homemade granola sprinkled on top. Store any leftovers in an airtight container in the fridge for 3 to 4 days.

Tip 1. To toast the almonds, preheat the oven to 325°F (160°C). Spread the sliced almonds over a small rimmed baking sheet and toast in the oven for 8 to 10 minutes, until lightly golden. 2. Don't want to steam the sweet potatoes? You can boil them instead.

FOR THE PUDDING

170g diced peeled sweet potato or yam

75ml pure maple syrup

75ml unsweetened almond milk

25g unsweetened cocoa powder

2 tablespoons raw or roasted smooth almond butter or raw cashew butter

1 tablespoon virgin coconut oil, softened

1 teaspoon pure vanilla extract

¼ teaspoon fine sea salt

TOPPING SUGGESTIONS

Coconut Whipped Cream (page 275)

Fresh berries or pomegranate arils

55g sliced almonds, toasted (see Tip)

Homemade granola (pages 33 and 71)

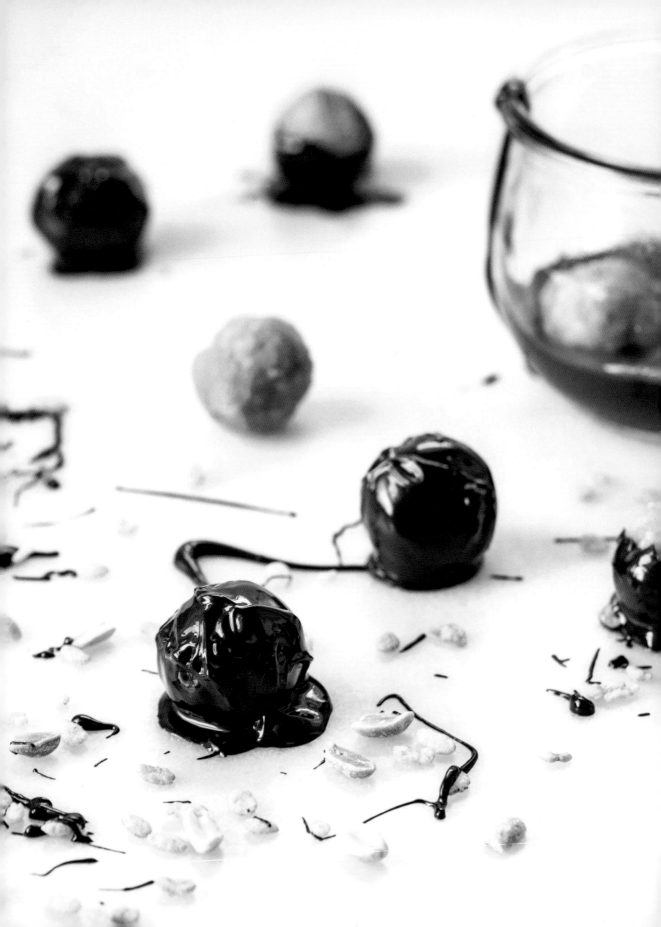

Peanut Better Balls

VEGAN, GLUTEN-FREE, NUT-FREE OPTION, SOYA-FREE OPTION,
FREEZER-FRIENDLY

MAKES 18 TO 20 BALLS

PREP TIME: **20 MINUTES**

FREEZE TIME: **25 MINUTES**

Traditional peanut butter balls are loaded with powdered sugar and butter, but my version is made with lighter ingredients and just a touch of unrefined sweetener. You'll wonder how you ever lived without them! As a child, I loved to help my mum make peanut butter balls each Christmas Eve, and now these 'better' balls are our new holiday favourite. Truthfully, though, I love to make these whenever the craving for peanut butter and chocolate strikes (which is often!). They are simple to throw together and are a terrific crowd-pleaser at parties—for a mess-free finger food, serve them in mini cupcake liners. I recommend using 100% natural peanut butter for this recipe. You want to see just roasted peanuts listed on the label (salt is fine, too, just reduce the amount of salt in the recipe to taste). Also, avoid using the thick peanut butter that often collects at the bottom of a jar; it's simply too dry for this recipe.

1. Stir the jar of peanut butter before using. Line a large plate or tray that will fit in your freezer with a piece of parchment paper.

2. In a large bowl, vigorously stir together the peanut butter, maple syrup, and salt for 30 to 60 seconds, until the mixture thickens. It's important to stir very well for the whole time so that the mixture thickens enough to shape into balls.

3. At this point, the 'dough' might be thick enough to skip the coconut flour. You want a cookie dough that rolls easily, but is neither too wet nor too dry. If the dough is still too sticky/runny, stir in 1 tablespoon of the coconut flour until thoroughly combined. Let it sit for a minute, as the coconut flour will continue to absorb moisture. If the peanut butter mixture is still too sticky, add a touch more coconut flour and mix again. The dough should hold together well and shouldn't crack. If by some chance it becomes too dry you can add a bit more maple syrup and mix again.

4. Add the cereal and use your hands to gently knead the cereal into the dough until combined.

5. Shape the dough into 18 to 20 balls (using about 1 tablespoon of dough each), rolling the mixture between your hands. Place each ball on the lined plate.

(recipe continues)

250g smooth or crunchy 100% natural peanut butter

60ml pure maple syrup

¼ to ½ teaspoon fine sea salt, to taste

1 to 2 tablespoons coconut flour, as needed

10g to 20g gluten-free crispy rice cereal (not puffed rice cereal), to taste

120g non-dairy chocolate chips

1 teaspoon virgin coconut oil

6. In the top of a double boiler, melt the chocolate and coconut oil together over low-medium heat, stirring frequently until smooth. (Alternatively, melt them in a small pot over low heat, stirring frequently.) Turn off the heat.

7. Place a ball into the melted chocolate. Roll it around with a fork until it's fully coated in chocolate. With the fork, lift the ball out of the chocolate and tap off any excess. Place the ball on the lined plate, being sure it isn't touching the other balls. Repeat to coat the rest. (It's okay if some chocolate pools underneath the balls—you can break it off after freezing or simply leave it as is—I know, extra chocolate, what a problem to have!) Save any leftover melted chocolate for drizzling on top of the balls later.

8. Place the balls in the freezer on a flat surface for about 10 minutes, until the chocolate is firm.

9. Using a spatula, scoop the leftover melted chocolate to one side of the pot. Dip a small spoon into the chocolate and drizzle it on top of the balls to create a 'fancy' design, if desired.

10. Freeze the balls for 10 to 15 minutes more, until the chocolate is completely set. Leftovers balls can be stored in an airtight container in the fridge for 5 to 7 days or in the freezer for about 1 month.

Tip 1. If you don't have any coconut flour on hand, you can use all-purpose gluten-free flour, all-purpose white flour or light spelt flour instead. Keep in mind that the latter two will add gluten to the recipe. 2. Try adding flaky sea salt or crushed salted peanuts to the top of the balls before freezing to enhance the flavors.

Make it nut-free Use sunflower seed butter instead of peanut butter.

Make it soya-free Use soya-free non-dairy chocolate chips, such as Enjoy Life brand.

Meyer Lemon Cheesecake with Strawberry-Vanilla Compote

VEGAN, GLUTEN-FREE, SOYA-FREE, GRAIN-FREE, ADVANCE PREP REQUIRED,
KID-FRIENDLY, FREEZER-FRIENDLY

SERVES 10

SOAK TIME: **1 TO 2 HOURS, OR OVERNIGHT**

PREP TIME: **35 MINUTES**

FREEZE TIME: **6 HOURS OR OVERNIGHT**

COOK TIME: **10 MINUTES (FOR THE COMPOTE)**

I created this almost raw cheesecake for a spring get-together last year, and it blew everyone away—even the self-proclaimed lemon haters in the group. The filling uses Meyer lemons, which have a distinctively sweet-tart flavour, but don't worry if you can't find them; regular lemons work, too. The crust is made up of almonds and coconut, and it's the perfect complement to the tangy lemon and lightly sweet strawberry compote. I recommend making the cheesecake and compote the day before, so they have ample time to chill, but if you make it in the morning it should be ready by dinnertime. I recommend using a Vitamix or Blendtec blender to achieve a super-smooth cheesecake filling.

1. Soak the cashews in a bowl of water overnight or for a minimum of 1 to 2 hours to soften. For a quick-soak method, soak the cashews in boiling water for 30 to 60 minutes. Drain and rinse before using.

2. Grease an 18cm/1.5l springform cake pan with coconut oil and then line the base with a circle of parchment paper cut to fit. You can use a 20- or 23cm (2 or 2.5l) springform pan, but just note that the cake won't have nearly as much height as the photographed cake. If you don't have a springform pan, feel free to use a greased pie or cake pan—you'll just need a bit more patience when removing the cake from the pan.

3. Make the crust In a food processor, process the almonds until a coarse meal forms. Add the shredded coconut, dates, oil, salt and 1 teaspoon water and process until the mixture comes together. It should stick together when pressed between your fingers. If for some reason it's dry or crumbly, add more water, a teaspoon at a time, and process again.

4. Set aside 80g of the crust mixture for later. Spoon the remaining crust mixture into the prepared pan. Spread it out evenly along the base and then press down firmly with your hands until smooth and even.

5. Make the filling In a high-speed blender, combine the cashews, lemon zest, lemon juice, maple syrup, melted coconut oil and salt. Blend on high until super smooth—you don't want any grittiness at all. Using a spatula, spoon the filling onto the crust and smooth it out evenly. Scatter the reserved crust mixture all over the top of the filling.

FOR THE CRUST

210g raw almonds

15g unsweetened shredded coconut

90g pitted Medjool dates

1 tablespoon virgin coconut oil, softened

Pinch of fine sea salt

1 teaspoon water

FOR THE FILLING

195g raw cashews

1 tablespoon lemon zest

125ml fresh lemon juice

30ml pure maple syrup

125ml virgin coconut oil, melted

Pinch of fine sea salt, or to taste

FOR THE STRAWBERRY-VANILLA COMPOTE

500g hulled fresh strawberries or thawed frozen strawberries

3 tablespoons pure maple syrup

1 teaspoon arrowroot powder

1 vanilla pod, seeds scraped, or 1 teaspoon pure vanilla extract

Fresh sliced strawberries, for garnish

(recipe continues)

6. Cover the pan with aluminium foil or plastic wrap and carefully transfer to a flat surface in the freezer. Freeze until solid, at least 6 hours or overnight.

7. **Make the strawberry-vanilla compote** If the strawberries are fresh, toss them into a food processor and pulse until coarsely chopped or smooth (your choice). (Thawed frozen strawberries are usually soft enough to mash directly in the pot using a potato masher.) Transfer the strawberries to a medium pot and set over medium heat. In a small bowl, whisk together the maple syrup and arrowroot powder until smooth. Stir this mixture into the strawberries until combined. Increase the heat to medium-high and bring the mixture to a simmer. Reduce the heat to medium and cook the compote, stirring every now and then, for 8 to 10 minutes, until it has thickened up a bit. Remove from the heat and stir in the vanilla pod seeds. Let cool to room temperature and then transfer to an airtight container and refrigerate until ready to serve.

8. Allow the frozen cheesecake to sit on the counter for 15 to 30 minutes before slicing (I like to slice the entire cheesecake at once and then freeze leftover slices).

9. Serve each slice with fresh sliced strawberries and a generous spoonful of compote over the top or swirled on the plate. This cake is best served cold, in a semi-frozen state, and it will soften greatly at room temperature. To freeze leftovers, wrap each frozen slice individually in clingfilm or foil and store in an airtight container in the freezer for 4 to 6 weeks. I recommend freezing the compote separately in its own small freezer-safe zip-top bag.

Tip If your blender has a hard time blending dates, soak the pitted dates in boiling water for 20 to 30 minutes, until softened. Drain well and proceed as directed.

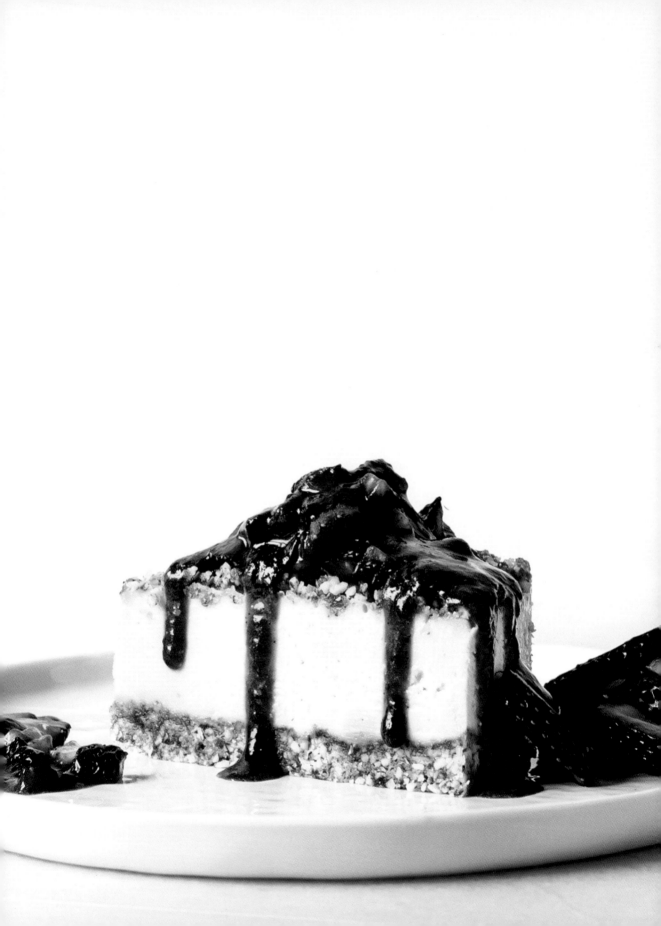

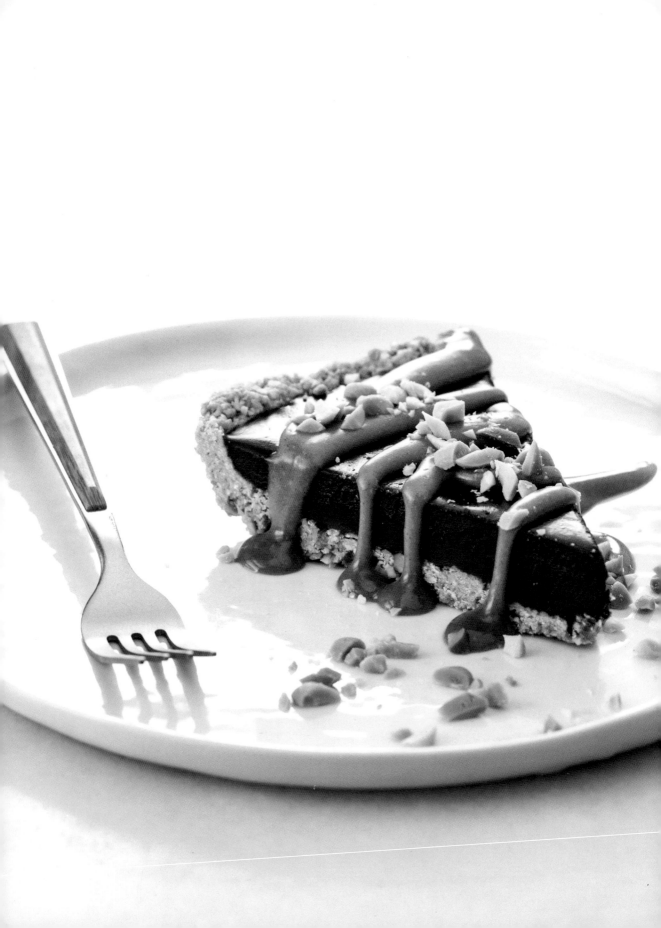

Peanut Butter Lover's Chocolate Tart

VEGAN, GLUTEN-FREE, SOYA-FREE OPTION, ADVANCE PREP REQUIRED,
KID-FRIENDLY, FREEZER-FRIENDLY

SERVES 10 TO 12

PREP TIME: **30 MINUTES**

BAKE TIME: **15 MINUTES**

FREEZE TIME: **4 TO 6 HOURS**

This pie is for all the peanut butter and chocolate lovers out there! The crust is made with salted, roasted peanuts and oats, which are a perfect complement to the creamy dark chocolate and peanut butter filling, and it's topped with my Magic No-Cook Caramel Sauce (page 253) to take it over the top. Yes, folks, this dessert is a game-changer! You can enjoy this pie frozen or let it sit on the counter until it softens; the choice is yours. Be sure to chill the can of coconut milk for at least 24 hours before you begin this recipe.

1. **Make the crust** Preheat the oven to 350°F (180°C). Lightly grease a 23cm glass pie dish. Cut two long, 5cm wide strips of parchment paper and place them over the pie dish in a criss-cross fashion. This will make it easy to lift out the tart after it freezes.

2. In a food processor, combine the peanuts, oats and salt and process into a coarse crumb. Add the oil and maple syrup and process until the mixture comes together into a dough. The dough should stick together when pressed between your fingers, but it shouldn't be super sticky. If it's still too dry, try adding the water and processing again.

3. Crumble the dough all over the bottom of the prepared pie dish in an even layer. Starting at the centre, press the dough into the pan with your fingers and work your way outwards and up the sides. If the dough starts to stick to your hands, lightly wet your hands and shake off the excess water. With a fork, prick the base of the tart seven or eight times to allow steam to escape while baking.

4. Bake the crust, uncovered, for 13 to 17 minutes, until lightly golden. Let cool completely on a cooling rack.

5. **Make the filling** Open the can of coconut milk and scoop all the solid white cream into a medium pot. Remove 75ml of the coconut water and discard it. Add the remaining coconut water to the pot. Turn the heat to medium. Add the chocolate and cook, stirring occasionally, until melted. Add the maple syrup, peanut butter and salt and whisk until completely smooth and uniform.

(recipe continues)

FOR THE CRUST

95g salted roasted peanuts

150g gluten-free rolled oats

¼ teaspoon fine sea salt

60ml virgin coconut oil, melted

3 tablespoons pure maple syrup

1½ teaspoons water, if needed

FOR THE FILLING

1 400ml can full-fat coconut milk, chilled for 24 hours

150g non-dairy dark chocolate (55 to 60% cocoa)

75ml pure maple syrup

85g natural smooth roasted peanut butter

Pinch or two of fine sea salt, to taste

FOR THE GARNISH

Peanut Butter Caramel Sauce (see page 253), for serving

85g salted roasted peanuts, chopped, for garnish

6. Pour the filling into the cooled crust. Carefully transfer the dish to a flat spot in the freezer and freeze, uncovered, for 4 to 6 hours, until solid. If you plan on freezing it longer, you can cover the tart with foil once the filling has firmed up.

7. Let the tart sit on the counter for a few minutes. Using the parchment 'handles', carefully lift the tart out of the dish (sometimes this takes a bit of wiggling back and forth). Slice the tart. Plate each slice and top with a generous drizzle of caramel and a tablespoon of peanuts. My mouth is watering just thinking about it! Store leftovers in an airtight container in the fridge for up to 5 days, or in the freezer for 4 to 6 weeks. I like to individually wrap frozen slices in foil and place them all in an airtight container.

Tip The photo of this pie (page 236) shows my Magic No-Cook Caramel Sauce, which has been chilled and piped on. This is why the caramel sauce has a thicker texture than when it's drizzled on warm, straight from the pot.

Make it soya-free Use a soya-free chocolate, such as Enjoy Life brand.

Mile-High Black-and-White Freezer Fudge

VEGAN, GLUTEN-FREE, SOYA-FREE, GRAIN-FREE, FREEZER-FRIENDLY

MAKES 24 SMALL SQUARES

PREP TIME: **30 MINUTES**

BAKE TIME: **10 TO 14 MINUTES**

FREEZE TIME: **1 TO 1½ HOURS**

This melt-in-your-mouth, two-layer freezer fudge is sweetened naturally and made up of a delightful vanilla-cashew fudge and a rich chocolate-almond fudge. I bet you won't be able to resist enjoying a spoonful as you make the recipe! The toasted almond and cashew topping adds a crunchy contrast to the creamy, rich fudge. Be sure to serve this treat straight from the freezer, as it melts quickly at room temperature.

1. Preheat the oven to 300°F (150°C). Line a 23 x 13cm (2l) loaf pan with a piece of parchment paper, leaving some overhang.

2. Roast the nuts Spread the almonds and cashews over a small rimmed baking sheet and roast for 10 to 14 minutes, until lightly golden and fragrant. Let cool.

3. Make the vanilla-cashew fudge In a bowl, stir together the coconut oil, cashew butter, maple syrup, vanilla pod seeds, vanilla extract and salt until well combined and completely smooth. If it's not getting smooth enough, you can use an electric mixer to help it along. With a spatula, spoon the mixture into the prepared loaf pan and spread it out evenly. Immediately sprinkle on about one-third of the roasted nuts. Gently press down on the nuts to adhere. Place the pan in the freezer.

4. Make the chocolate-almond fudge In the same bowl in which you made the vanilla fudge, combine the coconut oil, almond butter, cocoa powder, maple syrup, vanilla and salt and stir well until smooth and no clumps remain. If it's not getting smooth enough, you can use an electric mixer to help it along.

5. With a spatula, spoon the chocolate fudge mixture over the vanilla fudge layer and spread it evenly. Scatter the remaining nuts all over the top of the chocolate fudge and lightly press down to adhere. Freeze for 60 to 90 minutes, uncovered, or until completely solid.

6. Slice into small squares and serve immediately. Store any leftovers in an airtight container in the fridge for up to 1 week or in the freezer for up to 1 month. This fudge melts at room temperature, so I suggest not leaving it on the counter top for longer than 15 minutes or so.

(recipe continues)

FOR THE ROASTED NUTS

45g raw almonds, finely chopped

50g raw cashews, finely chopped

FOR THE VANILLA-CASHEW FUDGE

125ml plus 2 tablespoons virgin coconut oil, at room temperature

128g smooth raw cashew butter (see page 75) or store-bought

75ml pure maple syrup

1 vanilla pod, seeds scraped, or ½ teaspoon pure vanilla powder

½ teaspoon pure vanilla extract

Large pinch of fine sea salt

FOR THE CHOCOLATE-ALMOND FUDGE

125ml virgin coconut oil, at room temperature

60ml smooth Homemade Almond Butter (page 75) or store-bought

50g unsweetened cocoa powder or raw cacao powder, sifted

125ml pure maple syrup

1 teaspoon pure vanilla extract

Large pinch of fine sea salt

Tip 1. If you don't want to make a two-layer fudge, you can simply make one of the layers. 2. This fudge is extremely versatile, so feel free to vary the flavour by subbing in your favorite nut butter, nuts and extracts. 3. This recipe also halves well, so if you don't want a big batch, you can simply halve all the ingredient measurements. 4. Feel free to make fudge cups by layering the fudge into mini silicone cupcake moulds.

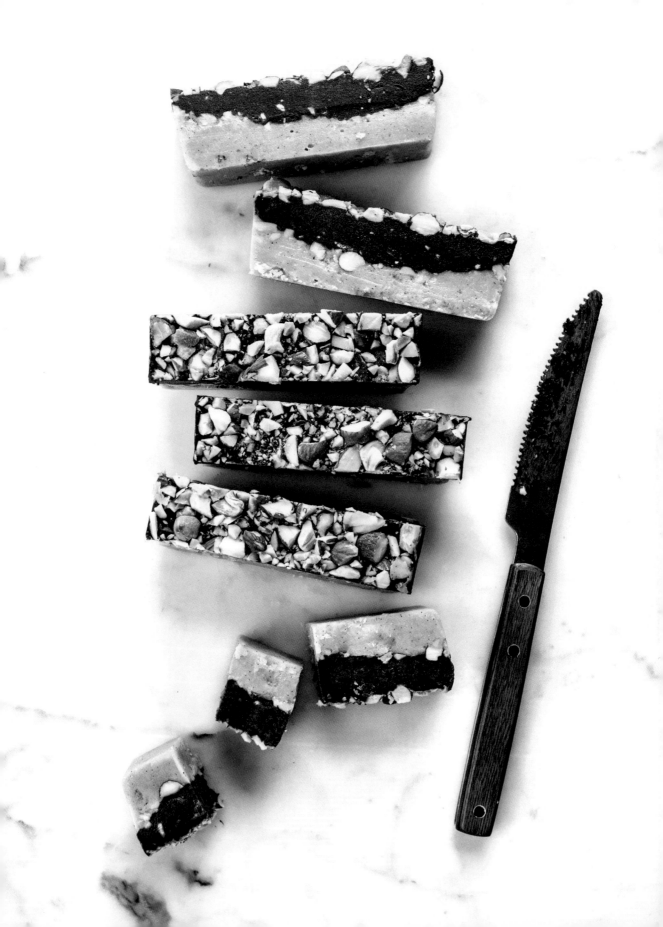

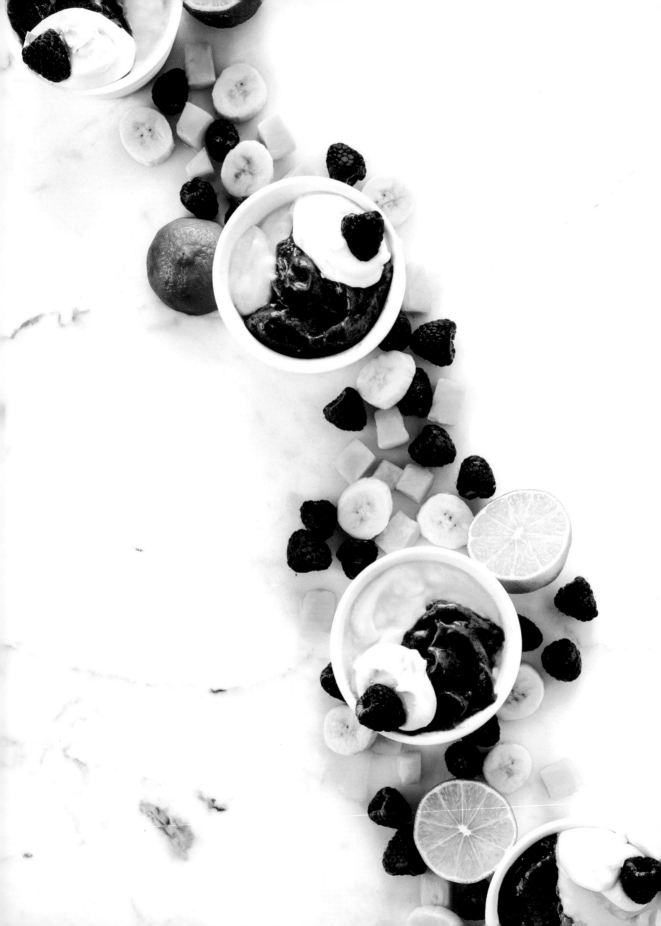

Mango-Coconut-Lime and Raspberry-Banana Sorbet

VEGAN, GLUTEN-FREE, NUT-FREE, SOYA-FREE, GRAIN-FREE, OIL-FREE,
ADVANCE PREP REQUIRED, KID-FRIENDLY OPTION, FREEZER-FRIENDLY

MAKES 500ML OF EACH FLAVOR

PREP TIME: **10 MINUTES**

Our whole family loves this healthy homemade sorbet! And you don't even need an ice cream maker to make it—a heavy-duty food processor will do the job. This sorbet is great to whip up on a hot summer day, and it comes together in a few minutes. The Mango-Coconut-Lime Sorbet is rich and full-bodied (thank you, coconut cream!), so it's a hybrid of fruity sorbet and traditional ice cream. It's smooth, naturally sweet, and luxurious, with a tangy kick from the lime juice. The tangy Raspberry-Banana Sorbet is intensely pigmented (no food colouring required) and banana and a touch of maple syrup give it a creamy, slightly sweet taste. Have fun experimenting with different frozen fruit blends; I also love swapping the frozen mango for frozen peaches and the frozen raspberries for frozen sweet cherries for a fun cherry-peach twist.

1. Chill the can of full-fat cocout milk for 24 hours before you begin.

2. Make the mango-coconut-lime sorbet In a heavy-duty food processor, process the frozen mango and coconut cream until creamy, 2 to 4 minutes, stopping to scrape down the bowl as needed. Add the lime juice to taste. Spoon the mango sorbet into a bowl and pop it into the freezer while you prepare the raspberry sorbet.

3. Make the raspberry-banana sorbet In the food processor, process the frozen raspberries and the banana until creamy, 2 to 4 minutes, stopping to scrape down the bowl as needed. Add the maple syrup and process again. Retrieve the mango sorbet from the freezer. Layer both sorbets in parfait glasses and serve immediately. This sorbet is best enjoyed right away, but you can spoon leftovers into ice pop moulds (being sure to press out air bubbles) and freeze for about 6 hours to make ice pops. Kids love these sorbet ice pops!

Tip 1. If you have leftover coconut cream, simply place it into a zip-top freezer bag and freeze it for up to 1 month. Thaw in the fridge or on the counter before using. 2. If you aren't a banana fan, you can swap the banana for coconut cream and 2 tablespoons maple syrup.

Make it kid-friendly While kids love the sorbet as it is, you can also turn it into ice lollies! Simply spoon the mixture into lolly moulds (being sure to press out any air bubbles), and freeze for about 6 hours.

FOR THE MANGO-COCONUT-LIME SORBET

300g frozen mango chunks (300g bag)

125ml full-fat canned coconut cream (white portion only)

1 to 2 teaspoons fresh lime juice, to taste

FOR THE RASPBERRY-BANANA SORBET

300g frozen raspberries

1 medium banana, at room temperature (see Tip)

1 tablespoon pure maple syrup, or to taste

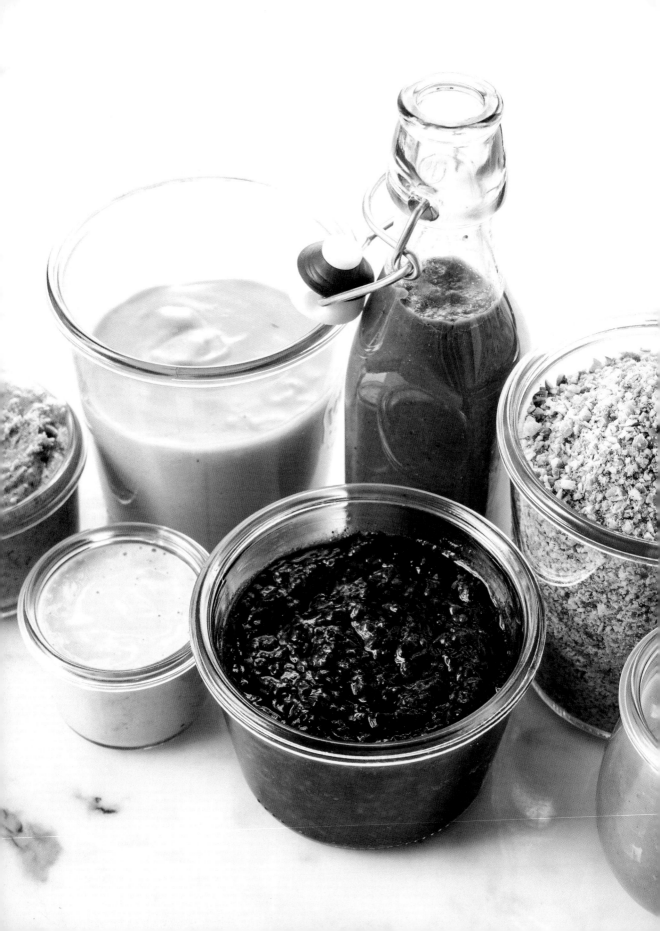

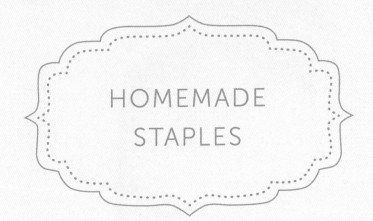

HOMEMADE STAPLES

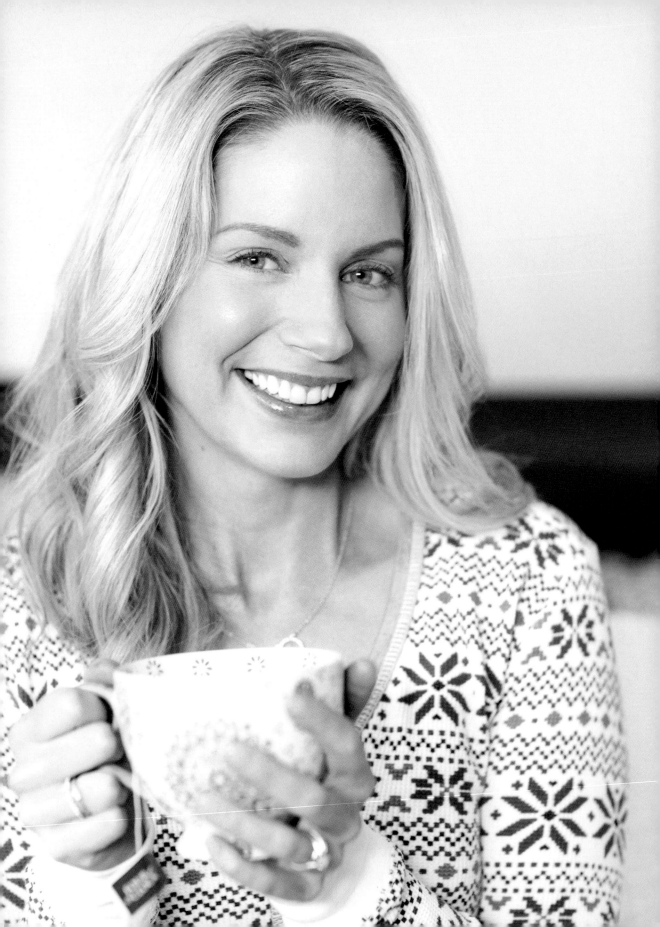

HOMEMADE STAPLES ARE so fresh and flavourful, and they often don't take more than ten minutes to whip up. Many of the recipes in this section can also be made a day or two before you need them, which can cut down on prep time when making a larger recipe. Store-bought versions will always work at a pinch (see The Oh She Glows Pantry, page 289, for some of my trusted brands), but it's nice to have an easy, wholefoods-based collection of staple recipes on hand to use whenever the inspiration strikes.

This chapter shares my go-to recipes and methods for creating easy, homemade versions of things you can often buy pre-packaged, such as sauces, flours, croutons, dressings, mayonnaise and more. It's often the case that preparing just one of these recipes along with your meal can transform the entire dish. For example, my Apple-Mango Chutney elevates my Comforting Red Lentil and Chickpea Curry (page 181) to a whole new level, adding a sweet tanginess that contrasts with the earthy, spicy curry. My Magic No-Cook Caramel Sauce is an absolute must drizzled over The Ultimate Flourless Brownies (page 199). The Easiest Garlic Croutons can complete a soup or salad, such as my Crowd-Pleasing Caesar Salad (page 107), providing rustic, chewy texture and comforting flavour. My All-Purpose Cheese Sauce is perfect on my Chilli Cheese Nachos (page 169), but once you've tasted it, I bet you'll find yourself inventing reasons to pour it on just about everything!

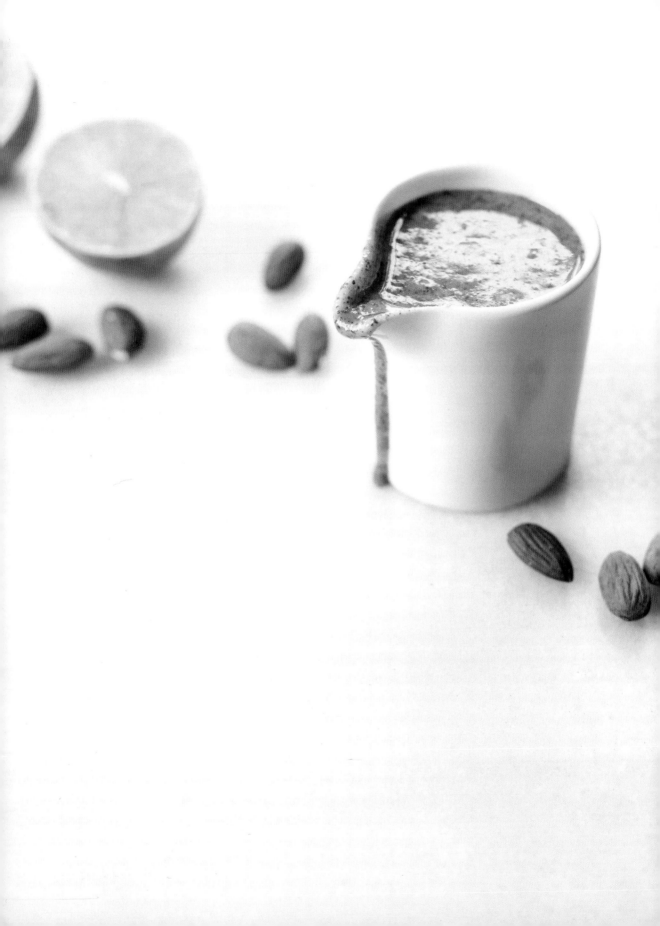

Thai Almond Butter Sauce

VEGAN, GLUTEN-FREE, SOYA-FREE OPTION, GRAIN-FREE, OIL-FREE,
KID-FRIENDLY

MAKES 325ML

PREP TIME: **10 MINUTES**

Warning: This almond butter sauce is seriously addictive! If you are anything like me, you'll be spooning it straight from the bowl. I recommend playing a bit with the exact amounts of the ingredients to suit your own taste buds—you might like yours a bit sweeter, or prefer to add an extra helping of fresh garlic, salt, lime, etc. If it turns out the dressing you create has too strong a flavour for your taste, simply thin it with some water and let it thicken in the fridge for a bit. Serve this dressing with my Thai Crunch Salad (page 101); it's also great mixed into warm soba noodles and sautéed veggies for an energizing entrée. This dressing will thicken when chilled, so you can leave it at room temperature to soften up or whisk in a touch of water to thin it.

1. In a food processor, process the garlic until finely chopped.

2. Add the rest of the ingredients and process until smooth. Add the water to thin the sauce to your desired consistency—start with 2 tablespoons and work from there. The sauce will keep in an airtight container in the fridge for up to 10 days.

Make it soya-free Use coconut aminos instead of tamari.

1 large or 2 small clove(s) garlic

2 to 3 teaspoons grated fresh ginger, to taste

175ml smooth Homemade Almond Butter (page 75) or store-bought

3 to 4 tablespoons fresh lime juice, to taste

2 tablespoons low-sodium tamari or coconut aminos, or more to taste

3 to 4½ teaspoons pure maple syrup, to taste

⅛ teaspoon cayenne pepper, or to taste (optional)

2 to 6 tablespoons water, as needed to thin

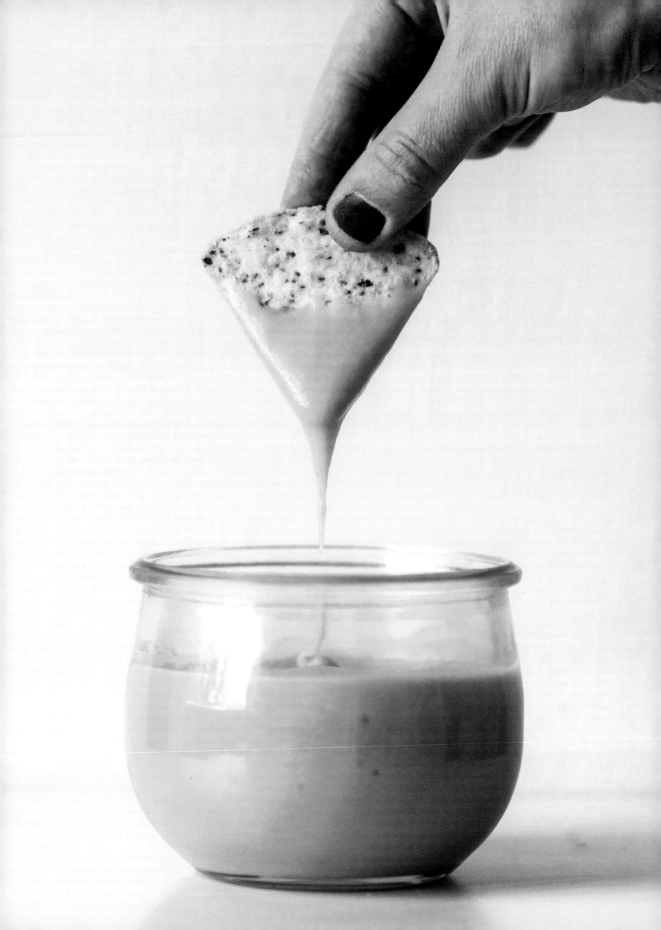

All-Purpose Cheese Sauce

VEGAN, GLUTEN-FREE, NUT-FREE OPTION, SOYA-FREE, GRAIN-FREE,
ADVANCE PREP REQUIRED, KID-FRIENDLY

MAKES 250ML

SOAK TIME: **1 TO 2 HOURS, OR OVERNIGHT**

PREP TIME: **10 MINUTES**

COOK TIME: **10 TO 15 MINUTES**

Here it is: my favorite vegan 'cheese' sauce that not only tastes amazing, but can be used in a wide variety of dishes! Who knew that just a few simple ingredients could create such a decadent, silky, pourable sauce? No, it isn't a dead ringer for traditional cheese sauce, but we think it's comforting in its own right. Use it in my Chilli Cheese Nachos (page 169) or Mac and Peas (page 177), or heat it up and use it as a nacho dip paired with salsa or as a spread on a wrap. It's also fantastic drizzled over roasted or steamed broccoli or cauliflower! I love to add my favourite Sriracha sauce to this to really amp up the flavours. A big thanks to Jennifer Houston and Ruth Tal's *Super Fresh* cookbook for inspiring this versatile and wallet-friendly recipe!

1. Soak the cashews in a bowl of water overnight or for at least 1 hour. Rinse and drain.

2. Put the potatoes and carrots in a medium pot and add water to cover. Bring to a boil over high heat, reduce the heat to medium, and simmer uncovered for 10 to 15 minutes, until fork-tender. Drain. (Alternatively, you can steam the veggies.)

3. Transfer the cashews, potatoes and carrots to a blender, add the nutritional yeast, coconut oil, water, lemon juice, ½ teaspoon of the salt, garlic and vinegar and blend until smooth. If using a Vitamix, use the tamper to help it blend. If it's too thick, you can add another splash of water or oil to help it along. Taste the sauce and add Sriracha and more salt, if desired. The sauce will keep in an airtight container in the fridge for up to a week.

Tip It's important to dice the potatoes and carrots small before measuring (about 1cm pieces); I recommend weighing the potato and carrot for the most accurate measurement.

Make it nut-free Simply omit the cashews. It won't be quite as rich, but it still tastes great!

40g raw cashews

190g diced peeled potatoes (see Tip)

55g diced carrots (see Tip)

2 to 3 tablespoons nutritional yeast, to taste

2 tablespoons refined coconut oil or other neutral-tasting oil, such as grapeseed oil

2 tablespoons plus 1½ teaspoons water

1½ teaspoons fresh lemon juice, or more to taste

½ teaspoon plus ⅛ teaspoon fine sea salt, or to taste

1 medium clove garlic

½ to ¾ teaspoon white wine vinegar, to taste

Sriracha or other hot sauce (optional)

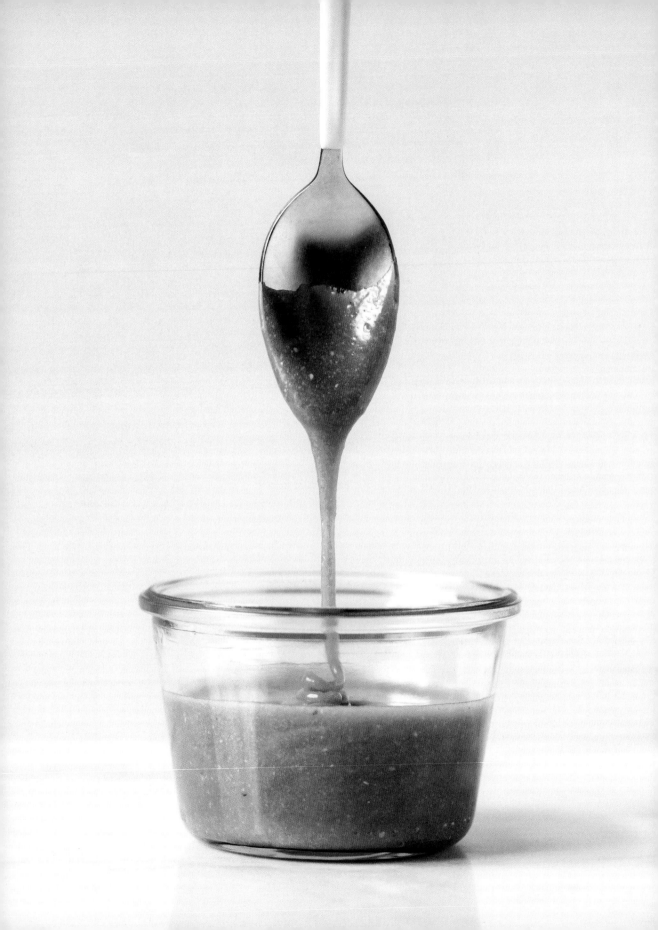

Magic No-Cook Caramel Sauce

VEGAN, GLUTEN-FREE, SOYA-FREE, GRAIN-FREE, FREEZER-FRIENDLY

MAKES 250ML

PREP TIME: **5 MINUTES**

CHILL TIME: **1 HOUR**

'When I die, I want to be buried in a vat of this caramel sauce.' That's what I told Eric when I made this the first time. I'm telling you, this caramel sauce is unbelievable. You'll be amazed that this sauce is thick just like traditional caramel, but it doesn't require hovering over a boiling pot on the stove or tedious stirring. Nope: Just a quick spin in the food processor is all it takes!

This is by no means a traditional caramel sauce—cashew butter gives it its creaminess and maple syrup and coconut nectar (both unrefined sweeteners) make it gently sweet and tangy—but if you ask me, it's even tastier than ultra-sugary versions. I don't recommend swapping the raw coconut nectar for any other sweetener, because the coconut nectar creates a fruity, caramel-like flavour and gives the sauce a deep amber hue (but if you absolutely must substitute, see my tip below). Serve this caramel drizzled over The Ultimate Flourless Brownies (page 199) or on High-Rise Pumpkin Cupcakes (page 224) with Spiced Buttercream Frosting (page 227) for a decadent treat. It works great as a fruit dip, too (I love apples paired with this caramel). If you don't care for a very light coconut flavour, be sure to use refined coconut oil rather than virgin coconut oil.

1. In a food processor, combine the coconut oil, maple syrup, cashew butter, and coconut nectar and process until smooth, stopping to scrape down the bowl as needed. Add the salt and process again until combined.

2. Using a spatula, spoon the caramel into a jar. You can use the caramel immediately or chill it in the fridge, covered, for about 1 hour. It will firm up when chilled. You can easily melt it over low heat on the hob, if desired. Leftovers can be stored in an airtight container in the fridge for up to 2 weeks, or you can freeze it in a freezer bag or freezer-safe container for 1 to 2 months. After thawing, beat the caramel briefly with electric beaters to combine.

Tip I recommend using coconut nectar in this recipe for the best flavour and caramel-like colour; however, you can substitute 2 tablespoons brown rice syrup and 1 teaspoon fresh lemon juice at a pinch.

For Peanut Butter Caramel Sauce Swap the cashew butter for an equal amount of smooth natural peanut butter.

75ml virgin coconut oil, softened

125ml pure maple syrup

60ml smooth raw cashew butter (see page 75) or store-bought

2 tablespoons raw coconut nectar (see Tip)

¼ to ¾ teaspoon fine sea salt, to taste

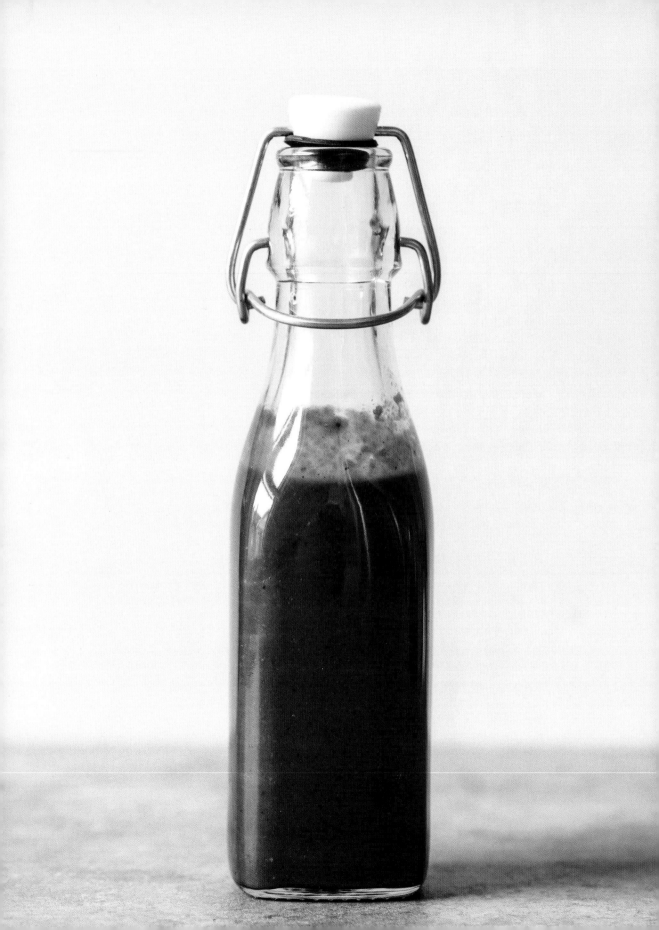

Easy Barbecue Sauce

VEGAN, GLUTEN-FREE, NUT-FREE, SOYA-FREE, GRAIN-FREE, FREEZER-FRIENDLY

MAKES 250ML

PREP TIME: **10 MINUTES**

COOK TIME: **10 MINUTES**

Is it just me, or is it challenging to find a good-tasting vegan barbecue sauce (at least, barbecue sauce that isn't loaded with sugar) at the store? As my dad always says, 'If you want something done right, you gotta do it yourself!' (Thanks, Dad. Your sayings are forever burned into my memory.) This barbecue sauce is smoky, sweet and deeply flavourful. If you have some on hand, adding a dash of liquid smoke to the sauce is a nice addition, too. Try using the sauce in my Oh Em Gee Veggie Burgers (page 159) or bring a Mason jar to your next barbecue event and use it to baste vegetables or tofu steaks. I recommend making this a day in advance if you can; allowing the sauce to sit overnight really helps the flavors blend.

1. In a medium saucepan, heat the oil over medium heat. Add the onion and garlic and sauté for 4 to 5 minutes, until the onion is translucent.

2. Stir in the tomato sauce, vinegar, maple syrup, molasses, salt, mustard powder, paprika, black pepper, Sriracha and cayenne (if using).

3. Simmer over low-medium heat for 5 to 10 minutes, until thickened.

4. Carefully transfer the sauce to a blender and blend on low until smooth.

5. This sauce will keep in an airtight container in the fridge for up to 2 weeks, or you can freeze it for up to 1 month. I like to portion it into a silicone mini ice cube tray, freeze it, and then pop the cubes out and store them in a freezer-safe container.

2 teaspoons extra-virgin olive oil

75g minced red or brown onion

2 cloves garlic, minced

250ml tomato sauce

2 tablespoons cider vinegar

1 to 2 tablespoons pure maple syrup, to taste

1 to 1½ teaspoons blackstrap molasses, to taste

½ to ¾ teaspoon fine sea salt, to taste

1 teaspoon mustard powder

¾ teaspoon smoked paprika, or to taste

½ teaspoon freshly ground black pepper

Sriracha or other hot sauce

Cayenne pepper (optional)

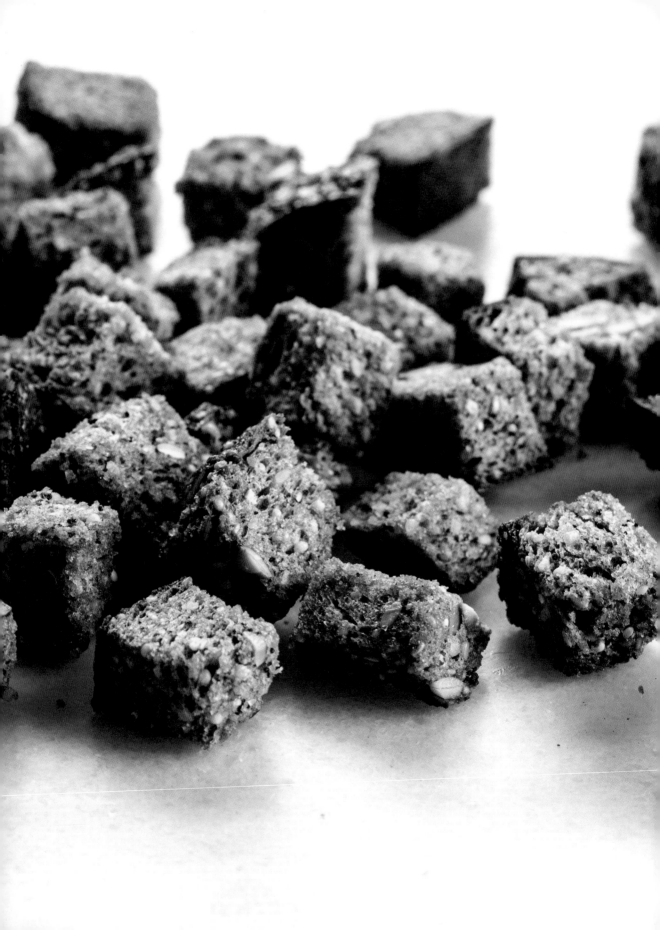

Easiest Garlic Croutons

VEGAN, GLUTEN-FREE OPTION, NUT-FREE, SOYA-FREE, KID-FRIENDLY OPTION

MAKES 375 TO 500ML

PREP TIME: **5 MINUTES**

COOK TIME: **14 TO 16 MINUTES**

These garlic croutons make a great topping for soup and salad such as my Go-To Gazpacho (page 147) or my Crowd-Pleasing Caesar Salad (page 107), and they can be thrown together in twenty minutes flat. Be generous with the garlic powder and salt, as they really make a difference to the overall flavour.

1. Preheat the oven to 400°F (200°C). Line a baking sheet with parchment paper.

2. Rub the cut sides of the garlic halves all over the bread slices to infuse them with garlic flavour.

3. Using a pastry brush, spread the oil over one side of each slice of the bread, being sure to spread it out to the edges.

4. Sprinkle a generous amount of garlic powder and salt on top of the oil.

5. Slice the bread into 2.5cm cubes and transfer them to the prepared baking sheet, oiled side up.

6. Bake for 14 to 16 minutes, until golden and firm (there's no need to flip them). The croutons will firm up as they cool. These croutons are best enjoyed immediately, but cooled leftovers can be stored in an airtight container on the counter for a few days. If they soften from storing, lightly toast them in a skillet over medium heat for a few minutes before serving.

Make it gluten-free Use gluten-free bread.

Make it kid-friendly Kids love the savoury flavours and crunch of these croutons. Make this recipe even more kid-friendly by slicing the bread into strips for dipping into various dishes!

2 or 3 slices bread (thick and hearty style preferred)

1 large clove garlic, halved lengthwise

3 to 4 teaspoons extra-virgin olive oil or avocado oil

Garlic powder

Fine sea salt

9-Spice Mix · MAKES ABOUT 2 TABLESPOONS PREP TIME: 5 MINUTES

VEGAN, GLUTEN-FREE, NUT-FREE, SOYA-FREE, GRAIN-FREE, OIL-FREE

1 teaspoon sweet paprika

1 teaspoon garlic powder

1 teaspoon dried minced onion

¾ teaspoon fine sea salt

½ teaspoon freshly ground black pepper

½ teaspoon dried oregano

¼ teaspoon ground turmeric

¼ teaspoon dried thyme

¼ teaspoon smoked paprika

This multi-purpose spice mix seems to steal the heart of every person who tries it. It's super flavourful and lightly sweet, and it pairs well with so many different dishes. It combines some familiar Latin flavours, such as oregano and paprika, lemony thyme and the pungent notes of onion, turmeric and garlic. I discover new uses for it all the time. Try it on my 9-Spice Avocado Hummus Toast (page 39), Oh Em Gee Veggie Burgers (page 159), 9-Spice Super-Seed Crackers (see page 82), Metabolism-Revving Spicy Cabbage Soup (page 139), Roasted Breakfast Hash (page 53), in pasta, soups, salad dressings and sprinkled on my Every Day Lemon-Garlic Hummus (page 91).

1. Combine all the spices in a small jar. Screw on the lid and shake to combine. Store in a cupboard for up to 2 months.

Large Batch 9-Spice Mix · MAKES 50g PREP TIME: 5 MINUTES

VEGAN, GLUTEN-FREE, NUT-FREE, SOYA-FREE, GRAIN-FREE, OIL-FREE

1 tablespoon sweet paprika

1 tablespoon garlic powder

1 tablespoon dried minced onion

2¼ teaspoons fine sea salt

1½ teaspoons freshly ground black pepper

1½ teaspoons dried oregano

¾ teaspoon ground turmeric

¾ teaspoon dried thyme

¾ teaspoon smoked paprika

This is simply a larger batch of my 9-Spice Mix above. I love to make a large quantity so I always have some on hand.

1. Combine all the spices in a small jar. Screw on the lid and shake to combine. Store in a cupboard for up to 2 months.

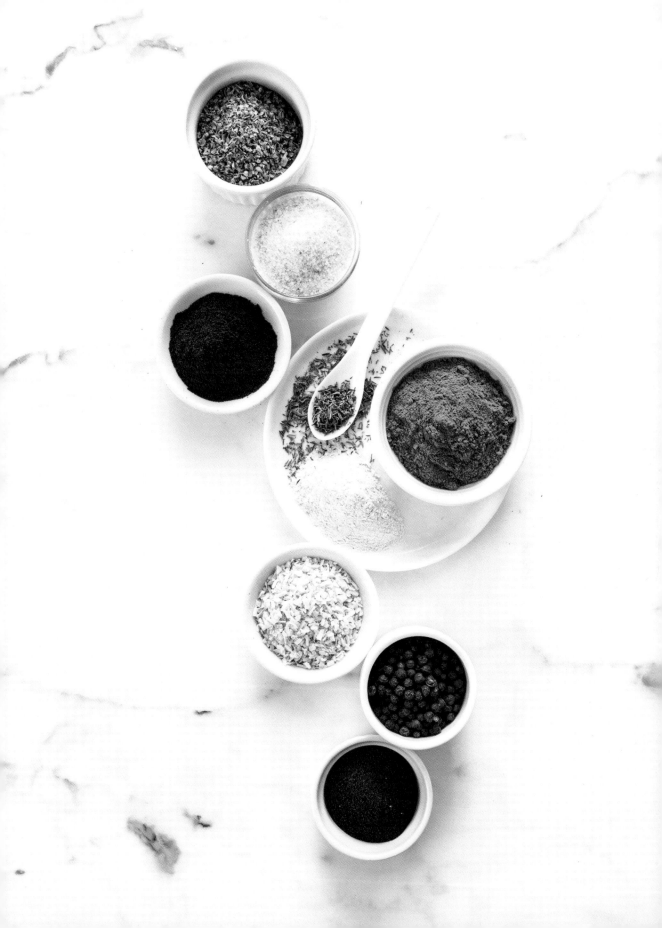

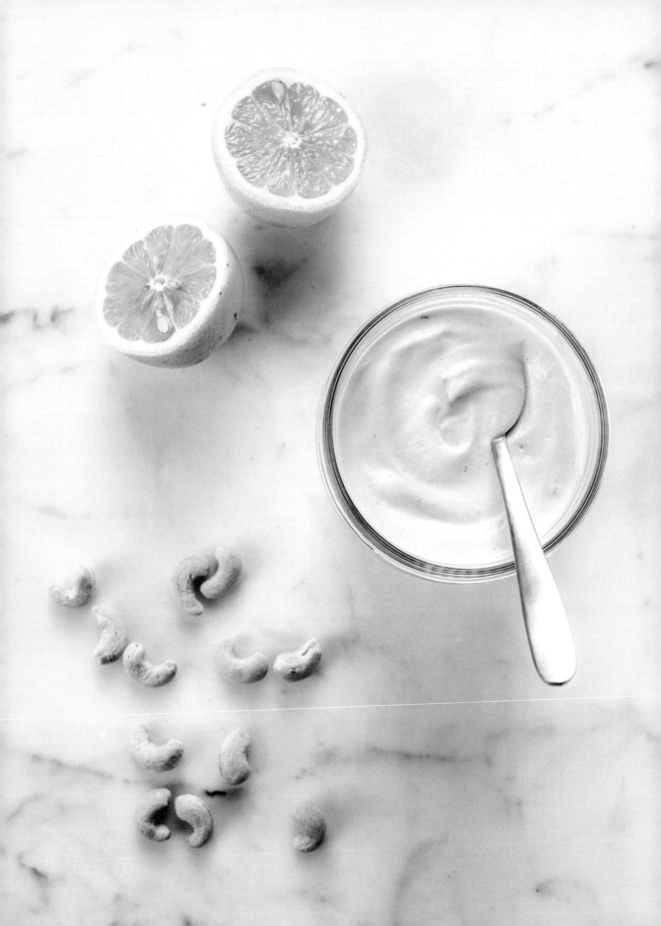

Cashew Sour Cream

VEGAN, GLUTEN-FREE, SOYA-FREE, GRAIN-FREE, OIL-FREE,
ADVANCE PREP REQUIRED, FREEZER-FRIENDLY

MAKES ABOUT 500ML

SOAK TIME: **1 HOUR (QUICK-SOAK
METHOD) OR OVERNIGHT**

PREP TIME: **5 MINUTES**

This multi-purpose cashew cream can be used in a variety of dishes, such as my Ultimate Green Taco Wraps (page 191) or Metabolism-Revving Spicy Cabbage Soup (page 139). The recipe prepares a generous amount, but don't worry if you have leftover cream, because it freezes and thaws beautifully! I love to freeze my leftover cream in a silicone mini muffin tray. That way, I have individual servings that I can thaw at a whim. You can use cashew cream leftovers on sandwiches or wraps, stirred into salad dressings, on vegan nachos, in chilli or soup, or you can even add a frozen cashew cream cube to a smoothie to make it extra decadent!

225g raw cashews

175ml water, or as needed

2 tablespoons fresh lemon juice

2 teaspoons cider vinegar

½ teaspoon fine sea salt, to taste

1. Place the cashews in a bowl and cover with 5cm of water. Soak for 8 to 12 hours, or overnight. (For a quick-soak method, cover with boiling water and soak for 30 to 60 minutes.) Drain and rinse.

2. Transfer the cashews to a high-speed blender and add the water, lemon juice, vinegar and salt. Blend on the highest speed until smooth, stopping to scrape down the blender container if necessary. You can add a splash more water if necessary to get it going. Transfer the cashew cream to an airtight container and refrigerate if you're not using it right away. It will thicken up as it chills. The cashew cream will stay fresh in an airtight container in the fridge for up to 1 week or in the freezer for 4 to 6 weeks. See the headnote for tips on freezing.

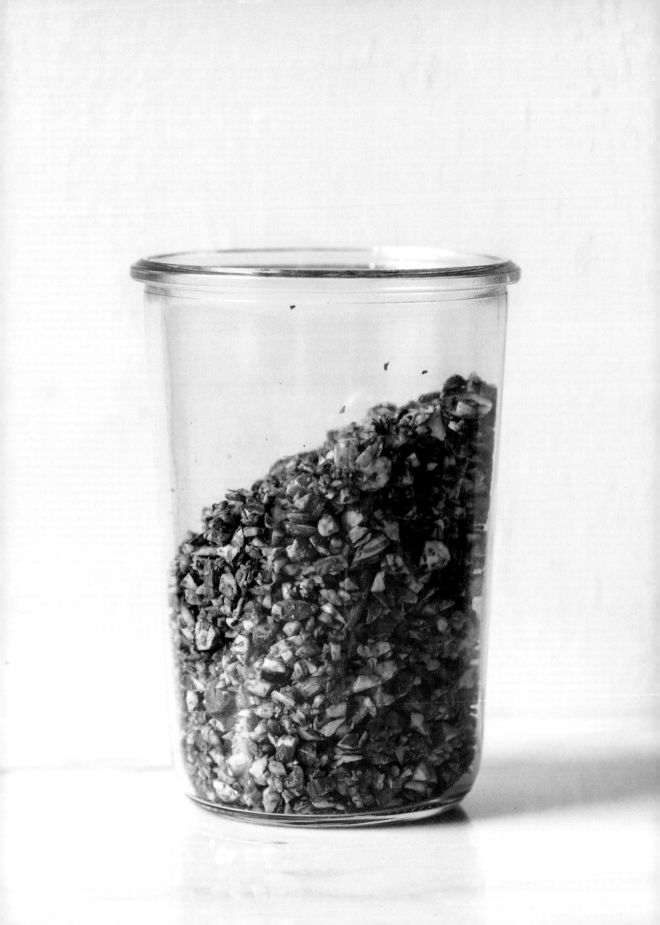

Roasted Tamari Almonds

VEGAN, GLUTEN-FREE, SOYA-FREE OPTION, OIL-FREE, GRAIN-FREE

MAKES 125ML

70g raw almonds, finely chopped

20ml low-sodium tamari or coconut aminos

This salty, crunchy, nutty topping is downright addictive! Finely chopped almonds are seasoned with low-sodium tamari and then roasted until they're golden and fragrant. After they cool, the almonds transform any soup, stew or salad into something extra special. I love them on top of my Creamy Thai Carrot Sweet Potato Soup (page 141), Every Day Glow salad (page 115), or Thai Crunch Salad (page 101)—but I've been known to enjoy them by the handful, too! They are also the perfect topping for any vegan bowl or salad recipe. A note for those of you with soya allergies: Low-sodium tamari is the most flavourful seasoning option, but if you're allergic to soya, you can use coconut aminos instead. Add a pinch of salt if the almonds taste a bit flat.

1. Preheat the oven to 325°F (160°C). Line a large baking sheet with parchment paper.

2. In a medium bowl, toss the almonds with the tamari until the almond pieces are fully coated. Spread the almonds over the prepared baking sheet in an even layer.

3. Roast the almonds for 9 to 12 minutes, until lightly golden. The tamari will have dried up.

4. Let cool completely on the pan. The almonds will harden up as they cool. Using a spoon, scrape the almonds off the parchment paper and enjoy! Leftovers can be stored in an airtight container at room temperature for a couple of weeks.

Make it soya-free Use coconut aminos instead of tamari.

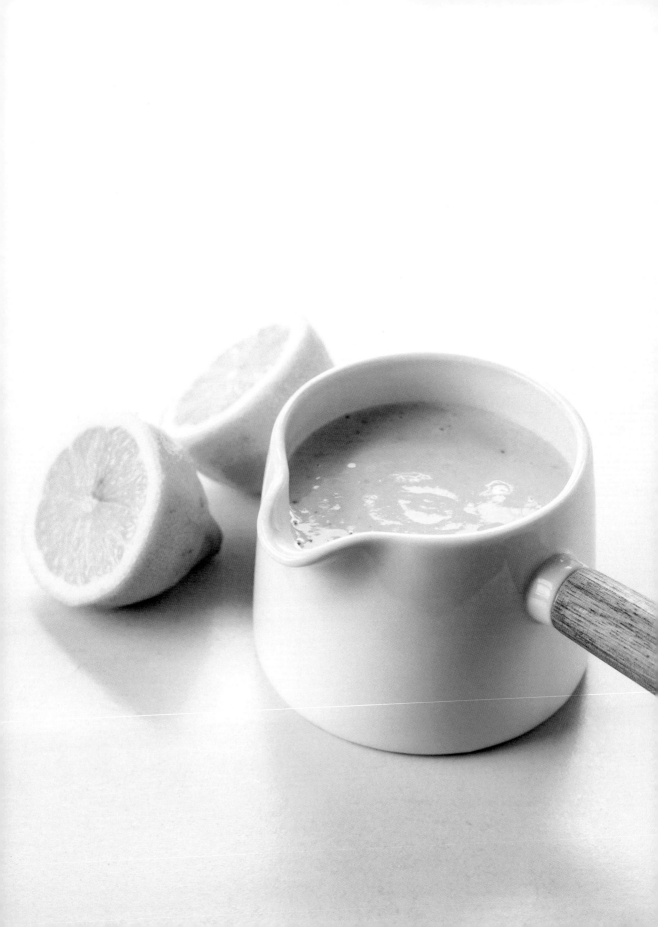

Lemon-Tahini Dressing

VEGAN, GLUTEN-FREE, NUT-FREE, SOYA-FREE, GRAIN-FREE,
FREEZER-FRIENDLY

MAKES 250ML

PREP TIME: **10 MINUTES**

After years of making half-cup batches of this dressing at a time, I said enough is enough and created a larger batch so I could have leftovers for the whole week. Afterward, I thought, *Why didn't I do this sooner!?* This lemon-tahini dressing is so good that you'll find yourself inventing new ways to use it again and again. Try it drizzled over The Big Tabbouleh Bowl (page 157), Every Day Glow Salad (page 115), Roasted Garlic Chickpeas (page 107), Cast-Iron Tofu (page 137), or yes, even on 9-Spice Avocado Hummus Toast (page 39)! One thing's for sure: you won't regret having some leftovers in the fridge all week long.

1. In a mini food processor, pulse the garlic until minced.

2. Add the rest of the ingredients and process until smooth. Taste and adjust the seasonings, if desired. The dressing will keep in an airtight container in the fridge for a week or a bit longer, and it will thicken as it sits. Stir well before use. You can also freeze it in a freezer-safe zip-top bag for up to 1 month.

1 large or 2 small cloves garlic

60ml tahini

125ml fresh lemon juice (from about 3 large lemons)

2 to 4 tablespoons nutritional yeast, to taste

75 to 125ml extra-virgin olive oil, to taste

1/2 to 3/4 teaspoon fine sea salt, to taste

Freshly ground black pepper

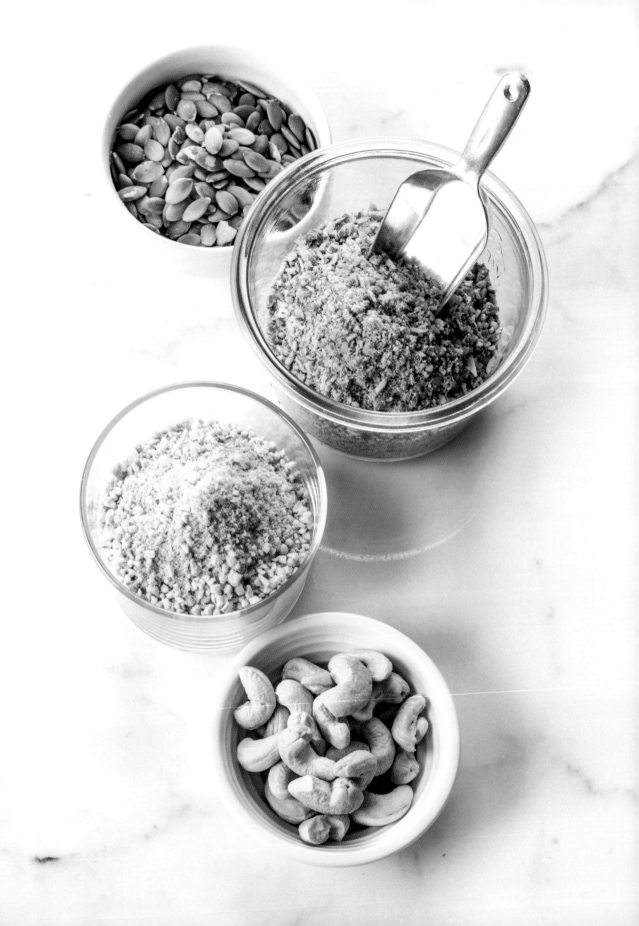

Vegan Parmesan Cheese: Two Ways

VEGAN, GLUTEN-FREE, NUT-FREE OPTION, SOYA-FREE, GRAIN-FREE, OIL-FREE   PREP TIME: **5 MINUTES**

MAKES 175ML

I offer two approaches to this wonderful vegan spin on parmesan cheese. Use pumpkin seeds for a delicious, nut-free option. For an extra 'cheesy' version, use raw cashews. I love both versions and alternate them frequently! I prefer to use raw garlic in this parmesan cheese recipe because it results in a bold, spicy flavour, but you can use garlic powder at a pinch. If you aren't a big garlic lover, start with a very small clove (or even half a clove) and add more to taste. (I love garlic, so I usually add one medium clove for a nice kick.) Sprinkle the topping over any recipe in which you might usually crave parmesan, like my Sun-Dried Tomato Pasta (page 185), Crowd-Pleasing Caesar Salad (page 107), Spiralized Courgette Summer Salad (page 103), or on any pasta dish, wrap or salad. The pumpkin seed version also serves as the delectable coating for my Aubergine Parmesan (page 173).

75g raw cashews or raw pumpkin seeds

2 tablespoons nutritional yeast

¼ to ½ teaspoon fine sea salt, to taste

1 clove garlic, or ¼ teaspoon garlic powder, or to taste

1. If using fresh garlic, mince it in a mini food processor. Add the cashews or pumpkin seeds, nutritional yeast, salt and garlic powder (if not using fresh garlic). Process until a coarse meal forms. The parmesan will keep in an airtight container in the fridge for up to 2 weeks.

Make it nut-free Use pumpkin seeds instead of cashews.

For a triple batch of pumpkin seed parmesan cheese (as used in Aubergine Parmesan, page 173) Use 145g raw pumpkin seeds plus 2 tablespoons nutritional yeast, ¾ to 1½ teaspoons fine sea salt and 3 cloves garlic or ¾ teaspoon garlic powder.

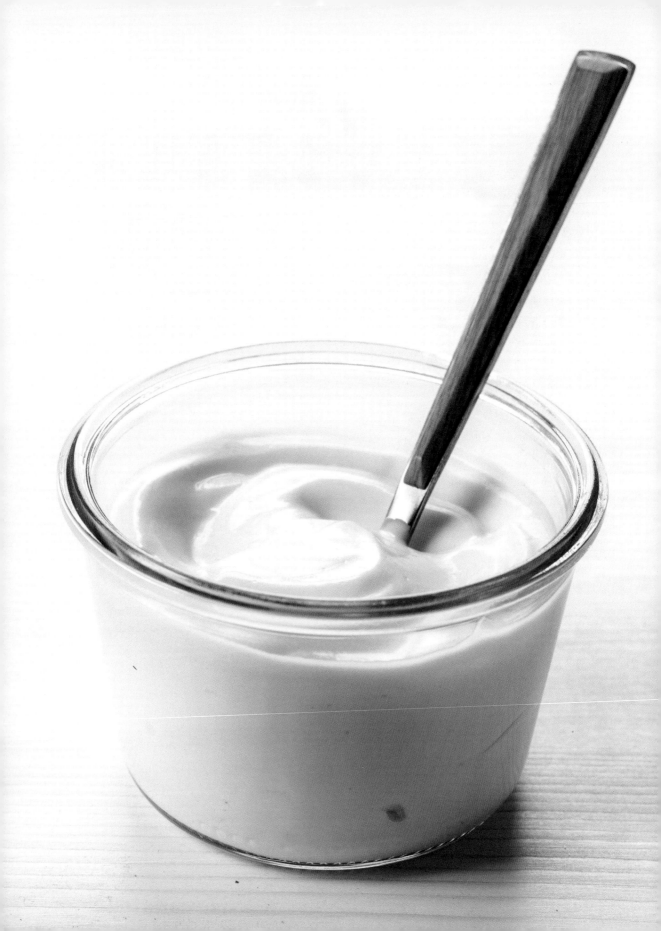

Homemade Vegan Mayo

VEGAN, GLUTEN-FREE, NUT-FREE, GRAIN-FREE, KID-FRIENDLY

PREP TIME: **5 MINUTES**

MAKES 425ML

In just five minutes, you can have creamy homemade mayonnaise that'll rival any store-bought brand. This mayonnaise is creamy, thick, a little tangy, and absolutely delicious. Use it in my Curried Chickpea Salad (page 113), Crispy Smashed Potatoes (page 123), or as a topping for my Oh Em Gee Veggie Burgers (page 159). You can also use it in any recipe in which you'd use traditional mayonnaise.

1. In a high-speed blender, combine the soy milk, lemon juice, vinegar, brown rice syrup, salt and mustard. Blend on low until smooth.

2. With the blender running on low-medium speed, very slowly stream in the oil. The mixture will thicken gradually into a white, fluffy mayo.

3. Transfer to an airtight container and store in the fridge for 3 to 4 weeks.

Tip I don't recommend substituting any other kind of non-dairy milk for the soya milk, as the protein content in soya is what thickens this mayo. I didn't have any luck using almond milk (it was a runny mess). If you need a soya-free mayonnaise, try Vegenaise brand.

125ml plain unsweetened soya milk (no substitutes; see Tip)

1 tablespoon fresh lemon juice

1 teaspoon cider vinegar

1 teaspoon brown rice syrup

¾ teaspoon fine sea salt

¼ teaspoon dry mustard

250ml grapeseed oil

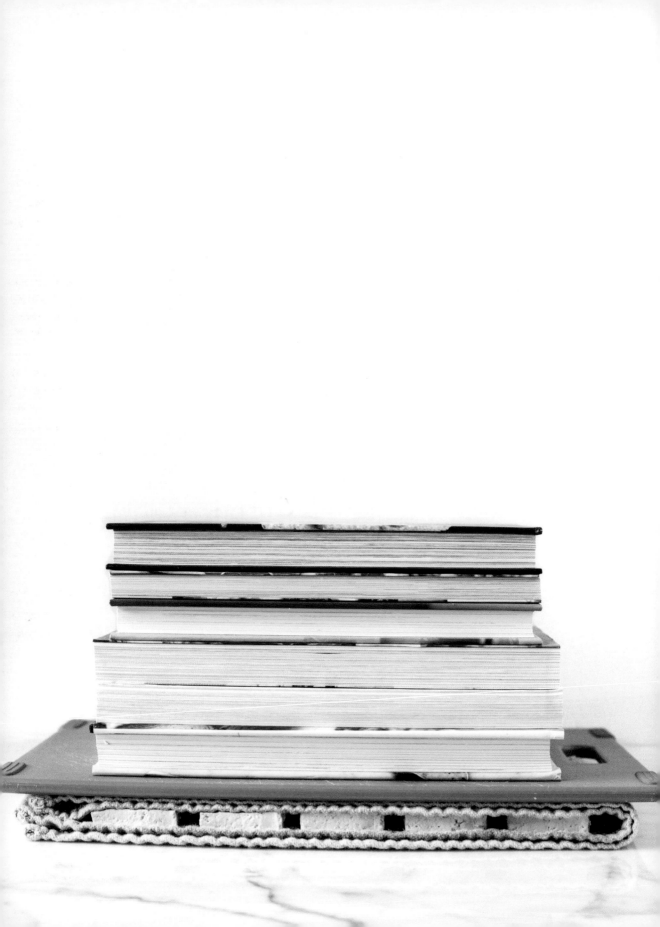

How to Press Tofu

When I first started to experiment with tofu, I had no idea what all of this 'pressing' talk was about. *Why do I need to press tofu? It looks pretty firm already!* Well, I soon found out that there's a lot of water hiding inside a block of tofu (yes, even in the firm and extra-firm varieties). Pressing the tofu helps release unnecessary water, resulting in a firmer, denser block and a more satisfying, chewy texture. Once you try pressing it, you won't go back!

BOOK-STACKING METHOD

If you don't have a tofu press, here's the old-fashioned (and free!) method of pressing tofu. It doesn't get out as much water as a tofu press, but it works at a pinch.

Rinse the tofu with water. Lay two thick dish towels on top of each other on the counter and place a few sheets of paper towel on top. Slice the tofu into 9 or 10 rectangles and set them on the paper towel in a single layer. Place two more thick dishcloths on top of the tofu slabs and place a cutting board on top. Set several heavy books on top of the cutting board. Let this sit for at least 20 to 30 minutes to allow the weight of the books to press out the water.

TOFU PRESS

After a couple of years of using the book-stacking method, I finally bought a tofu press. It changed everything! The tofu press gets out much more water, and I don't have to fuss with books and towels. I love to press tofu overnight in the fridge for a super-duper firm tofu. The press collects the water at the bottom, and I'm always shocked by how much it presses out. If you eat tofu regularly, it's a great investment and won't take up much space at all. You can find tofu presses online and in some speciality health food stores. I use the Tofu Xpress brand.

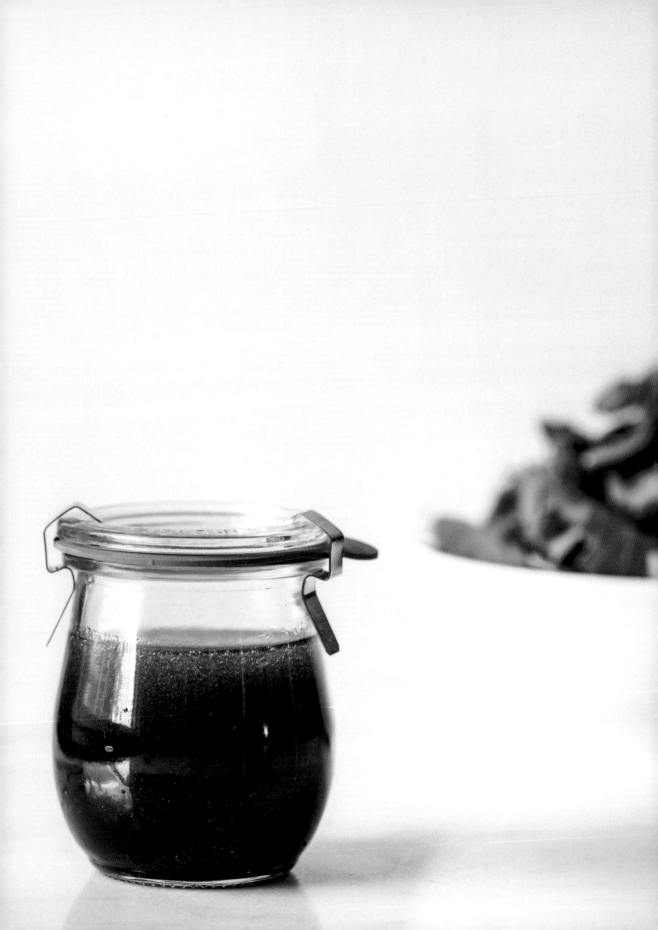

Shake-and-Go Balsamic Vinaigrette

VEGAN, GLUTEN-FREE, NUT-FREE, SOYA-FREE OPTION, GRAIN-FREE

MAKES 150 TO 250ML

PREP TIME: **2 MINUTES**

This is the easiest vinaigrette I've made to date. Just toss it into a jar, screw on the lid, and shake! Don't let the short ingredient list deceive you: The dressing is incredibly flavourful. But feel free to adjust the acidity, sweetness, and/or saltiness to your taste and make it your own. Try adding a dash of liquid smoke, paprika, and thyme for a 'smoky' dressing, a pinch of dried or fresh herbs (such as oregano and basil) for an Italian vinaigrette, or dashes of cumin, coriander and turmeric for a slight Indian flair.

1. Combine all the ingredients in a small Mason jar, seal, and shake vigorously. Store in the fridge for up to a couple of weeks. Shake before each use.

Make it soya-free Swap the tamari for 2 to 4 tablespoons coconut aminos, to taste.

75 to 150ml extra-virgin olive oil, to taste

75ml balsamic vinegar

4½ teaspoons low-sodium tamari

1 large clove garlic, minced

1 teaspoon pure maple syrup, or to taste

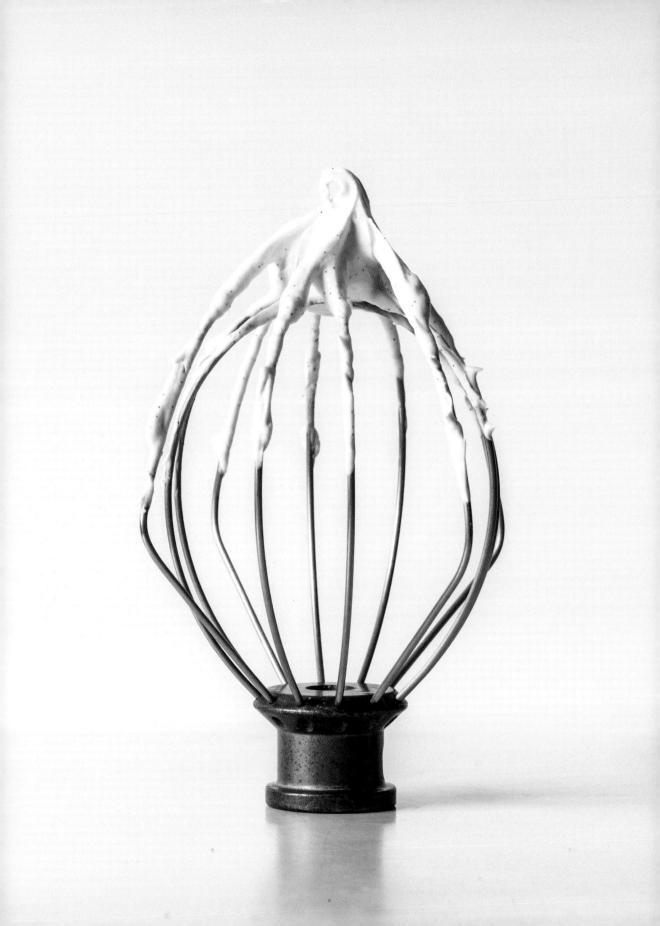

Coconut Whipped Cream

VEGAN, GLUTEN-FREE, NUT-FREE, SOYA-FREE, GRAIN-FREE, OIL-FREE,
ADVANCE PREP REQUIRED, FREEZER-FRIENDLY

MAKES 175 TO 250ML

PREP TIME: **5 MINUTES**

CHILL TIME: **24 HOURS**

You can easily create a decadent, fluffy whipped cream by using a can of full-fat coconut milk. Not only is the technique simple, but it's easily the best-tasting whipped cream I've tried. You can use this whipped cream just like regular whipped dairy cream. I like to use it in desserts such as my Pillowy Pumpkin Snacking Cookies (page 217), and it's also amazing with a bowl of fruit, on top of a fruit crisp or stirred into banana soft serve. The options are really endless! One important tip: You'll want to chill the can of coconut milk for at least twenty-four hours before you whip the cream, to ensure that the white coconut cream solidifies. I like to keep a few cans in the fridge at all times so I don't have to wait. Be sure to read all my tips on how to buy the right coconut milk for this recipe.

1. Chill the can of coconut milk in the fridge for at least 24 hours.

2. About 1 hour before making the whipped cream, chill a mixing bowl or the bowl of a stand mixer in the freezer.

3. Open the can and scoop the solid white coconut cream into the chilled bowl. Discard the coconut water or save it for another use (such as coconut water ice cubes).

4. Using an electric whisk or a stand mixer fitted with the whisk attachment, beat the cream until fluffy and smooth. Add the sweetener and vanilla bear pod seeds (if using), and beat again.

5. Cover the whipped cream and return it to the fridge until ready to use. It will firm up when chilled and soften at room temperature. The whipped coconut cream will keep in an airtight container in the fridge for up to 1 week, or you can freeze it in a freezer bag for up to 1 month. After chilling in the fridge, let sit at room temperature until it softens slightly and then rewhip it as needed.

1 400ml can full-fat coconut milk (see Tip)

1 to 2 tablespoons sweetener (maple syrup, powdered sugar, cane sugar, etc.), to taste

1 vanilla pod, seeds scraped, or ½ teaspoon pure vanilla extract (optional)

Tip Some brands of canned coconut milk are better than others for making whipped cream, and some cans of the same brand may even vary quite a bit. For whatever reason, the cream and water in some brands or cans does not separate. A few of the most consistent brands for making coconut whipped cream are: Thai Kitchen full-fat coconut milk, Trader Joe's Coconut Cream and Native Forest. I keep a few cans of full-fat coconut milk in my fridge at all times so I have backups in case I get a 'dud'. If you happen to get a dud, don't be discouraged. Try out one of the brands I've listed here, and be sure to chill it for at least 24 hours. If all else fails, So Delicious Coco Whip is a handy store-bought alternative to homemade coconut whipped cream. You can find it in the freezer section of some grocers, such as Whole Foods.

For Orange-Maple Coconut Whipped Cream Use 1 400ml can full-fat coconut milk (chilled for 24 hours), 60ml pure maple syrup, pinch of fine sea salt, ½ teaspoon orange zest. Omit the vanilla.

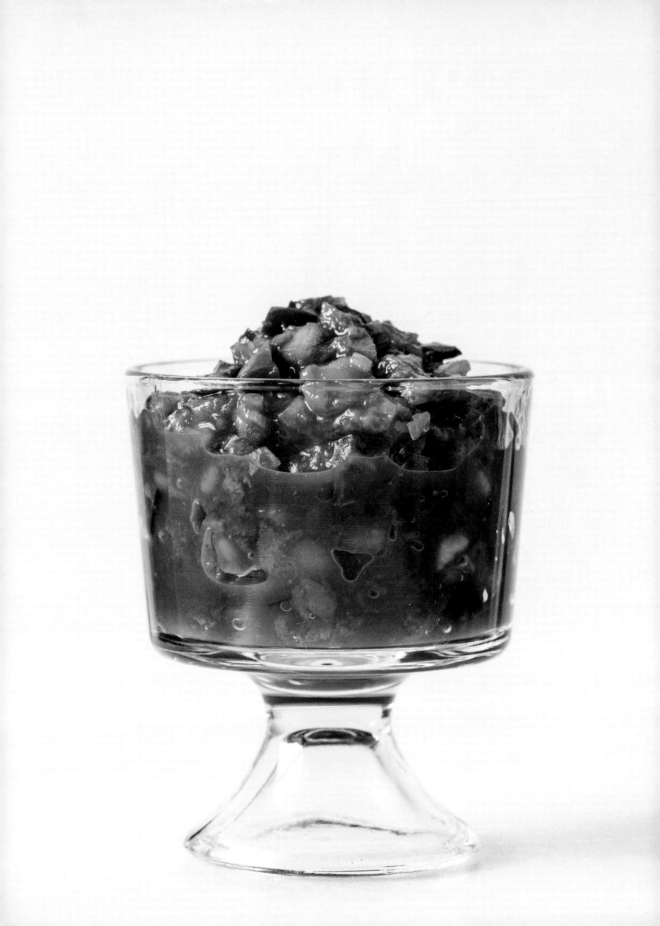

Apple-Mango Chutney

VEGAN, GLUTEN-FREE, NUT-FREE, SOYA-FREE, GRAIN-FREE, OIL-FREE

MAKES 375ML

PREP TIME: **15 MINUTES**

COOK TIME: **15 MINUTES**

This sweet, savoury and tangy apple-mango chutney is essential when you're making my Comforting Red Lentil and Chickpea Curry (page 181), providing a delightful sweet contrast to the spicy curry. I like to prepare the chutney a day in advance, which cuts down on prep time when the time comes to make the curry.

1. In a medium saucepan, stir together the apple, mango, bell pepper, onion, sugar, vinegar and ginger and bring to a simmer over medium-high heat. Simmer, stirring frequently, for about 15 minutes, until the fruit is soft and the mixture has thickened. Reduce the heat if necessary to keep the mixture from sticking to the bottom of the pot.

2. Add the lemon juice and salt and stir to combine. Cook for another minute or two and then remove from the heat. Let cool, then store in an airtight container in the fridge for 4 to 5 days.

150g diced peeled apple (about 1½ medium apples)

330g diced peeled mango (about 1 large mango)

90g diced red bell pepper

75g finely chopped onion

100g coconut sugar or natural cane sugar

60ml distilled white vinegar

1 tablespoon grated fresh ginger

1 to 1½ teaspoons fresh lemon juice, to taste

¼ teaspoon fine sea salt, or to taste

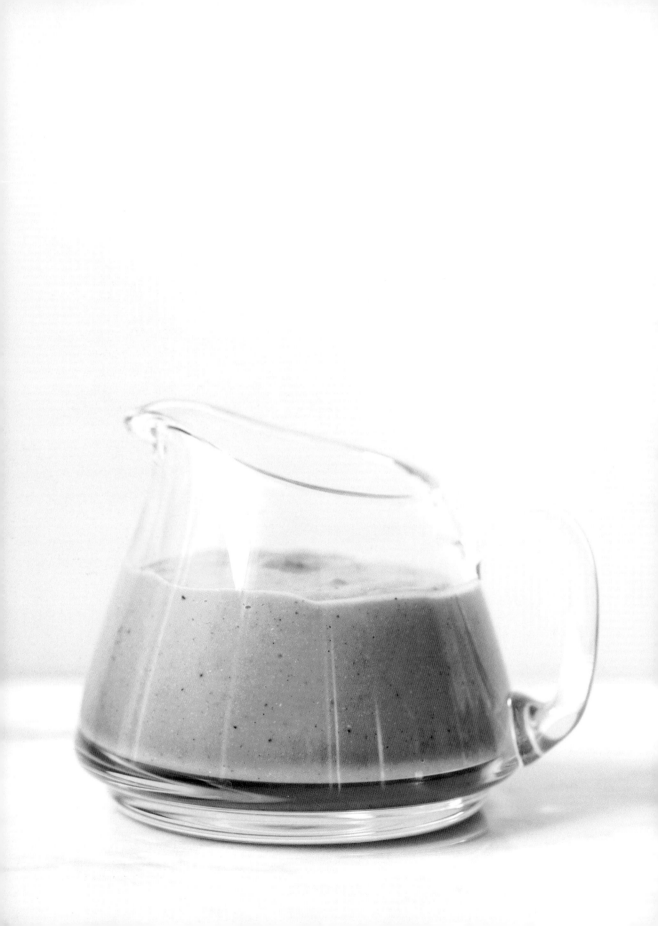

Cosy Gravy

VEGAN, GLUTEN-FREE OPTION, NUT-FREE, KID-FRIENDLY

MAKES ABOUT 500ML

PREP TIME: **5 TO 10 MINUTES**

COOK TIME: **10 MINUTES**

This is a simple and healthy yet decadent-tasting gravy that comes together in less than twenty minutes. Serve it with my Marinated Portobello Mushroom Bowl (page 187) with cauliflower mashed potatoes (page 187), or Shepherd's Pie (page 167). It's also amazing drizzled over a simple baked sweet potato!

1. In a medium saucepan, heat the oil over medium heat. Add the onion and garlic and sauté until softened, 4 to 5 minutes.

2. In a medium bowl, whisk together the broth and flour until no clumps remain. Pour the broth mixture into the pan with the onion and stir until combined. Add the tamari, nutritional yeast and pepper and stir again. Simmer for a few minutes, whisking frequently, until the gravy thickens. Reduce the heat if necessary to keep the mixture from sticking to the bottom of the pan.

3. Carefully transfer the gravy to a blender and blend on medium speed until smooth. (Alternatively, use a stick blender to blend the gravy directly in the pot.) Transfer the gravy back to the pot and add the vinegar and salt (if using) to taste. Simmer over low-medium heat, stirring frequently, until thickened. If the gravy is still too thin, whisk a tablespoon of flour with a tablespoon of water in a small bowl and then whisk this mixture into the gravy until smooth. If it's too thick, you can thin it with a splash of broth and stir. It will thicken up more as it cools.

4. Leftover gravy can be stored an airtight container in the fridge for a few days.

Make it gluten-free Use gluten-free plain flour.

2 tablespoons extra-virgin olive oil

150g diced onion

5 or 6 medium/large cloves garlic, minced (2 tablespoons minced garlic)

500ml low-sodium vegetable broth, plus more if needed

45g plain flour, white spelt flour, or gluten-free plain flour, plus more if needed

60ml low-sodium tamari

2 tablespoons nutritional yeast

½ teaspoon freshly ground black pepper

½ teaspoon white wine vinegar

Fine sea salt (optional)

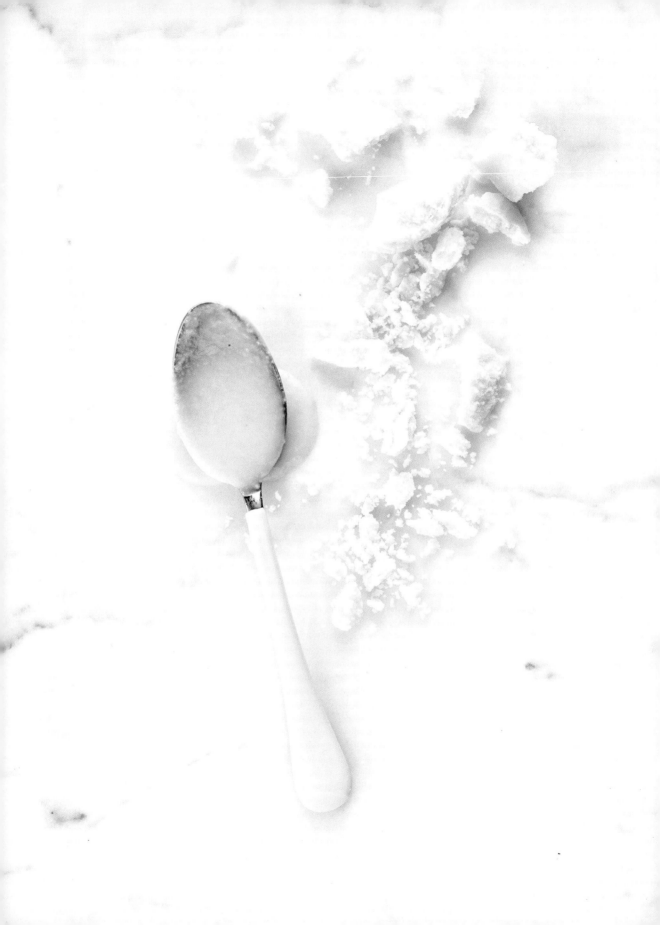

Homemade Coconut Butter

VEGAN, GLUTEN-FREE, NUT-FREE, SOYA-FREE, GRAIN-FREE, OIL-FREE

MAKES 400ML

PREP TIME: **1 MINUTE**

PROCESSING TIME: **5 TO 8 MINUTES**

I will never understand why store-bought coconut butter is so expensive. It's so incredibly easy to make at home and relatively inexpensive, too—especially if you buy shredded coconut in bulk. I buy a bag of No Name unsweetened medium-shredded dried coconut, toss it in the food processor and process away. It's super easy to make, with a rich buttery texture and light coconut flavour. Use this coconut butter in my Chocolate-Dipped Vanilla Macaroons (page 201). Be sure to use unsweetened medium-shredded coconut (not sweetened or large-flake coconut).

1. In a heavy-duty food processor, process the coconut until liquid and smooth, 5 to 8 minutes. Leftover coconut butter can be stored in an airtight container at room temperature for at least 1 month.

180 to 240g unsweetened medium shredded coconut

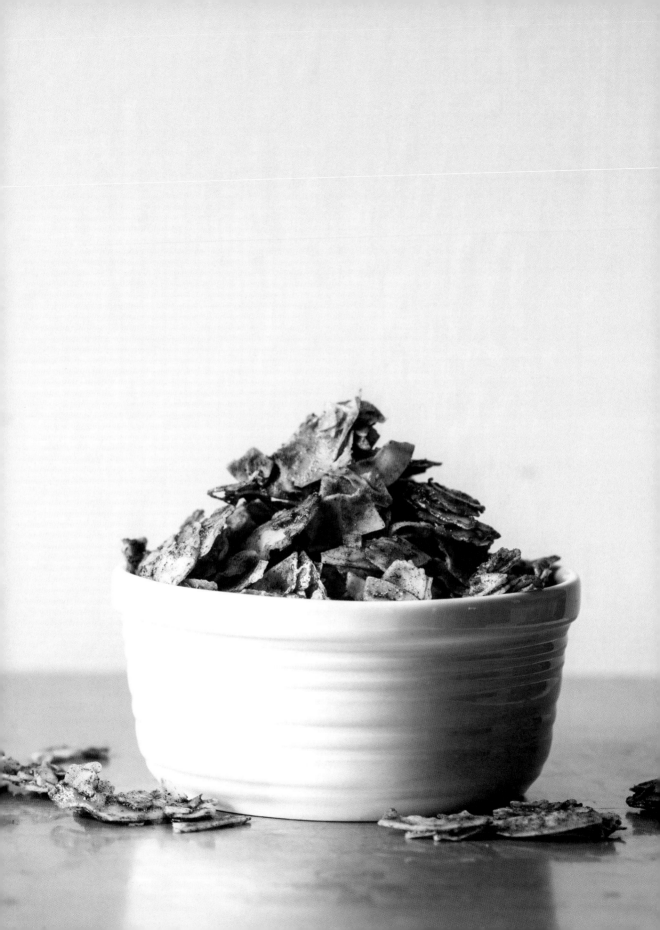

Maple Cinnamon Coconut Chips

VEGAN, GLUTEN-FREE, NUT-FREE, SOYA-FREE, GRAIN-FREE, OIL-FREE,
FREEZER-FRIENDLY

MAKES 250ML

PREP TIME: **3 MINUTES**

BAKE TIME: **9 TO 12 MINUTES**

These baked coconut chips are a perfect topping for desserts, hot
porridge or overnight oats (such as my Apple Pie Overnight Oats,
page 55). The recipe is so simple: Large coconut flakes are tossed in a
maple, cinnamon and sea salt mixture and baked until lightly golden.
After cooling, the flakes get crispy and clump together (similar to
granola). They are just such fun to eat straight from the pan.

1. Preheat the oven to 300°F (150°C). Line a large baking sheet with
parchment paper.

2. In a medium bowl, stir together the coconut, maple syrup, cinnamon
and salt until thoroughly combined.

3. Spread the coconut mixture over the prepared baking sheet in a thin,
uniform layer.

4. Bake for 9 to 12 minutes, until golden.

5. Let cool completely on the baking sheet. It will harden as it cools. The
coconut chips will keep in an airtight container in the fridge for at least
1 week or in the freezer for 2 to 3 weeks.

75g unsweetened large-flake coconut
(coconut chips)

2 tablespoons pure maple syrup

1 teaspoon ground cinnamon

Small pinch of fine sea salt

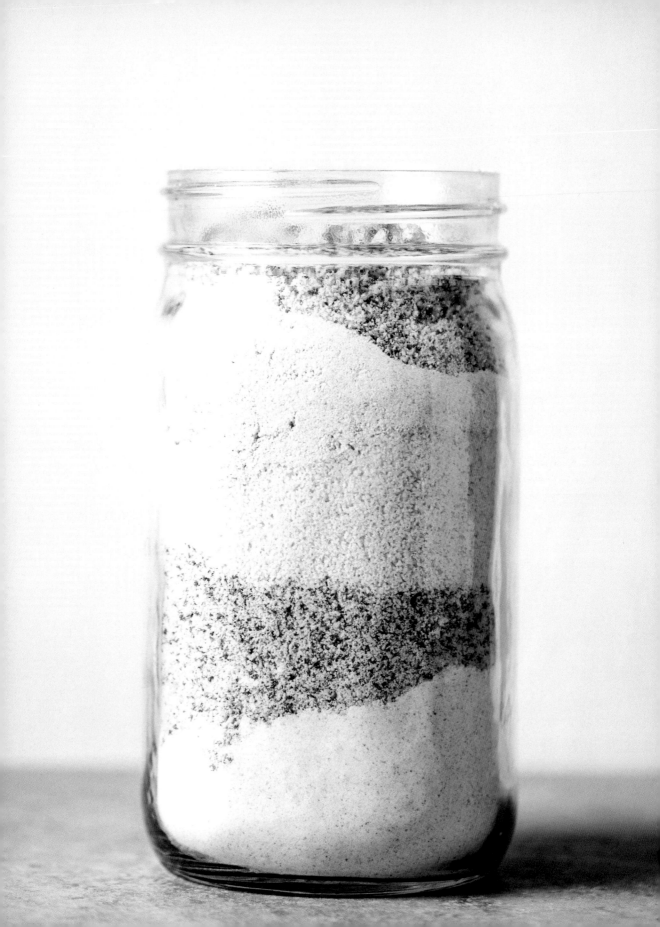

Homemade Flours and Meal

I love to make homemade flours as often as possible. It's easy to do with a high-speed blender, and the flour tastes much fresher than if you were to buy it from a store. Making almond meal is also a breeze—I just toss whole almonds into my food processor and process until they've been trans-formed into fine crumbs. Freshly made flours and especially almond meal have a shorter shelf life than commercial ones. I recommend storing flours in an airtight container in the refrigerator for up to four months, and almond meal for up to two months. Truthfully, I usually prefer to grind them fresh before each use.

ALMOND FLOUR
In a high-speed blender, blend 110g blanched slivered almonds on high speed until a flour forms. Be sure not to blend for too long or the oils will be released and the flour may clump together. Sift out any clumps or large almond pieces before using.

ALMOND MEAL
In a food processor, process 140g whole almonds (with the skin left on) into fine crumbs (you can use a blender if you prefer).

OAT FLOUR
In a high-speed blender, blend your desired amount of rolled or steel-cut oats on high speed for several seconds until they have a fine, flour-like consistency.

RAW BUCKWHEAT FLOUR
In a high-speed blender, blend your desired amount of raw buckwheat groats on high speed until they have a fine, flour-like consistency. Be sure to use *raw* buckwheat groats and not kasha or toasted buckwheat, as the latter have a much more earthy and pronounced flavour, which tends to stand out in baked goods.

Basics of Cooking Grains

While this is not intended to be a complete guide to cooking grains or legumes, these are the varieties that I cook with most frequently.

General cooking guidelines for grains: I suggest rinsing grains in a fine-mesh sieve before cooking. This removes debris and prevents unwanted particles from getting into the cooking water. Place the grain and fresh water (or vegetable broth, if desired) in a medium pot and bring to a low boil over high heat. Reduce the heat to medium-low, cover with a tight-fitting lid, and simmer for the suggested time, or until the grain is tender enough for your liking. Cooking times may differ depending on the heat level and how fresh the grains are, so I suggest keeping an eye on them until you are familiar with your hob. Quinoa, millet and rice benefit from a five-minute steam after cooking. To do this, simply remove the pan from the heat and let it sit with the lid on for five minutes. Fluff the grains with a fork after steaming.

Last, I included green lentils at the bottom of this chart. Follow the same procedures as above except simmer the lentils *uncovered* and drain any excess water after cooking.

GRAINS & LENTILS	DRY AMOUNT	WATER AMOUNT	TIPS	TIME
Basmati rice	100g	200 ml	Watch closely after 10 minutes.	10 to 15 minutes
Millet	100g	200 ml	Lightly toast millet in 1 tablespoon oil before adding water to enhance flavor.	20 minutes, plus 5 minutes steaming
Quinoa	100g	200 ml	Cook in vegetable broth to enhance flavour.	15 to 17 minutes, plus 5 minutes steaming
Short-grain brown rice	100g	300 ml	Steam for 5 minutes off heat.	40 minutes
Sorghum	100g	300 ml	Cook in vegetable broth to enhance flavour.	50 to 60 minutes
Spelt berries	100g	250 ml	For chewier spelt berries, reduce cooking time as needed.	35 minutes, or until water is absorbed
Wild rice	100g	300 ml	Steam for 5 minutes off heat.	40 minutes
Green lentils	100g	300 ml	Simmer lentils uncovered and drain excess water after cooking.	20 to 25 minutes

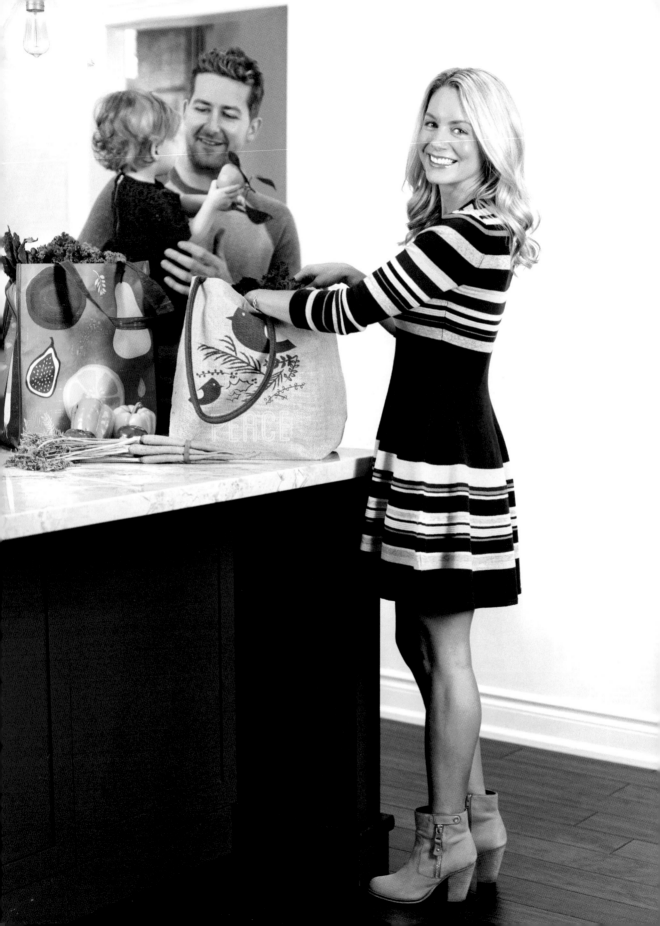

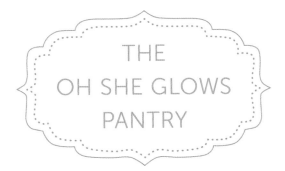

THE OH SHE GLOWS PANTRY

The number one item on my house wish list came true when we moved. Yes, I now have a pantry. A glorious pantry! Eric still jokes that the pantry was what sold me on our house, and he's right. I remember that on the first walk-through of the house, I lit up when I saw the pantry. I probably would have inked the deal right then and there.

Even though I'm no longer storing bags of flour in the TV cabinet like I was guilty of in our last place, I'm now ramming every ingredient I can into a pantry that looks like a bomb went off in it. So it appears that the problem is not the space (or lack thereof)—it's the person *in* the space. Or so I'm told. The bright side is that if there's ever a food shortage, I'm pretty sure my pantry could feed the entire neighborhood. Come one, come all!

This chapter gives you the most up-to-date list of the pantry staples I use these days. I'll describe each ingredient and give you advice on how to select, store, and prepare it. But I'm not going to give you tips on how to organize your pantry (I know my limits!). Maybe someday. I hope this detailed chapter will help you cook confidently with my favourite ingredients and also encourage you to add a few new things to your own arsenal.

Whole Grains, Flours, and Starches

GROUND ALMONDS AND ALMOND FLOUR

Using ground almonds in baked goods can create a rich, buttery texture and a pleasant, nutty fragrance. It is important to understand the distinction between ground almond and almond flour before using either ingredient in baking. Almond meal (ground almonds) is more coarsely ground than almond flour, and it contains the skins of the almonds (so you may see specks of brown in it). Almond flour is more finely ground and is made from blanched (i.e., skinless) almonds, so it has a white, refined appearance. Almond meal can work nicely in quick breads and cookies (such as my Chocolate-Almond Espresso Cookies, page 207) where a hearty texture is desirable, while almond flour is best for lighter baked goods, like cupcakes or cake.

Selection, Storage and Preparation: It is easy to create almond meal at home using a food processor (see page 285). You can also purchase almond meal and almond flour in health food stores or online. For delicate baking, be sure to buy almond flour made from blanched almonds. Almonds are prone to rancidity, so almond meal and flour should be stored in a tightly sealed container in a cool, dark place, or ideally in the refrigerator. Refrigerated almond flour and meal will keep for up to 6 months; check manufacturers' 'best by' dates when storing, and replace almond products often.

ARROWROOT POWDER

Arrowroot powder, which is derived from the roots of various tropical plants such as cassava, has been cultivated and used as a thickener for thousands of years. It was popular in the Victorian era for jellies and puddings, and it can be used in sauces, desserts, gravies and soups. If you're accustomed to using cornflour as a thickener, you may appreciate the more natural results of arrowroot: It preserves the lustre of foods and doesn't have the characteristic 'chalky' texture that can result from other thickening agents.

Selection, Storage and Preparation: When using arrowroot, it's best to create a slurry before adding the powder to hot liquid. Add the arrowroot to a small amount of cool liquid (you don't need much more than the quantity of arrowroot you're using). Whisk it together until the arrowroot is smooth, and then add it to the recipe as directed. This will prevent clumping. Arrowroot should be stored in an airtight container in a cool, dry place. It has a shelf life of about a year.

MILLET

Millet is a pearl-shaped yellow seed that is native to arid climates, including many parts of Asia and Africa. It boasts a pleasantly nutty and slightly sweet flavour. The texture of millet varies quite a bit with the amount of liquid used to cook the grain. Less liquid produces millet with a chewy texture. Add more water or broth, and the grain begins to resemble a soft polenta.

Selection, Storage and Preparation: Like all whole grains, millet should be purchased fresh and stored in an airtight container in a cool, dry place. It will keep for 3 to 4 months. Millet can be slightly difficult to cook, as it is prone to being either too dry or too wet. I recommend a ratio of 200g millet to 550ml liquid (broth or water) if you're aiming for the millet grains to be distinct and fluffy. Prepared this way, millet can be used in grain salads or for serving under stews and curries. If you'd like your millet to resemble porridge or polenta, use 750ml liquid for every 200g millet. Soft, stewed millet makes for a lovely breakfast, especially when paired with dried fruit and toasted nuts or seeds.

POTATO FLOUR

The challenge of gluten-free baking is to bind or thicken ingredients without gluten, which adds a sticky quality to dough. This challenge becomes much easier when you combine gluten-free flours with starches, such as potato or tapioca flour. Potato flour has an incredibly light texture, and it creates a lovely crumb when used in proper ratios with other flours. My favourite way to use potato flour is in my Shepherd's Pie (page 167); it thickens the sauce perfectly without the need for any flour.

Selection, Storage and Preparation: Potato flour should be stored in an airtight container in a cool, dry place for up to several months.

QUINOA

Quinoa is often classified as a whole grain, but it is actually a pseudograin, or an edible plant seed. It is wildly popular, with good reason: It cooks quickly and

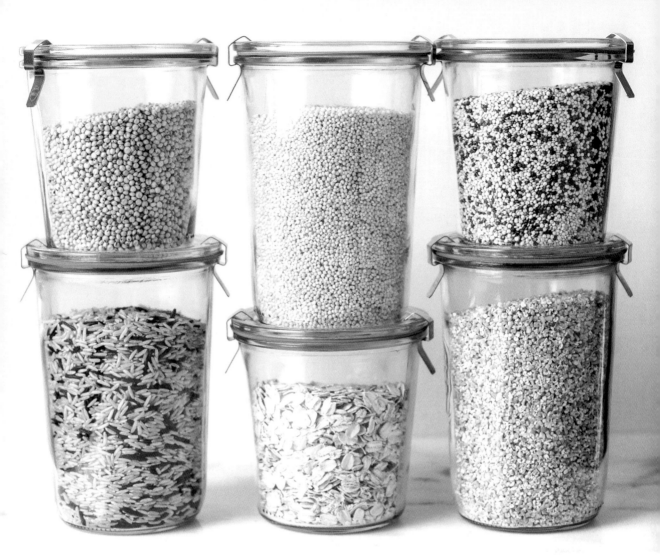

requires no soaking beforehand, which makes it a convenient option for weeknight dinners. It has a distinctive, nutty aroma and taste, but it absorbs flavours well, making it a perfect canvas for a wide variety of dishes. It is light, easy to digest, and naturally gluten-free.

Selection, Storage and Preparation: Raw quinoa has a natural coating of chemical compounds called saponins, which can create a bitter flavour, so it's important to rinse quinoa thoroughly in a fine-mesh sieve under cold water prior to cooking. A ratio of 110g dry quinoa to 375ml water works well for cooking, which should only take 15 minutes or so. I like to fluff quinoa with a fork and allow it to steam with the lid on for a few minutes before serving. Raw quinoa should be stored in an airtight

container in a cool, dry place for up to several months.

ROLLED OATS AND OAT FLOUR

It's hard not to love oats. They have a chewy, toothsome texture, they're easy to cook, and most of us associate them with the comfort of porridge and oatmeal raisin cookies. I love oats because of their tremendous versatility: rolled oats can be used not only for porridge, but also to add texture and bind vegan burgers, loaves, pie crusts, snack bars and baked goods. Oat flour has a soft texture and sweet taste, and it is an ideal addition to gluten-free baking so long as the brand you purchase is certified gluten-free. For the purposes of this book, recipes containing oats that don't contain other sources of gluten are labelled as gluten-free.

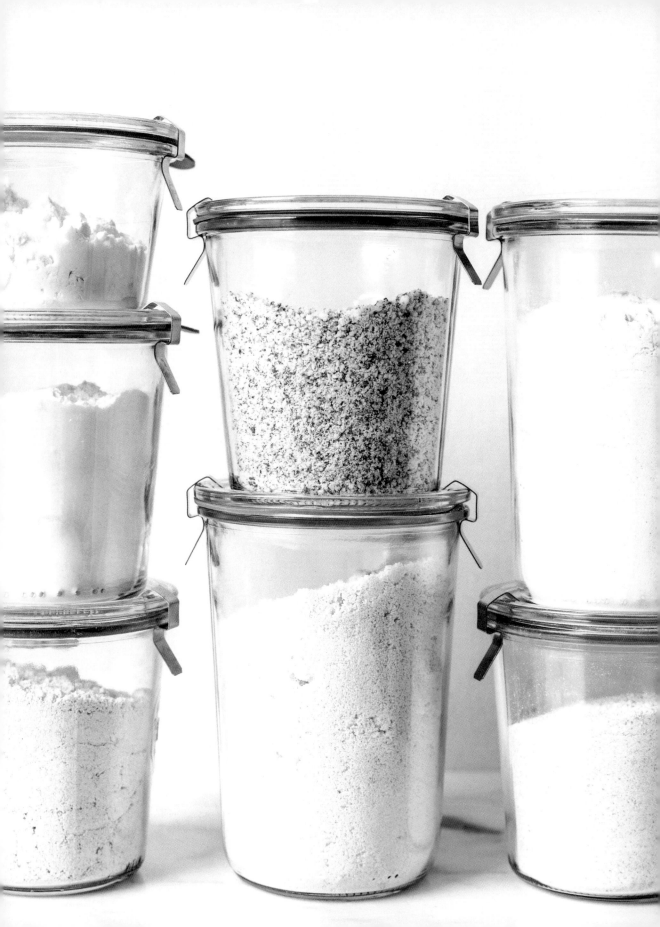

Selection, Storage and Preparation: If you have coeliac disease or strictly avoid gluten, it's important to purchase oat products that are certified gluten-free. Oats are slightly higher in fat than other grains, which means they can go rancid if stored for long periods of time. They should be stored in an airtight container in a cool, dry and dark place for up to 3 months. A word about oat flour: Like rolled oats, oat flour has a relatively short shelf life. It should be protected from heat and light and stored in an airtight container for up to 2 months.

SORGHUM

Sorghum is a relatively unfamiliar whole grain in North America, but its popularity is growing, thanks to the rise of food allergies and a demand for more gluten-free, wheat-free grain options. Sorghum is a staple crop in Africa and India, in part because it's hardy and resistant to drought. Sorghum is known for its chewy, plump texture, which makes it a wonderful, gluten-free substitute for wheat berries or barley. It has a sweet, neutral flavour, and it works especially well in grain salads.

Selection, Storage and Preparation: Sorghum flour should be stored in an airtight container in a cool, dry place for up to 6 months. Whole sorghum can be boiled until tender (about 1 hour) and used in grain salads, or the grain can be popped in a skillet.

SPELT FLOUR, WHOLE-GRAIN AND WHITE

Spelt flour has a slightly nutty flavour and a dense, hearty texture. It adds both protein and minerals to traditional baked goods when substituted for conventional wheat flour. Wholegrain spelt flour has a heartier texture, which works well in denser baked goods such as muffins, while white (or light) spelt flour is more similar to plain flour and is great in cakes and other delicate baked goods.

Selection, Storage and Preparation: Spelt flour can be found in health food stores and some grocery stores, or ordered online. It should be stored in an airtight container in a cool, dry place for up to 3 months, or in the freezer for up to 6 months.

STEEL-CUT OATS

Those of us who are accustomed to rolled or instant oats may forget that oats originate as whole oat groats (which resemble wheat berries, but are slightly longer and more tapered). When oat groats are split into pieces, they are called steel-cut oats. Steel-cut oats take longer to cook than rolled oats, but their chewy texture and creamy consistency make the cooking time well worth it.

Selection, Storage and Preparation: Steel-cut oats can take up to 45 minutes to simmer, but you can reduce that cooking time significantly if you soak the oats overnight, prior to cooking. Even if you aren't short of time, you must try The Fastest Sprouted Steel-Cut Oatmeal (page 37) for steel-cut oatmeal porridge that comes together in just 10 minutes.

WHOLESOME GRAIN FLOURS

There are many plain gluten-free flour blends on the market now, which begs the question: Why not simply use a store-bought mix? Well, I find homemade blends to be more reliable. Baking, especially vegan and gluten-free baking, is definitely not a one-size-fits-all process. This is exactly why I prefer to create my own unique flour blends for my gluten-free recipes rather than simply ask you to use any gluten-free mix. Store-bought gluten-free flour blends can vary dramatically in absorbency, texture and taste, and it's not always easy to predict how they'll behave when you use them. Because of this, I always recommend that you follow the recipe as written, especially when it comes to gluten-free flour blends that I've developed for specific recipes. This isn't to be a pain in the butt; I just truly want you to have the same results as I do!

Beans and Legumes

All dried beans and legumes have a very long shelf life if stored in a cool, dark place. After 1 to 2 years, dried beans will begin to lose moisture, and as a result they will take longer to soak and cook.

BLACK BEANS

Black beans are one of the most accessible and familiar members of the bean family. They are used in dishes around the world, and especially in Mexican, Indian and Brazilian cooking. I love the flavour, texture, and dramatic colour of black beans, and I use them in enchiladas, soups, casseroles and salads.

Selection, Storage and Preparation: As with most legumes, it's easiest to soak dried black beans prior to cooking them (at least 4 hours and up to 12). After soaking, black beans should cook for about 1 hour. It's also easy to find cooked black beans at the grocery store; just try to find BPA-free cans and packaging.

CHICKPEAS

Chickpeas (also known as garbanzo beans) are one of the most popular legumes around the world. Chickpeas are remarkably versatile: Whip them up into creamy hummus, use them in curries, blend them into soups or stews for texture and added protein, roast them for a crispy snack, or simply pile them onto fresh salads. What can't they do?

Selection, Storage and Preparation: Prior to cooking, pick over dried chickpeas to remove grit or any beans that appear discolored (black, grey or green) or shrivelled. Chickpeas demand a slightly longer cooking time than smaller legumes (60 to 90 minutes on average); however, you can reduce this time by soaking the uncooked chickpeas in water for 12 hours or so. (Of course, you can stock canned beans in your pantry for those times when you need beans in a hurry. My go-to brand of canned beans is Eden Organic.) Removing the skins from cooked chickpeas will create exceptionally creamy hummus (something I mention in my first book) or other blended dishes, though it's certainly not necessary to do so if you have a good blender or food processor. If you do wish to remove the skins, submerge cooked chickpeas in a large bowl of water and gently rub until the skins rise to the top and can be skimmed off and discarded.

FRENCH GREEN LENTILS

French lentils—also known as Puy lentils or *lentilles de Puy*, for the region in France from which they originate—have a sturdy texture and plenty of chew. They retain their shape well after cooking, which means they're perfect for lentil salads or for sprinkling onto grain dishes. They have a distinctive, speckled green-grey color and a smaller circumference than brown or green lentils. Be sure to try them in The Best Marinated Lentils (page 129).

Selection, Storage and Preparation: Pick over dry lentils prior to cooking to remove grit or debris. They will cook in 15 to 30 minutes.

GREEN OR BROWN LENTILS

No matter how small and humble, lentils are one of the most powerfully nutritious and versatile plant-based ingredients. Sauces, burgers, beef-like crumbles, loaves, salads, soups and more—there's almost nothing the lentil can't do. As if their nutrition profile and culinary range isn't enough, lentils are also a remarkably inexpensive and sustainable protein source, which may explain their popularity in so many global cuisines. I'm also quite proud to say that Canada is the world's largest producer of lentils. How cool is that?

Selection, Storage and Preparation: Prior to cooking, pick through dried lentils to remove any pieces of grit or debris. It's widely thought that lentils do not need to be soaked, and this is true if you're in a hurry, but a quick soak (2 to 4 hours) will reduce cooking time and may make your lentils slightly easier to digest. Once you're ready to cook them, cover the dry lentils with a few centimetres of water, bring to a boil, and simmer for 20 to 30 minutes, or until the lentils are tender but still hold their shape.

KIDNEY BEANS

Kidney beans—so called because of their characteristic shape—are wonderfully dense and substantial, which make them a perfect addition to chillis or stews. They probably originated in Peru, and they are a traditional component of many South and Central American dishes. They make perfect baked beans, and they're also a good addition to hearty pasta bakes and casseroles.

Selection, Storage and Preparation: Before cooking, pick over dried kidney beans to remove grit or damaged/misshapen beans. Kidney beans should be soaked for 8 hours or overnight prior to cooking, and the cooking time will vary between 75 and 90 minutes.

RED LENTILS

Unlike green, brown, black, or French lentils, red lentils don't hold their shape when cooked. Instead, they soften and break down, resulting in a thick texture

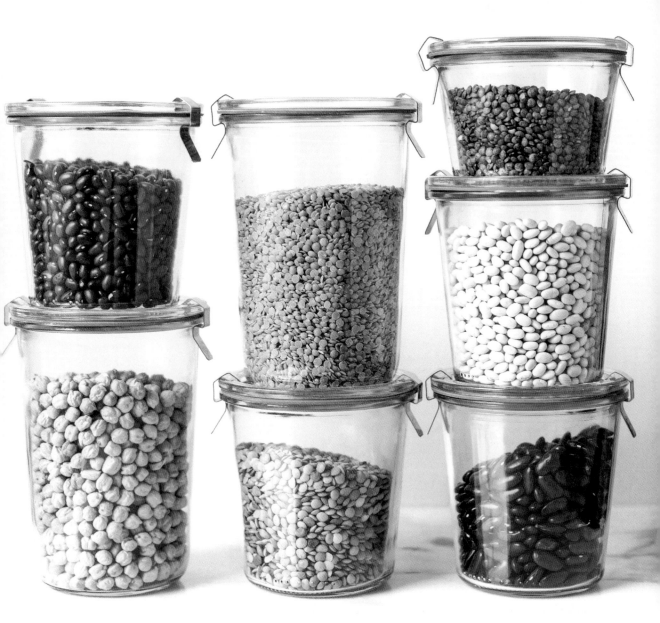

somewhat similar to a purée. For this reason, they are a perfect addition to soups or stews, adding thickness along with plenty of nutrition.

Selection, Storage and Preparation: Because they're split, red lentils cook more quickly than any other lentil variety. Twelve to 15 minutes of simmering will do the trick. To cook, simply place 200g lentils and 375ml water or broth in a medium saucepan and bring to a boil. Reduce the heat to maintain a simmer and cook until the lentils are soft, 12 to 15 minutes.

WHITE BEANS

Three popular white beans—great northern, haricot, and cannellini—have a pleasant, mild flavor. Haricot beans and great northern beans have a slightly grainy texture, while cannellini beans have a creamier consistency. Great northern beans are had to find in the UK but you could substitute butter beans. All three add texture and taste to soups, stews, grain dishes, or casseroles.

Of the three, haricot beans are smallest, great northern beans are slightly larger, and cannellini beans are the largest. If you're using precooked beans in a recipe, you can usually use these beans interchangeably.

I often blend white beans into creamy sauces or use them for herb dip (white beans and rosemary are a classic flavour pairing).

Selection, Storage, and Preparation: Before cooking, pick over dried white beans to remove grit or damaged/misshapen beans. Haricot beans can be soaked for 4 to 6 hours prior to cooking; great northern beans and cannellini beans should be soaked for 8 hours or overnight. Haricot beans should cook in about 45 minutes, whereas cannellini beans will need between 60 and 90 minutes to finish.

Nuts and Seeds

ALMOND MILK

Almond milk has become one of the most popular non-dairy milk alternatives. Its pleasantly nutty, mildly sweet flavour makes it ideal for smoothies, porridges (see Apple Pie Overnight Oats, page 55) and other breakfast dishes, but it can also be used in soups or any other creamy dishes. Almond milk is easy to prepare at home in a blender, but it is also widely available in grocery stores.

Storage, Selection and Preparation: When selecting commercial almond milk, be aware that there is some controversy surrounding carrageenan, a food thickener and stabilizer that is derived from seaweed. While the research on this ingredient is far from conclusive, there is some evidence that carrageenan may promote inflammation. Some commercial almond milks are made with sunflower lecithin instead of carrageenan, so it is possible to avoid it if you wish to. I am a fan of Whole Foods 365 brand organic almond milk.

ALMONDS

Almonds are one of the healthiest, most convenient, and most versatile tree nuts. The mild flavour of raw almonds becomes bolder and more distinctive when they are roasted or toasted, but I enjoy using both raw and roasted almonds in various recipes. Raw almonds are particularly good for making homemade almond milk (see page 35) or snacking, while toasted/roasted almonds make incredible, nutrient-dense nut butter and an ideal topping for grains and roasted vegetables (see my Roasted Tamari Almonds, page 263).

Selection, Storage and Preparation: Like all nuts, almonds should be purchased fresh. Look for a mildly sweet and nutty fragrance, which signals freshness. Almonds can be stored in an airtight container in a cool, dry place; if you plan to store them for more than a few months, it is best to keep them in the fridge or freezer. If you're purchasing roasted almonds, it's best to use dry-roasted almonds (rather than oil-roasted), and be sure to avoid almonds with added sweeteners.

CASHEWS

Cashews may be the single most versatile tree nut, thanks to their buttery texture and mild, subtly sweet flavor. They can be blended into sauces, dressings, nut milk or nut cheeses, or toasted and added to stir-fries, salads or grain dishes. I love blending soaked cashews into pasta sauces and soups; they add the richness that many of us associate only with cream. Cashew butter, which is made from ground cashews, is a good alternative to peanut or almond butter.

Selection, Storage and Preparation: It's best to purchase cashews fresh and replenish them often. Cashews should be stored in an airtight container in a cool, dry place. If you don't plan to eat them right away, storing them in the fridge is best. Cashew butter should be stored in the fridge after opening.

CHIA SEEDS

Though their popularity has boomed in the last decade, chia seeds have been a part of Central American diets for centuries. They were a staple food in the Mayan and Aztec empires, prized for their energy-sustaining nutrition. Chia seeds can be added to smoothies or puddings, or sprinkled onto fresh fruit or salads, and they can add texture to porridge or baked goods.

Selection, Storage and Preparation: Chia seeds can be ground and used as a binder in baked goods or as a thickener for smoothies and sauces. They do not, however, need to be ground in order to be digested, and they can be added directly to porridges or cereals. The most common preparation method for chia seeds is to allow them to plump up in liquid, which makes them take on a texture similar to tapioca pudding. See my Coconut Chia Seed Pudding (page 67) for a healthy snack!

The omega-3 fatty acids in chia seeds can easily go rancid, so it is important to store them in a cool, dry

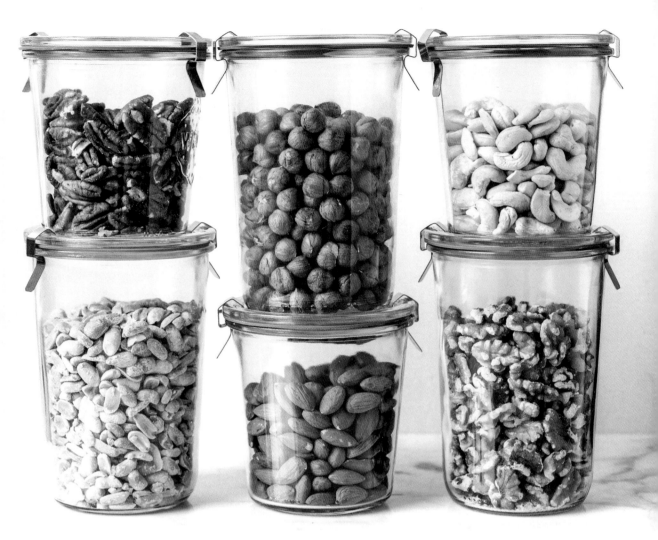

place. I recommend storing chia seeds in an airtight container in the refrigerator for up to 8 months.

LINSEED AND MILLED LINSEED
Linseed is known for both its nutrient density and its utility in vegan dishes. It acts as an excellent binder in baked goods and crackers. Ground linseed can also thicken and enrich porridges, breads and smoothies.
Selection, Storage and Preparation: The delicate omega-3 fatty acids in linseed can turn rancid when exposed to heat or light. It's best to store it in an airtight, opaque container in the refrigerator or freezer for up to 6 months. It can be purchased ground or whole; if you wish to grind it yourself, you can do so with a spice grinder or food processor. Whole linseed will pass through the digestive tract undigested, so it's important to grind them before eating in order to reap the fullness of their nutritional benefits.

HAZELNUTS
The rich, nutty flavour and buttery texture of hazelnuts make them a wonderful choice for homemade desserts. They are a classic dessert ingredient, appearing in such time-honoured recipes as Linzer torte, Linzer cookies, biscotti and many varieties of shortbread. You can try them in my Roasted Hazelnut-Almond Granola Clusters (page 71), Roasted Hazelnut-Almond Butter (page 77) and Coffee Shop-Worthy Hazelnut Milk (page 35).
Storage, Selection and Preparation: Shelled hazelnuts should be purchased fresh and have uniform shape and size. Raw hazelnuts should be

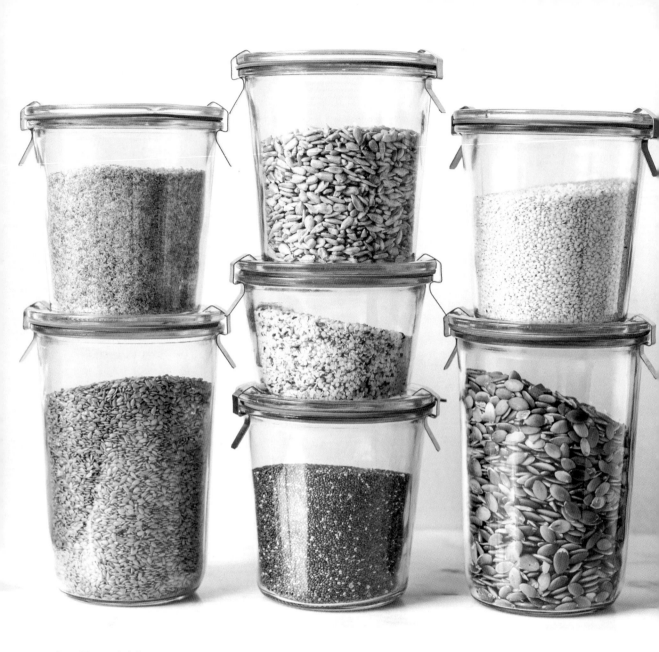

stored in an airtight container in a cool, dry place for up to 6 months. Most people prefer the taste of roasted hazelnuts, which can be easily prepared by baking whole shelled hazelnuts at 300°F (150°C) for 12 to 14 minutes, or until fragrant. Roasted hazelnuts should be stored in the fridge for up to 3 months, or frozen for up to 1 year.

HEMP HEARTS

Hemp hearts (hulled hemp seeds) are a quick, convenient and complete source of plant-based protein, which makes them ideal for sprinkling onto salads or roasted vegetables, blending into smoothies or dressings or adding to porridge. I recommend purchasing hulled hemp seeds, which can be used immediately in any recipe.

Selection, Storage and Preparation: The high omega-3 and omega-6 content of hemp seeds makes them prone to rancidity, so it is best to store them in an airtight container in the fridge for up to a year.

NUT BUTTERS

Nut butters add delicious flavour and a dose of healthy fat to toast, fruit, porridge and even raw vegetables (if you've never tried carrots and almond butter, now is the time!). They also serve as a base for delicious salad dressings and sauces, such as my Thai Almond Butter Sauce (page 249). There is an extensive variety of nut butters available in grocery stores these days, from almond butter to cashew butter to coconut butter to hazelnut butter, which means that you can pick and choose the flavours you love, but I also offer simple recipes for these butters (see pages 75, 77 and 281).

Storage, Selection and Preparation: Many nut butters are shelf stable in a cool, dry place, but others should be refrigerated. Check the individual nut or seed butter for storage directions and 'best by' dates.

PEANUTS

Though we often think of them as tree nuts, peanuts are actually a member of the legume family. Like many legumes, they are rich in protein, as well as B vitamins and minerals. Peanut butter is a comfort food for many of us. It is of course a perfect topping for sandwiches or toast, but it can also add a unique flavour to chillis or stews. Chopped peanuts, meanwhile, are a perfect topping for Asian-inspired salads, slaws, curries and stir-fries.

Selection, Storage and Preparation: Conventional peanuts are often treated heavily with pesticides, so it's best to purchase peanut butter and peanuts that are certified organic. When buying peanut butter, also be sure to look out for excess sweeteners or sodium. Shelled peanuts should be stored in an airtight container in the fridge for up to 3 months, or in the freezer for up to 6 months.

PECANS

Pecans are a traditional ingredient in many classic American dishes, and they're particularly beloved in Southern American cooking. Their high fat content and buttery flavour make them ideal for desserts and sweets. Toasted with sweet potatoes, they add a particularly nutty aroma and flavour, but I love using raw pecans in homemade energy bars and balls. Pecans are also useful for making creamy, homemade nut milk.

Storage, Selection and Preparation: Pecans should be purchased fresh and be relatively uniform and smooth in size and shape. They can be stored in an airtight

container in a cool, dry place for up to 6 months.

PUMPKIN SEEDS

Hulled pumpkin seeds make a cheap, inexpensive and delicious addition to your diet. They have a pleasant crunch (especially when roasted!) and mild flavour, as well as a myriad of health benefits.

Selection, Storage and Preparation: Pumpkin seeds can be toasted and added to salads or slaws, sprinkled on top of a hot bowl of chilli, ground up in place of pine nuts in pesto, and even blended into soups or sauces. They should be stored in an airtight container in the fridge for up to a year.

SESAME SEEDS AND TAHINI

The characteristically nutty flavour of sesame seeds and sesame paste (better known as tahini) brightens up a good many Asian and Middle Eastern recipes. Hulled sesame seeds add subtle crunch to salads, stir-fries, noodle dishes, and even baked goods, while tahini is an outstanding base for salad dressings (see my Lemon-Tahini Dressing, page 265) and even stirred into pasta dishes (see my Fusilli Lentil-Mushroom Bolognese, page 161).

Selection, Storage and Preparation: Sesame seeds are less prone to rancidity than hemp hearts, pumpkin, or sunflower seeds, but they should still be stored in an airtight container in a cool, dry place. Stored this way, they will keep for up to a year. Tahini can be kept in an airtight container in a cool, dry place for up to several months.

SUNFLOWER SEEDS AND SUNFLOWER SEED BUTTER

Inexpensive, easy to find, and nutritious, sunflower seeds make a wonderful healthy snack or addition to salads. Sunflower seeds can be purchased hulled (without the shell) or in the shell, but for the purposes of snacking and cooking, it's usually easiest to purchase hulled seeds. You can find hulled seeds raw or roasted and/or salted. Sunflower seed butter is made from ground seeds, and it is an ideal replacement for almond or peanut butter if you have nut allergies. See my Homemade Sunflower Seed Butter (page 79) recipe to make some in your own kitchen.

Selection, Storage and Preparation: Sunflower seeds are prone to rancidity, so it's best to store them in an airtight container in the refrigerator for up to 8 months. They can be blended into creamy salad dressings, sprinkled onto salads or whole grains, or added to porridges. You can also try blending them into your smoothies for a healthy dose of vitamin E. Sunflower seed butter is best stored in a cool, dry place for up to a few weeks, or refrigerated for several months.

WALNUTS

Walnuts are a common ingredient in quick breads, granolas, oatmeal dishes and other breakfast foods, but they make a wonderfully nutritious addition to any savoury dishes (see my Ultimate Green Taco Wraps, page 191) or snacks. More than any other tree nut, walnuts are known for their remarkable range of potential health benefits, from cardiovascular support to brain health.

Selection, Storage and Preparation: Thanks to their high omega-3 content, walnuts do go rancid quickly. It's best to store them in an airtight container in the fridge for up to 6 months, or to freeze them for up to 1 year. I find it easiest to purchase shelled walnuts, so I can avoid having to remove their thick, tough shells.

Coconut

Coconut-derived ingredients are rich in lauric acid, a medium-chain fatty acid that may have antibacterial properties. Coconut milk is exceptionally high in saturated fat, which is unusual for a plant-based ingredient. However, most research demonstrates that populations who consume significant amounts of coconut products do not seem to be at a higher risk of chronic disease. Given the scarcity of saturated fat in plant-based diets, most vegans and vegetarians can safely consume coconut foods in moderation. Coconut flesh and coconut products are also rich in antioxidants, which may have a protective effect against aging and disease.

CANNED FULL-FAT COCONUT MILK

Canned full-fat coconut milk adds unmistakable richness and subtle hints of coconut flavour to soups, stews, and especially to curries. It is a potent ingredient; because the fat content of full-fat coconut milk is so high, a small amount can go a very long way in cooking. I use it to transform my Sweet Potato, Chickpea and Spinach Coconut Curry (page 179).

Selection, Storage and Preparation: Canned full-fat coconut milk is easy to locate in the Asian aisles of most grocery stores. It is a unique ingredient, and it cannot be replaced with the coconut milk beverages sold in cardboard cartons. When full-fat coconut milk is left in the fridge, a thick layer of solid cream will rise to the top and congeal. This cream (known as coconut cream) can be whipped into a silky topping or used to thicken desserts. See page 275 for my Coconut Whipped Cream recipe and tips for selecting brands suitable for the job.

COCONUT AMINOS

Coconut aminos is a salty seasoning made from fermented coconut sap. It is comparable to soya sauce, tamari or nama shoyu, but it is both wheat- and soya-free, which makes it a wonderful option for those with food allergies. It has a sweeter taste and more mild saltiness than soya sauce. It can be added to dressings or stir-fries, and it can be sprinkled directly onto salads or fresh vegetables.

Selection, Storage and Preparation: At the moment, the most readily available brand of coconut aminos is Coconut Secret brand. You can find it in health food stores, at Whole Foods, or online at coconutsecret.com.

COCONUT BUTTER

Coconut butter is a heavenly ingredient. It is rich, fragrant, and luxurious, with hints of vanilla. It tends to be somewhat expensive, and it can be difficult to find, but it's incredibly easy and cost efficient to make at home (see page 281). A very small amount can transform a hot bowl of oats, a thick slice of toast or a roasted sweet potato. Coconut butter is a mixture of coconut oil and coconut solids. At room temperature, it is solid, but it melts when added to hot food, emitting a delightful aroma and flavor.

Selection, Storage and Preparation: Coconut butter should be stored in a cool, dry place for up to 6 months. It can become very solid in a cold cupboard, but once you add a little heat, it will melt partially and become silky smooth.

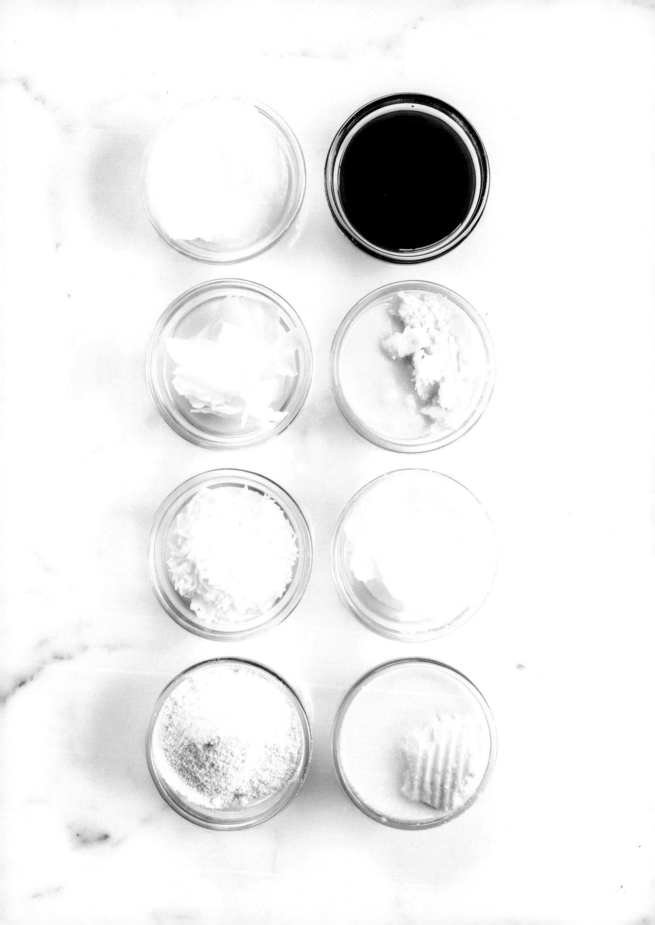

COCONUT FLOUR

Though it has become mainstream only recently, coconut flour is already a popular option among health-conscious foodies. It is high in fibre and free of wheat, gluten, soya, legumes and grains, which makes it a good option for those with food allergies or sensitivities. I love to use a small amount in my Peanut Better Balls (page 231) to slightly thicken the dough.

Selection, Storage and Preparation: Coconut flour can be found in most health food and grocery stores and online. It absorbs moisture easily, so it should be stored in an airtight container in the fridge or freezer immediately after opening. Because coconut flour is a 'thirsty' flour (it absorbs a lot of liquid in recipes), you'll have the best results when you mix it with other flours, like brown rice or sorghum.

REFINED COCONUT OIL

Refined coconut oil has a milder and less distinctive flavour than virgin coconut oil. It is usually extracted from the coconut fruit with the use of certain chemicals and heat, which means that it retains less of the coconut's naturally occurring polyphenols than virgin coconut oil. It has a high smoke point, which means that it's a good choice for baking or roasting up to temperatures of 400°F (200°C). I use it whenever I don't want a coconut flavour in my recipes, such as in my Sweet Potato Casserole (page 133).

Selection, Storage and Preparation: Once again, try to select an organic brand of refined coconut oil. Coconut oil will be solid at room temperature and liquid above room temperature, and it should be stored in a cool, dry place.

UNSWEETENED LARGE-FLAKE COCONUT

Large-flake coconut has a taste similar to shredded coconut, and it can similarly be used in porridges or desserts. The texture, though, is different: Large-flake coconut is more substantial and toothsome than shredded coconut. It's a perfect topping for morning oats or a hearty curry, for adding texture to granolas or cereals, or for afternoon snacking (unlike shredded coconut, you can eat it right out of the bag).

Selection, Storage and Preparation: Be sure to purchase unsweetened coconut flakes. Store them in an airtight container in a cool, dry place for up to 6 months.

UNSWEETENED SHREDDED COCONUT

Shredded coconut (also sometimes labelled as desiccated coconut) is a classic addition to desserts, breakfast porridges, granolas and cookies. It adds chewy texture and a delightfully tropical hint of coconut flavour.

Selection, Storage and Preparation: Much of the shredded coconut on the market has been sweetened, so it is important to select unsweetened varieties. Unsweetened coconut can be found in most health food stores or ordered online. Shredded coconut should be stored in an airtight container in a cool, dry place for up to 6 months. It can be added directly to recipes or blended with water to create quick, easy and inexpensive homemade coconut milk.

VIRGIN COCONUT OIL

Virgin (also called unrefined) coconut oil is extracted directly from the coconut fruit, without excess processing or heat. Virgin coconut oil contains more beneficial polyphenols than refined coconut oil, which has been extracted with the use of both heat and chemicals, and is prized for its heart-healthy, antibacterial and antifungal properties. I love to cook and bake with it, as it adds a wonderful, sweet aroma to vegetable dishes and has a distinctly coconutty flavour. I think it pairs particularly well with sweet, roasted root vegetables.

Selection, Storage and Preparation: It can be difficult to select coconut oil in the stores, as there are so many different varieties available nowadays. If you're looking for virgin coconut oil, be sure to select an organic brand, as the integrity and quality of the product will be higher. Virgin coconut oil is suitable for medium-heat cooking, such as sautéing. As an added bonus, it can also be used as a natural skin moisturizer. Coconut oil will be solid at room temperature and liquid above room temperature, and it should be stored in a cool, dry place. You can melt it prior to using by running the jar under hot tap water or in a small saucepan over low heat on the hob. Occasionally, in my recipes I call for 'softened' coconut oil. This means that the coconut oil should have a very soft, spreadable texture, but it shouldn't be completely liquid.

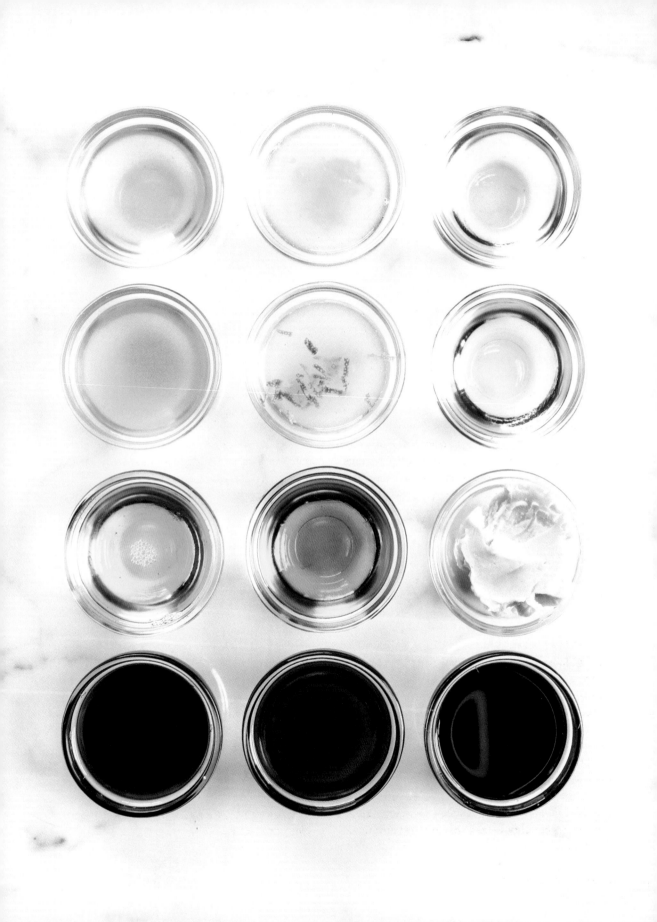

Oils and Fats

AVOCADO AND AVOCADO OIL

In the nineties, when low-fat dieting was all the rage, avocados were feared for their high fat content. Today, it's widely recognized that the polyunsaturated fats in avocado help to lower LDL cholesterol and protect the heart. This is good news for avocado lovers every-where, and what's not to love? Avocados have delightfully creamy yet firm flesh. They can be used in guacamole or as a fat source in dressings, but they can also be spread on toast, used as a topper for chilli, and mixed into salads. For any recipes where you crave creaminess, avocados are a perfect choice! I love them whipped up in smoothies, or in savoury creams such as my Avocado Coriander Crema (page 165). I recently started cooking with expeller-pressed naturally refined avocado oil. I love its light and neutral flavour (try it in my Every Day Lemon-Garlic Hummus, page 91), and the fact that it has a high smoke point (over 500°F/260°C), which makes it great for high-heat cooking.

Selection, Storage and Preparation: Avocados should be purchased at the peak of their freshness or just before. I like to buy them when they are just soft to the touch, but not yet mushy or tender. The skin of avocados should be even, not dappled or cracked. One great trick for determining if your avocado is fresh is to take a peek under the stem; if it's black, the avocado will be bruised and rotten. If it's still slightly green, it's almost ready to enjoy. If your avocados are underripe, you can ripen them by placing them in a paper bag for a night or two. If you have leftover avocado you can freeze the flesh for smoothies (I like to portion leftovers in 2- to 4-tablespoon amounts).

COLD-PRESSED EXTRA-VIRGIN OLIVE OIL

Olive oil has played a central role in the Mediterranean diet for thousands of years, and nowadays it is one of the most popular oils for cooks around the world. It is made by crushing or grinding the fruit of olive trees and has a mildly fruity flavor. It is a versatile oil, equally good for salad dressings and for roasting or sautéing.

Selection, Storage and Preparation: Grocery stores are flooded with fine olive oils from around the world. It is possible to find good olive oil on even a modest budget, but I do recommend purchasing cold-pressed extra-virgin olive oil if possible. Cold-pressed olive oil is prepared with a time-honoured process of pressing olives between stone slabs, although it can be made using stainless steel, too. The oil created with this method retains more of its nutrients and polyphenols than refined olive oil, and it also has a more delicate and fruity flavour.

Good olive oil should be stored in an opaque or semi-opaque container in a cool, dry place. Stored properly, good olive oil will typically remain fresh for up to a year.

SESAME OIL, TOASTED OR UNTOASTED

Toasted sesame oil has a nutty aroma and an incredibly potent sesame flavour, while untoasted sesame oil is much more mild in flavour and doesn't tend to overpower other flavours. Both can be used in stir-fries, soba noodle bowls (such as my Soba Noodle Salad, page 183), and other Asian dishes, and they can also be used to flavour dressings and sauces.

Selection, Storage and Preparation: Sesame oil should be refrigerated or stored in a cool, dry place after opening.

DAIRY-FREE SPREAD

We are lucky to live in an era when so many innovative vegan products are available in grocery stores. While I try to cook most things from scratch, I do have a few favorite vegan products that help to add flavour and authenticity to my food. Dairy-free spread is one such product that I use occasionally. It tastes amazingly like butter, and it works perfectly in dishes like my Sweet Potato Casserole (page 133) where I like a subtle butter flavour; otherwise, I prefer to use coconut oil for its health benefits.

Selection, Storage and Preparation: There are a few different dairy-free spread brands on the market. I tend to purchase the soya-free Earth Balance brand of buttery spread. Store the spread in the fridge for the duration suggested by the manufacturer.

Sweeteners

BLACKSTRAP MOLASSES

Blackstrap molasses is a uniquely nutritious option within the world of liquid sweeteners. It undergoes more reduction and caramelization than other forms of molasses (sulfured or unsulfured), which means that it is thicker, darker, slightly lower in sugar, and richer in minerals. It is potent, but when used in small amounts it will add a lovely molasses flavour to baked goods, chillis and homemade barbecue sauce (page 255).
Selection, Storage and Preparation: It's best to purchase organic blackstrap molasses. Blackstrap molasses should be stored in a cool, dry place for up to 6 months. It can be added to cookies, muffins or quick breads, but don't overlook its potential for adding flavour and character to chilli or barbecue dishes, too.

BROWN RICE SYRUP

Brown rice syrup has a mild, lovely sweetness and a light brown colour. It is a very thick and sticky liquid sweetener, and as a result, it works well for binding ingredients such as in my Mocha Empower Glo Bars (page 69). Brown rice syrup has a relatively low glycemic index and it's thought to deliver a consistent and steady energy supply.
Selection, Storage and Preparation: Buy organic brown rice syrup when possible. Brown rice syrup can be stored in an airtight container in a cool, dry place for up to 6 months.

COCONUT SUGAR AND COCONUT NECTAR

Coconut sugar (sometimes labelled as coconut crystals) and coconut nectar have appeared on the market only recently, but they have already gained tremendous popularity, thanks to their lovely flavour and their low glycemic ranking (which means that they tend not to spike blood sugar as dramatically as other sweeteners). Both coconut sugar and coconut nectar have a GI rating of only 35, which is relatively low for liquid or crystal sweeteners. Neither one tastes like coconut; rather, they both have a pleasant, burnt-sugar flavour (with coconut nectar tending to fall on the 'tangy' side) and a lovely caramel hue.
Selection, Storage and Preparation: Coconut sugar and coconut nectar can be found in most health food stores and healthy grocery stores, as well as online. Coconut sugar and nectar should be stored in airtight containers in a cool, dry place for up to several months. Coconut sugar can be quite drying in baked goods, so if I use cane sugar in a recipe and you're wondering why I didn't just use coconut sugar, it's because coconut sugar doesn't give a moist enough result!

MEDJOOL DATES

Medjool dates are sometimes called 'nature's candy', and once you experience their taste and texture for the first time, it isn't hard to see why. These luscious, creamy dates—not to be confused with the smaller and firmer neglet dates—have a taste that is almost similar to caramel. They add sweetness, as well as some naturally occurring minerals and fibre, to desserts and baked goods. Medjool dates blend easily, thanks to their tender texture, which means that you can seamlessly incorporate them into nut milks and sauces.
Selection, Storage and Preparation: Medjool dates can be stored in an airtight container in a cool, dry place for a couple of months. They will last even longer in the refrigerator and can be frozen for up to 1 year. If I'm chopping up dates for a recipe, I'll often refrigerate them first, as a firm texture makes it easier to chop them evenly.

ORGANIC BROWN SUGAR

Brown sugar is a time-honoured sweetener of choice for cookies and quick breads. Its rich flavour is reminiscent of molasses, which makes good sense, since molasses is mixed with regular sugar to produce brown sugar. Brown sugar has a moist texture and a lovely amber colour. It is particularly good in granolas, sprinkled on top of hot cereal, or used in baking, such as in my Chewy Molasses Spelt Cookies (page 219).
Selection, Storage and Preparation: Be sure to purchase organic brown sugar, to ensure that it is free of pesticide residues and potential animal by-products. Brown sugar should be stored in an airtight container in a cool, dry place, separated from any odorous foods or other ingredients. It can be stored for many months, but it will dry out gradually.

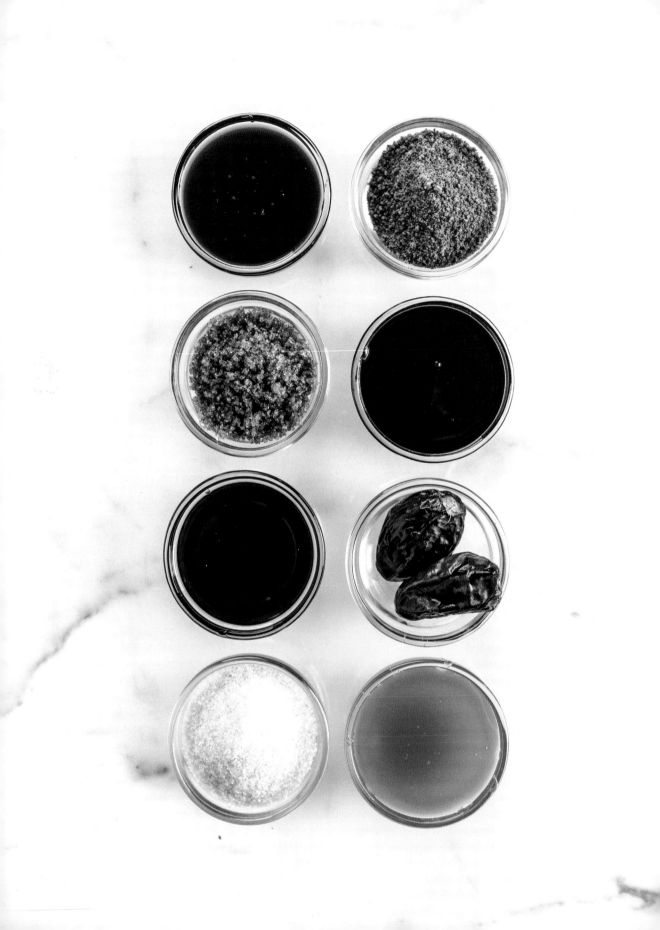

ORGANIC CANE SUGAR

Organic cane sugar is an excellent sweetener for authentic baked goods. Of all the vegan sweetening options, it is the most similar to white sugar.

Selection, Storage and Preparation: Cane sugar can be substituted for white sugar in recipes in a 1:1 ratio. Be sure to purchase an organic brand to ensure that it is free of pesticide residues and potential animal by-products. Store cane sugar in an airtight container in a cool, dry place, away from odorous foods. Stored this way, it will keep for many months.

PURE MAPLE SYRUP

With its distinctive flavour and cherished place in North American cooking, maple syrup is one of the most popular natural sweeteners. Most of us have enjoyed the syrup, which is made from the sap of red, black or sugar maple trees, along with pancakes, waffles or oatmeal. But maple syrup is also tremendously versatile, and it works well as a sweetener for desserts and breakfast foods, as well as some savoury dishes.

Selection, Storage and Preparation: Maple syrup is usually sold in glass, tin or plastic containers. It will have the longest life in tin or glass, because plastic packaging 'breathes', and exposure to air can ultimately cause the syrup to spoil or allow mould to form. Maple syrup should be stored in the fridge after opening. Syrup from a tin or glass container will keep for 11 to 12 months, while syrup in plastic packaging will keep for 3 to 6 months.

You may see maple syrup labeled as 'grade A' or 'grade B'. This grading system is based on the color of the syrup (grade A is a lighter amber color, while grade B is darker). Grade A medium amber and dark amber as well as grade B are thought to have more characteristic 'maple' flavour.

Because I often use maple syrups in dessert recipes along with coconut oil, which can harden at cool temperatures, I tend to store my maple syrup at room temperature (and I tend to go through it quickly).

Salt

FINE SEA SALT

Sea salt is produced from evaporated seawater. It contains trace minerals in addition to sodium chloride, and it is a favourite ingredient among chefs, as the taste and texture is superior to that of table salt. Sea salt is sold in both coarse and fine form; coarse sea salt will absorb into food gradually, so it can be difficult to season accurately. For this reason, fine sea salt yields more predictable results in recipes.

Selection, Storage and Preparation: Sea salt should be stored in an airtight container in a cool, dry place. It is nonperishable.

FLAKED SEA SALT

Flaked sea salt is a coarser form of sea salt. It is ideal for sprinkling onto vegetables for a bit of crunch and texture in addition to seasoning. It's also heavenly sprinkled on top of desserts, such as The Ultimate Flourless Brownies (page 199).

Selection, Storage and Preparation: Flaked sea salt should be stored in an airtight container in a cool, dry place and will keep indefinitely.

HERBAMARE (HERBED SALT)

Herbamare is a wonderful herbed salt. It has been manufactured by the A. Vogel company for decades, and it is now popular and widely available. It features a blend of celery, leek, watercress, onions, chives, parsley, lovage, garlic, basil, marjoram, rosemary, thyme and kelp. It is especially good for spring recipes, and it works beautifully sprinkled on salads or in vinaigrettes.

Selection, Storage and Preparation: Herbamare should be stored in a sealed container in a cool, dry place and will keep indefinitely.

HIMALAYAN PINK SALT

Himalayan pink salt is mined from the Punjab region of Pakistan. It is minimally processed and contains trace minerals in addition to sodium chloride (pure sodium chloride is table salt). I always use Himalayan pink salt in my recipes, but you can substitute fine sea salt in similar proportions (you may need to taste to adjust seasoning as you go along).

Selection, Storage and Preparation: Pink salt can be found in health food stores and online. It should be stored in an airtight container in a cool, dry place and will keep indefinitely.

Herbs and Spices

I consider the use of fresh herbs and spices an essential component of healthful, creative cooking, and I use them generously in my recipes. Herbs and spices add variety and layers of flavour to food, and they reduce the need for excess fat and salt in cooking. They are also a vital component of a food culture, serving as a calling card for a particular cuisine. Who among us doesn't associate the pungent smell of curry with Indian food, the taste of Chinese 5-spice with Asian dishes, or the smell of fresh basil and oregano with Italian fare? No matter where you are in the world, there is a set of herbs and spices that embodies the character of local food.

I recommend using fresh herbs whenever possible, in accordance with the seasons. However, dried herbs are great in a pinch, adding quick flavour to even the most humble of pantry meals (such as my Fusilli Lentil-Mushroom Bolognese, page 161). It's normal for novice home cooks to feel shy with herbs and spices, but I encourage you to be bold and courageous with your spice rack, taking chances and determining which flavours and combinations suit your palate!

Fresh herbs can be divided roughly into two categories: soft herbs and hard herbs. Soft herbs have soft, pliable stems and include basil, parsley, coriander, and tarragon. They can be stored like flowers, by snipping off the base of their stems and placing the whole bunch in a Mason jar or tall glass filled halfway with water. They'll keep for at least half a week this way, and can be washed and dried prior to use. Hard herbs have thick, woody stems and include rosemary, oregano and thyme. They should be wrapped in a damp (not dripping-wet) paper towel, then wrapped loosely in plastic wrap prior to refrigeration. Keep them in a warm part of the fridge (like in the door).

It is often said that ground spices are only good for 6 months; after that, they lose potency as their essential oils are exposed to heat and air. That said, if you store your spices in a cool, dry place, they can probably stretch quite a bit further than 6 months (think a year or two). Many cooks keep the spice rack near a toaster, a coffee maker or an oven, which are all warm spots in a kitchen. It's best to keep them in a dry, cool pantry drawer, or in the fridge or freezer if your kitchen tends to be on the warm side. They

should be sealed tightly and protected from too much sun. Whether you store spices for 6 months or longer, it is important to remember that they will not retain their flavour indefinitely. Replace spices that you suspect are losing their lustre.

If you really want to optimize the strength of spices like star anise, mustard seeds or cardamom pods, buy them whole and grind them as you need them in a spice mill or coffee grinder (both of which are inexpensive purchases). You'll still need to keep the whole spices in an airtight container in a cool, dry spot.

BAY LEAVES

Bay leaves have a long history in Mediterranean cooking, dating back to Ancient Greece. They have bitter and sweet notes, which can highlight the taste of other spices, such as mint, oregano and coriander. They are often added to soups and stews, either dry or fresh, and also to pasta sauces or legume dishes. They don't have the same intensity as basil, mint or thyme, but they do complement and enhance the flavours of those herbs.

BLACK PEPPERCORNS

Black pepper adds warmth and aroma to food. It is nearly ubiquitous in recipes, but is essential for most vinaigrettes, many pasta dishes, and roasted vegetables. For optimal freshness, I recommend purchasing whole peppercorns and grinding them in a pepper mill when needed.

CAYENNE PEPPER

Cayenne pepper is bold and hot, adding a burst of spicy flavour to food. It is common in Mexican dishes and Cajun cuisine. If you are sensitive to spice, it's best to get to know this type of pepper slowly, adding it to food by the dash. A small amount of cayenne goes quite a long way.

CHILLI POWDER

Chilli powder is made from a mixture of ground, dried chilli peppers and other spices. Depending on the blend, it may contain allspice, cumin, coriander, cloves or cayenne. Because there are many types of chilli powder blends, it's wise to explore a few and see which level of spiciness and pungency suits your taste. Chilli powder is a natural complement to Mexican

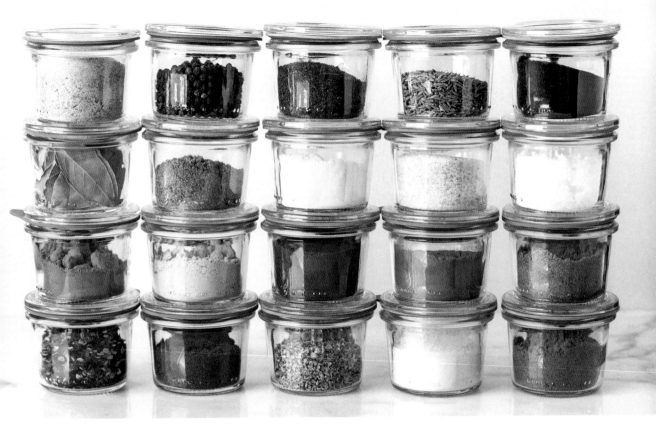

dishes, Cajun dishes, and some Indian and Middle Eastern dishes as well.

CINNAMON

Sweet, aromatic and slightly woody, cinnamon is an essential ingredient in baking. Its usefulness, however, is not limited to sweet dishes. Cinnamon plays a prominent role in Mexican, Indian and Middle Eastern dishes, from mole to tagines to chillis.

Most imported cinnamon is Indonesian cinnamon or Chinese cinnamon (cassia). Ceylon cinnamon, which is the cinnamon that I now use, is imported from Sri Lanka, and is sweeter and more refined. It is 'true cinnamon,' and it's well worth seeking it out for its superior flavour.

CORIANDER

Coriander has a bright, fragrant, and slightly sweet taste with hints of citrus. Both the fresh leaves and the seed pods are used in dishes, and one can detect the same astringent notes in both ingredients.

CUMIN AND CUMIN SEEDS

Cumin is the world's second most popular spice (behind black pepper). It plays a prominent role in North African, Indian, Mexican and Middle Eastern cuisines. Its earthy, nutty and smoky notes make it an appropriate addition to many recipes, including hummus, curry, chilli, salsa and baba ghanoush, to name only a few. Cumin has a strong flavour and can easily overpower other spices, so it's important to use it with some subtlety. Ground cumin makes for an easy addition to soups and stews, but for the boldest flavour, try toasting whole cumin seeds in a pan prior to adding them to your dish (such as in my Sweet Potato, Chickpea, and Spinach Coconut Curry, page 179).

CURRY POWDER

Curry powder is pungent and aromatic, and it can range from mild and sweet to quite hot, depending on the blend you select. Powdered curry blends may contain spices such as turmeric, cardamom or saffron. As with all other spice blends, it's wise to taste a few and develop a sense of what you like. I love Simply Organic brand.

Curry powder can be used in a wide variety of soups, stews and curries (though many curries are prepared with curry paste, which contains garlic, ginger and kaffir lime in addition to curry, and is quite distinct from the powder). It is fabulous in chickpea or tofu salads.

GARLIC POWDER

Fresh garlic adds bold, pungent flavor to food, but when you happen to run out of cloves (or if you're in a rush), garlic powder is a good substitute. I always purchase garlic powder, rather than granules. And be sure not to buy garlic salt, which could result in overly salty food!

GINGER

Sweet, pungent and warm, ginger is one of the oldest spices, and it plays a prominent role in cuisines and in medicinal applications around the world. It has a sweet, pungent and spicy flavour, and it is equally well suited to sweet and savoury dishes.

My preference is always to use fresh ginger for its unmistakable vibrancy of flavour. I keep ground ginger in my pantry at all times, however, so I can easily add it to baked goods, stews, soups, dressings and more.

ONION POWDER

The taste of sautéed onion is almost always preferable in cooking, but—as with garlic powder—it helps to have a shortcut at your fingertips if you happen to run out of onions or find yourself in a rush. You can find both onion powder and granulated onion for your spice rack.

OREGANO

Oregano, with its bitter, pungent, and spicy over-tones, is a cherished medicinal herb and a common ingredient in Mediterranean (especially Greek) cooking. It can be purchased fresh or dried, and it is a wonderful addition to pasta dishes and sauces. It is also used frequently in Mexican and Middle Eastern cooking.

RED PEPPER FLAKES

Red pepper flakes can quickly add heat and texture to a dish. They embolden chillis and soups and make a perfect topping for roasted vegetables or a humble plate of avocado toast. Like other peppers, they contain capsaicin, a compound that may help to fight pain and inflammation.

SMOKED PAPRIKA

Smoked paprika can be a superstar ingredient in plant-based cooking, thanks to its remarkable ability to create smoky flavour where ham or bacon might traditionally be used. It is one of many varieties of paprika, the national spice of Hungary and also a very significant spice in Spanish cuisine. (Spanish paprika, also called pimentón, is generally less intense than Hungarian paprika.) Paprika is made by grinding the pods of various kinds of peppers; smoked paprika is created by smoking pepper pods over wood fires, then grinding them. It is delicious and vibrant, and will quickly add smoky flavor to soups, stews, chillis, and grilling marinades.

SWEET PAPRIKA

Sweet paprika has a rich, earthy pepper flavour and hints of sweetness. It is excellent in pasta dishes and casseroles, and it pairs well with garlic, root vegetables, tomatoes and beans. I also love to sprinkle it over my Every Day Lemon-Garlic Hummus (page 91).

TURMERIC

Turmeric is a traditional ingredient in Middle Eastern, Indian and Southeast Asian cuisines. It has a bitter-sweet, peppery flavour and a brilliant orange colour. It is similar to ginger in that it is a root, which can be chopped or grated directly into food or purchased in dried, ground form. Turmeric adds a characteristic yellow colour to tofu scrambles and flavour to curries, soups and stews.

In recent years, more attention has been paid to turmeric's strong anti-inflammatory properties. Its orange pigment, curcumin, is a potent anti-inflammatory agent, which may help to provide relief from such conditions as inflammatory bowel disease and rheumatoid arthritis. Curcumin also has antioxidant activity that may help to fight chronic disease and perhaps even slow tumour growth. In addition, turmeric provides iron, potassium and vitamin B_6. Try it in my Golden French Lentil Stew (page 145) or my Miracle Healing Broth (page 151).

Soya Products

LOW-SODIUM TAMARI

Like soy sauce, tamari is a product of fermented soybeans, and it can add salty flavour to dishes, sauces and dressings. Whereas soy sauce is prepared with wheat, tamari is made with little or no wheat, and the certified gluten-free brands are suitable for those who follow gluten-free diets. For the purpose of this book, the tamari I use is always gluten-free (and thus, the recipe will be labelled as such unless it includes other ingredients containing gluten). I use San-J brand.

Selection, Storage and Preparation: As mentioned, if you do follow a gluten-free diet, it is crucial to read tamari labels, as not all brands are strictly wheat-free. I prefer low-sodium tamari to regular tamari, as it gives me more direct control of the seasoning in my recipe.

TOFU

Tofu, which originated in China some thousand years ago, is one of the most versatile protein sources for a plant-based diet. It can be blended, crumbled, cubed, shaped into cutlets, or cut into strips. You can turn tofu into vegan 'cheese', grill it as you would chicken or meat, marinate and bake it, crumble it into a delectable 'scramble', or blend it into smoothies. There's not much you can't do with tofu, and while you enjoy its many applications in recipes, you can also savour its myriad health benefits.

Selection, Storage and Preparation: There are two principal types of tofu in grocery stores: silken and firm. Silken tofu is great for blending into sauces or dressings or smoothies, but it won't hold its shape well for baking, sautéing, or grilling. Firm tofu, on the other hand, holds up well to all these preparation methods. I like to purchase extra-firm tofu and to press it overnight (or for an hour at a pinch) before preparing it in order to remove extra moisture. See how I press tofu on page 271. When purchasing tofu, it's best to shop organic. This won't be too much of a challenge, as most tofu on the market is organic already.

Chocolate

Rich, bitter, and slightly nutty, chocolate adds bold flavor and decadence to desserts of all kinds—not to mention snack foods, breakfasts, and even savoury dishes. Dark (non-dairy) has both a sophisticated taste and health benefits.

Cocoa, one of the main components of chocolate, is exceptionally high in antioxidants called flavonoids, which are associated with cardiovascular health and proper insulin management. The more bitter chocolate is—in other words, the higher the percentage of cocoa—the more antioxidant density it has. I tend to use 55 to 70% cocoa dark chocolate. As an added benefit, chocolate may help to control cortisol, a stress hormone that is associated with weight gain and inflammation.

NATURAL UNSWEETENED COCOA POWDER

I prefer to use natural, unsweetened cocoa powder in my recipes. It is labelled as 'natural' to distinguish it from Dutch process cocoa powder, which has been treated with a potassium solution to help neutralize some of the natural acidity in the chocolate. Natural cocoa powder consists simply of roasted and ground cocoa beans. It has a light colour and can sometimes have a bitter flavour. Adding a pinch of baking powder to recipes that call for a large amount of cocoa powder can help to neutralize its slightly acidic flavour.

Selection, Storage and Preparation: Try to seek out natural, unsweetened cocoa powder that is labelled as fairtrade and organic. Cocoa powder should be stored in an airtight container in a cool, dry place. Avoid refrigeration, as refrigerators are too humid and can promote spoilage of the powder. Stored properly, cocoa powder has a shelf life of up to 3 years.

NON-DAIRY CHOCOLATE CHIPS

Dark chocolate chips are perfect for cookies, brownies, snack bars and other treats. They melt quickly in a double boiler, which means that you can conveniently use them in pudding, cake and desserts that call for melted chocolate. Look for chocolate chips that are dairy-free; there's a good chance that dark chocolate marked as 70% cocoa or higher will be free of milk or milk powder, but it is wise to read labels.

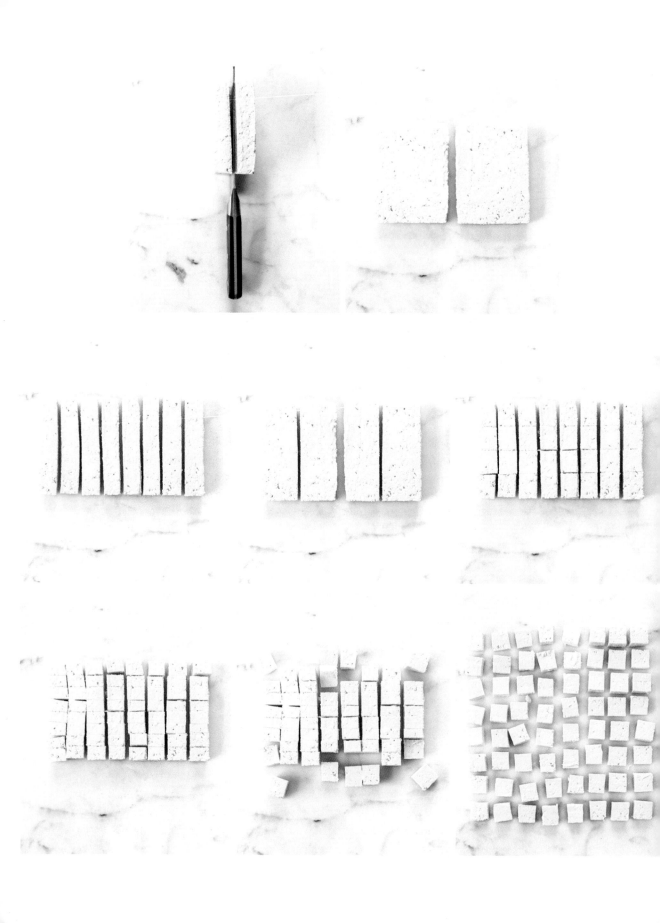

Selection, Storage and Preparation: When selecting dark chocolate, it is best to support bars that are labelled as fairtrade and organic; these labels suggest that the chocolate was harvested ethically. Dark chocolate should be stored in an airtight container in a cool, dry place (65 to 75°F/18 to 24°C is ideal). If your living space is significantly warmer, you can keep chocolate in an airtight container in the refrigerator instead. The shelf life of most dark chocolate is up to 2 years—but really, who has that kind of restraint?

Other

ALUMINIUM-FREE BAKING POWDER

Baking powder is usually a mixture of sodium bicarbonate and a weak acid. It is used to leaven baked goods, from muffins and quick breads to cookies and cakes. Unlike yeast, it requires no leavening time or kneading to take effect.

Selection, Storage and Preparation: Some brands of baking powder contain aluminium. It is an unnecessary additive that can create a slightly metallic flavour, so it is best to purchase aluminium-free baking powder. Baking powder should be kept in a very dry, cool place. It will lose effectiveness between 6 months and a year after opening, so do try to replace it regularly.

BAKING SODA

Baking soda, like baking powder, is used to leaven and lighten recipes. Unlike baking soda, it is pure sodium bicarbonate, so it is sometimes best to add a touch of acid to recipes in which it is included in order to neutralize its bitter flavour. It is especially useful in helping to make cookies 'spread' as they bake. Because it starts to work immediately, it is important to transfer dough or batter that contains baking soda to the oven as quickly as possible.

Selection, Storage and Preparation: Baking soda should be stored in an airtight container in a cool, dry place. It can lose its effectiveness over time, but there is a simple way to test it for activity if you're not sure whether it's still good: simply add a teaspoon of vinegar to a teaspoon of baking soda. If it bubbles immediately, then the baking soda is still active. You can also use the 'best by' date to gauge how much life is left in your baking soda.

In addition to its culinary uses, baking soda is a household superstar. It can be used for cleaning, for keeping the refrigerator smelling fresh, for homemade toothpaste or facial scrub, and more!

CAPERS

With their briny flavour and tart, salty qualities, capers make a flavourful addition to pastas, salads and more. They are perfectly suited to Mediterranean dishes, and they can also add character to dressings (such as my Crowd-Pleasing Caesar Salad, page 107) or marinades.

Selection, Storage and Preparation: Capers can be purchased pickled, in jars. They have a long shelf life (check the manufacturer's date) and should be stored in the refrigerator after opening.

DRIED KOMBU

Kombu is a type of seaweed that is typically sold in dried strips. It can be used to create umami-rich dashi (a traditional, mineral-rich broth in Japanese cooking), vegetable broth or soup. It is also useful in preparing beans from scratch, as the amino acids in kombu can help to neutralize the difficult-to-digest compounds in beans as they cook.

Selection, Storage and Preparation: Kombu can be purchased in dried strips. It has a long shelf life—up to several years—so long as it is stored in an airtight container in a cool, dry, and dark place. To use it in bean preparation, simply add a strip of kombu to a pot of simmering beans. When the beans are tender, use a slotted spoon to remove the kombu before draining them.

JARRED ROASTED RED PEPPER

Having a few jars of roasted red pepper in your pantry is a great way to add liveliness to sauces, dressings, pasta dishes and more at a moment's notice. Roasted red peppers add wonderful sweet-tart flavour to salads, grain dishes, soups and hummus. While it is undoubtedly rewarding to roast peppers in the oven or on the grill, especially in summer months, jarred peppers are a highly convenient and flavourful alternative, especially when peppers are out of season.

Selection, Storage and Preparation: Jarred red peppers can be purchased in various marinades (which may contain garlic, oil or herbs) or in a simple brine. I like to purchase simple, jarred peppers so I can create flavour according to my tastes. It is best to purchase organic jarred peppers when possible, as sweet peppers are on the Environmental Working Group's Dirty Dozen list. My go-to brand is Mediterranean Organic. After opening, jarred peppers should be sealed tightly and stored in the refrigerator. Prior to opening, they have a shelf life of many months; check the manufacturer's 'best by' date to ensure freshness.

LOW-SODIUM VEGETABLE BROTH OR LOW-SODIUM VEGETABLE BOUILLON POWDER

Having a few cartons of low-sodium vegetable broth or low-sodium bouillon cubes in one's pantry is a must if you plan to explore plant-based cooking. Vegetable broth will add flavour to soups, stews, grain dishes, chillis and countless other recipes. If you're new to whole-grain cooking, try simmering rice or quinoa in vegetable broth, rather than water; you will be pleasantly surprised at the flavour that a good broth adds to the grain! Vegetable bouillon cubes can be dissolved in water to make a quick, easy broth substitute, and they have the advantage of a long shelf life and light, compact packaging (which makes them much easier to carry home from a grocery store than several cartons of broth). If you'd like to make your own broth from scratch, you can find my recipe for homemade vegetable broth in *The Oh She Glows Cookbook* on page 299.

Selection, Storage and Preparation: Look out for a vegetable broth that is low-sodium and organic if possible. Broth can usually be stored in a cool, dry place for at least several months; check the 'best by' date on individual packages for storage directions.

MATCHA POWDER

Matcha is a fine powder made from green tea leaves. It can be added directly to hot water to create a particularly flavourful, potent cup of green tea. In addition to this traditional preparation, matcha powder can be added to non-dairy lattes, to smoothies (try my Green Matcha Mango Ginger Smoothie, page 17), or to baked goods and desserts.

Selection, Storage and Benefits: Matcha powder is potent, so it is best to add it to recipes in small quantities. A half teaspoon may be enough for tea or smoothies, though if you build up a taste for it, you may wish to add a little more than that. It can also be added to muffins or quick breads for a cool, bright green hue and a healthy infusion of antioxidants. Matcha is highly sensitive to light and heat, so it should be stored in an airtight container in a cool, dry place. The back of a dry, dark pantry is ideal. It will keep for 6 to 12 months.

NUTRITIONAL YEAST

The name certainly does it no favours, but nutritional yeast is a game-changing ingredient for vegan home cooks. A powder harvested from inactive yeast that has been grown on molasses, nutritional yeast is exceptionally nutrient-dense. It is sometimes described as nutty and frequently described as being 'cheesy'—which is why nutritional yeast is a staple in vegan cheese sauces (see my All-Purpose Cheese Sauce, page 251) and pasta dishes.

Selection, Storage and Preparation: Nutritional yeast can almost always be found in health food stores and natural groceries. It can also be ordered online, in bulk or in 450g bags. It can be stored in a cool, dry place for up to 1 year. In addition to its 'cheesy' flavour, you can use nutritional yeast to create umami flavour in savoury stews, sauces, and casseroles. You can also sprinkle it on whole grains, salads or soups for a quick and easy dose of protein and nutrition.

RED CURRY PASTE

I always have a couple of small jars of red curry paste on hand. It makes curry dishes come together in a snap! My go-to brand is Thai Kitchen, and it combines lemongrass, Thai ginger, and fresh red chilli along with other aromatic spices. Use it in stir-fries, soups and curries. Note that red curry paste, which is common in Thai dishes, imparts a very different flavour from curry powder, which is used more frequently in Indian cuisine. The two cannot be interchanged or substituted for each other.

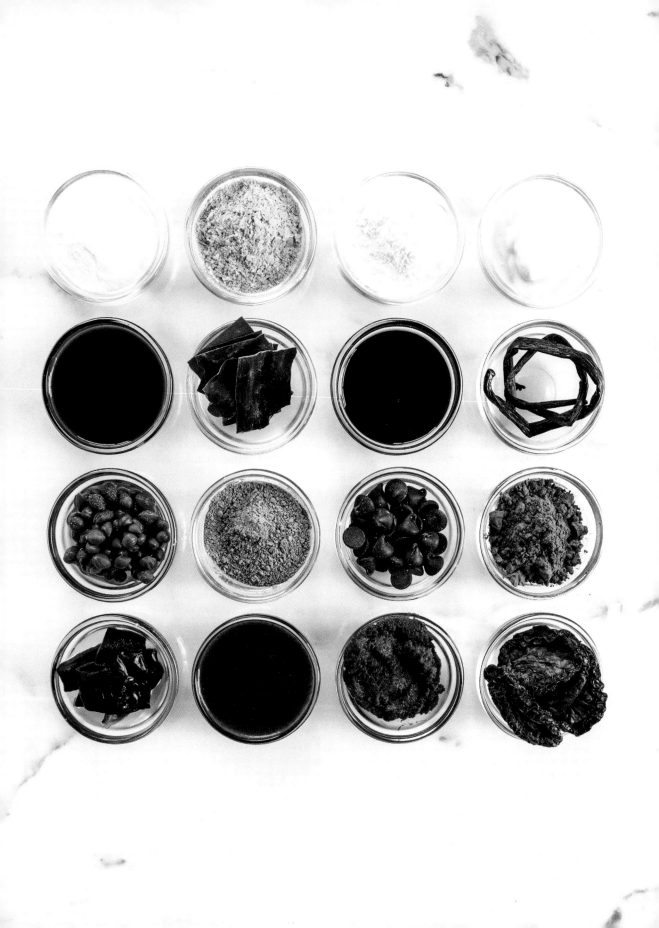

Selection, Storage and Preparation: Refrigerate after opening, and follow the manufacturer's instructions on shelf life.

SRIRACHA

Sriracha (pronounced 'see-rah-cha') is a type of hot sauce made with red chilli and garlic. It's a bit sweeter and less overwhelming than traditional hot sauces, and I use it liberally in my Mac and Peas (page 177) and Chilli Cheese Nachos (page 169), as well as a flavourful topping for steamed broccoli or roasted vegetables.

Selection, Storage and Preparation: Before purchasing Sriracha, check the label to be sure that it's vegan (some brands contain fish). Some are not gluten free, so if you avoid gluten, it's also worth checking your Sriracha brand for a certified gluten-free label. My favourite brand is Paleo Chef. Sriracha can be stored for short periods of time in a cool, dark pantry, but if you purchase a larger container and don't use it frequently, the safest bet is to store it in the fridge.

SUN-DRIED TOMATOES

Sun-dried tomatoes appear in many pasta recipes, tapenades, and Italian dishes, but I use them in salads, grain dishes and a wide variety of savoury meals as well. They add a hint of tartness and saltiness, as well as umami and texture.

Selection, Storage and Preparation: Sun-dried tomatoes can be bought either dry or oil-packed. The dry tomatoes can be tender when you buy them, but usually they are tough and you will need to rehydrate them before use. To rehydrate, simply pour hot or boiling water over the tomatoes and allow them to sit for 20 to 30 minutes before draining and using. Dry tomatoes can be stored in an airtight container in a cool, dry pantry for many months.

Oil-packed sun-dried tomatoes have a wonderful flavour and a tender texture, which means that they can be added directly to salads and pasta dishes. I usually default to using the oil-packed variety (except for in my Sun-Dried Tomato and Garlic Super-Seed Crackers, page 81) because I adore the herbed olive oil 'marinade' that engulfs them in flavor! They are also so quick and easy—no rehydrating necessary—which cuts down on prep time. Store them in the refrigerator after opening and use before the manufacturer's 'best by'

date. My preferred brand of oil-packed sun-dried tomatoes is Mediterranean Organic.

VANILLA PODS, PURE VANILLA EXTRACT, PURE VANILLA POWDER

Vanilla is an essential ingredient for baking and desserts, and I use it liberally. It has a complex flavour with sweet and floral notes. There are many ways to add vanilla to recipes; vanilla extract is the most common, but using fresh vanilla, straight from the pod, will add incomparable richness of flavour to your food. Pure vanilla powder, which is growing in popularity, is another flavourful alternative to vanilla extract, and it's often more cost effective than purchasing vanilla pods.

Selection, Storage and Preparation: Most vanilla is sourced from Madagascar, Tahiti or Mexico, though it is also grown in Bali, China, and Indonesia. It tends to be expensive, but it is worth purchasing a high-quality, pure vanilla extract. Be sure to check bottles for added sweeteners and to avoid 'vanilla flavour', which is very different from extract. You may also wish to seek out a vanilla extract that is fairtrade and organic in order to ensure it has ethical origins. Vanilla extract can be stored in a cool, dark place for up to 1 year.

You can also find whole, organic vanilla pods in most speciality grocers or health food stores. To use them, simply split the pod lengthwise down the centre and use a spoon to scrape out the tiny black seeds. The seeds of one vanilla pod can generally be substituted for ½ to 1 teaspoon high-quality vanilla extract. Vanilla powder is made from ground vanilla beans, and it can be added directly to baked goods, smoothies, ice creams, and other sweet treats. A half teaspoon vanilla powder can be substituted for 1 teaspoon vanilla extract. Vanilla powder can be stored in an airtight container in a cool, dry place for up to 1 year.

VEGAN MAYONNAISE

Vegan mayonnaise is one of a select group of store-bought products that I use to create authenticity in my cooking. It bears an uncanny resemblance to traditional mayonnaise and can be substituted in any recipe that calls for mayo, including dressings, pasta salad, or potato salad. Try it in my Curried Chickpea Salad (page 113).

Selection, Storage and Preparation: My go-to brand is Vegenaise, and there are several varieties of Vegenaise available. I like to purchase the soya-free version, but I also make a homemade soya-based version (page 269). Vegenaise should be stored in the refrigerator. Check the 'best by' date to be sure of its shelf life.

VEGAN WORCESTERSHIRE SAUCE

In spite of the fact that it is a traditional accompaniment to meat or to steak, Worcestershire sauce is also a wonderful addition to many vegan recipes, including barbecue sauces, vegan Caesar dressing, tempeh or tofu marinades, and more. A mixture of vinegar, molasses, salt, sugar, chilli, and sometimes tamarind, it has a rich, earthy, salty-sweet flavour.

Selection, Storage and Preparation: Vegan Worcestershire sauce can be found online or through health food stores. Some Worcestershire sauce that is not specifically labelled as vegan may actually have a vegan ingredient list, but it is important to read labels as many brands contain anchovy paste. Whole Foods 365 brand makes a vegan version. Worcestershire sauce can be stored in a tightly sealed bottle in a cool, dry place for up to 6 months.

Acids

CIDER VINEGAR

Cider vinegar is made from fermented apple cider or from apple must (crushed and aged apples). It is very tart, with a slight hint of sweetness from the apples, and it works well in any recipe or dressing that calls for wine vinegar.

Selection, Storage and Preparation: When you buy cider vinegar, it's best to choose an unpasteurized brand, so it has the healthy bacteria associated with the fermentation. Stored in a cool, dry place guarded from direct light, apple cider vinegar has a shelf life of 3 to 5 years.

BALSAMIC VINEGAR

Balsamic vinegar has a rich, complex flavour and a thicker, more viscous texture than other types of vinegar. Traditional balsamic vinegar is made from grape must or grapes that have been pressed along with their juice, skin and stems. The vinegar is aged in a process that is similar to the ageing of sherry or port. Really fine balsamic vinegar has a texture that is slightly syrupy, as well as a deep brown colour. In addition to being an excellent salad dressing, it also reduces beautifully when heated, creating a thick, sweet glaze, and it can work well as a marinade.

Selection, Storage and Preparation: While you don't need to purchase the finest balsamic vinegar, it is worth investing in a bottle that has been prepared traditionally. Look for bottles that are labeled 'Aceto Balsamico Tradizionale.' Bottles labeled as 'Balsamic Vinegar of Modena' are usually prepared with a base of wine vinegar rather than grapes. This keeps the cost of production low, but it does not give it the same flavor or mouthfeel as traditional balsamic vinegar. A good balsamic vinegar can be used over time in small doses; even a drizzle will transform fruit or salad. Be sure to try my Shake-and-Go Balsamic Vinaigrette (page 273).

Balsamic vinegar should be stored in a sealed container in a cool, dry, and dark place. It will keep indefinitely.

LEMON JUICE AND ZEST

Acid is essential for brightening and adding contrast to recipes, and the floral, bright tartness of lemon is one of the most universally appealing and versatile sources of acid. Lemon pairs beautifully with almost everything: soup, grains, salad, vegetables, dressings, marinades. It can even add subtle flavour and leavening to baked goods, as well as a hint of tartness to puddings and cheesecakes and other desserts. I love to use both lemon juice and lemon zest (which provides intense lemon flavour without sourness) in my cooking. One of my favourite ways to use lemon zest is in my Sun-Dried Tomato Pasta (page 185).

Selection, Storage and Preparation: Lemon juice should always be freshly squeezed. There is simply no substitute! Lemons should be stored in the refrigerator, where they will last for 2 to 3 weeks.

LIME JUICE AND ZEST

Lemons and limes both add tartness and acidity to recipes, and they both hail from the citrus family. It can be tempting, then, to wonder whether or not they are interchangeable. For the most part, the two fruits have distinctive tastes and characteristics. Limes are slightly more acidic and sour than lemons (which are thought to be slightly more bitter). Their sour taste makes them an ideal addition to guacamole, slaws, salsas and other Mexican fare, as well as to dressings and chilled soups.

Selection, Storage and Preparation: Limes should be stored in a tightly sealed bag or airtight container in the refrigerator for up to several weeks. Always use freshly squeezed lime juice and freshly grated zest in recipes.

RED OR WHITE WINE VINEGAR

Red and white wine vinegars tend to be more tart than either rice or balsamic vinegar. They work very well in vinaigrettes and other dressings, and they tend to pair nicely with Italian dishes and sauces (such as my All-Purpose Cheese Sauce, page 251).

Selection, Storage and Preparation: Like balsamic vinegar, wine vinegar can vary dramatically in price, though it is arguably less important to purchase a top-of-the-range brand. Wine vinegar will keep indefinitely if stored in an airtight container in a cool, dry, and dark place.

RICE VINEGAR

Rice vinegar, a staple in Asian cooking, is made from fermented rice or rice wine. It has a slightly sweet flavour, and it is generally less acidic than red or white wine vinegar. It is an excellent addition to stir-fries, slaws, sushi rice, dressings and dipping sauces.

Selection, Storage and Preparation: There are several types of rice vinegar, including white, brown, black and red. I like to use the white vinegar in my cooking, as it has the mildest flavour. You may also come across seasoned rice vinegar, which is sometimes used to prepare sushi rice. Seasoned rice vinegar can be quite flavourful, but it is seasoned with sometimes substantial amounts of salt and sugar. I prefer to buy plain rice vinegar and control the seasoning on my own.

ACKNOWLEDGEMENTS

I can't believe how many incredible people my blog and cookbooks have brought into my life since I started blogging in 2008. I'm so grateful to each and every one of you. Every time you make a recipe, tell others about my blog and cookbooks, leave a comment, or bump into me and say hello, it really makes my day. I wake up every morning feeling truly excited about the work I do, and I'm filled with gratitude for the wonderful people I've met along the way.

Eric, the love you give to our family and the people in your life is a beautiful thing. I don't think I've ever met someone who is so selfless, thoughtful and caring. You are the best father to Adriana, and the best spouse and business partner I could hope for. I couldn't have created this cookbook without your help. To my daughter, Adriana, thank you for making me a mother, and for showing me how to live in the moment. I'll never forget when we fed you your first food (puréed avocado) and the priceless (albeit horrified) reaction you had on your face. To my loving and supportive family and friends: I love you all so much!

I'm so thankful for my dedicated group of recipe testers. The amount of time, energy, and passion you poured into this cookbook simply blew me away, and I have no doubt that your feedback, tips and ideas improved it in countless ways. Tana Lise Gilberstad, you are a rock star. The fact that you tested 146 of my recipes (despite being incredibly busy) is just mind-boggling! Thank you for everything. Nicole White, thank you for sharing all of my recipes with your daycare children and parents, as well as your own family. The feedback you all provided has been absolutely invaluable to this cookbook, and allowed me to include oodles of kid-friendly tips, which will help so many families. My immense gratitude also goes out to Laura Beizer, Maren Williams, Nicolle Picou Thomas, Samantha Haas, Alison Scarlett, Carin Crook, Vanessa Gilic, Jane Airey, Anna Gunn, Camille Wright Hardy, Jessica Kennedy, Lisa Dickinson, Audrey Singaraju, Elaine Trautwein, Bridget Rosborough, Tammy Root, Katie Hay, Tracy Walter, Beth Erman, Kirsten Tomlin, Lisa Schiavi, Laura Houliaras, Andrea Bloomfield, Heather Bock, Stephanie Scilingo, Lori Stevens, Kristi Eskit, Magen Lorenzi, Heather Lutz, Lindsay Vyvey, Jillian Hylton-Smith, Dawn Vickers and Nikki Tews. I'm indebted to all of you for so selflessly giving your time and feedback over the past year.

To Lucia Watson, my editor at Avery, and Andrea Magyar, my editor at Penguin, thank you both for your passion and excitement for this second cookbook. Your enthusiasm and positivity kept me going on days when I didn't know if I could juggle everything, and I'm so proud that we've created such a stellar second cookbook. A huge thanks to the entire team at Avery and Penguin for all of your work on this cookbook.

To my friend and food photographer, Ashley McLaughlin, thank you for the countless hours you spent photographing the recipes in this book. I appreciated the fact that you were open to my ideas, feedback and suggestions during the entire process. Thanks for being so awesome.

To my friend and blogging colleague, Gena Hamshaw, thank you for lending your editorial and research talents to this book. I simply couldn't have done it without you!

Sandy Nicholson, thank you for coming into our house and photographing the candid lifestyle photos of our family. You and your team are so professional, down to earth, and just plain fun! I look forward to us working together again in the future.

SELECT BIBLIOGRAPHY

Berley, Peter, with Melissa Clark. *The Modern Vegetarian Kitchen*. New York: ReganBooks, HarperCollins, 2000.

Chaplin, Amy. *At Home in the Whole Foods Kitchen*. Boulder, CO: Roost Books, 2014.

Davis, Brenda, and Melina, Vesanto. *Becoming Vegan: The Complete Reference to Plant-Based Nutrition (Comprehensive Edition)*. Summertown, TN: The Book Publishing Company, 2014.

Haas, Elson, and Levin, Buck. *Staying Healthy with Nutrition: The Complete Guide to Diet & Nutritional Medicine*. Berkeley, CA: Celestial Arts, 2006.

Madison, Deborah. *Vegetable Literacy: Cooking and Gardening with Twelve Families from the Edible Plant Kingdom, with over 300 Deliciously Simple Recipes*. Berkeley, CA: Ten Speed Press, 2013.

Messina, Virginia, and Norris, Jack. *Vegan for Life: Everything You Need to Know to Be Healthy and Fit on a Plant-Based Diet*. Berkeley, CA: Da Capo Press, 2011.

Page, Karen. *The Vegetarian Flavor Bible: The Essential Guide to Culinary Creativity with Vegetables, Fruits, Grains, Legumes, Nuts, Seeds, and More, Based on the Wisdom of Leading American Chefs*. New York: Little, Brown and Co., 2014.

Palmer, Sharon. *The Plant-Powered Diet: The Lifelong Eating Plan for Achieving Optimal Health, Beginning Today*. New York: The Experiment, 2012.

Pitchford, Paul. *Healing with Whole Foods: Asian Traditions and Modern Nutrition*. Berkeley, CA: North Atlantic Books, 1993.

Whitney, Eleanor Noss, and Rolfes, Sharon Rady. *Understanding Nutrition, 14th Edition*. Independence, KY: Wadsworth Publishing, 2015.

INDEX

Mango-Coconut-Lime and Raspberry-Banana
    Sorbet, 243
mango(es)
    and apple chutney, 277
    Coconut Chia Seed Pudding, 67
    coconut lime and raspberry-banana sorbet, 243
    and green matcha ginger smoothie, 17
    Morning Detox Smoothie, 11
Maple Cinnamon Coconut Chips, 283
maple syrup, about, 308
Marinated Italian Tofu, 135
Marinated Portobello Mushroom Bowl, 187–88
matcha powder, about, 314
mayonnaise
    vegan, 269
    vegan, about, 316–17
Metabolism-Revving Spicy Cabbage Soup, 139
Compote, 233–34
Mile-High Black-and-White Freezer Fudge, 239–40
milk, hazelnut, 35
millet
    about, 290
    cooking, 287
mint
    Hemp Heart and Sorghum Tabbouleh, 105
    pear vanilla smoothie, 21
    Reset Button Green Smoothie, 25, 27
Miracle Healing Broth, 151
Mocha Empower Glo Bars, 69–70
molasses
    about, 305
    and spelt cookies, 219
Morning Detox Smoothie, 11
mushroom
    and fusilli lentil bolognese, 161–62
    marinated portobello bowl, 187–88
    Shepherd's Pie, 167–68

N
nachos, 169–70
9-Spice Avocado Hummus Toast, 39
9-Spice Mix, 258
noodles, soba salad, 183
nut butters, about, 298–99
nut milk bags, xvi
Nut-Free Dream Bars, 211–12

nutrional information, about, xiii
nutritional yeast, about, 314
nuts and seeds, about, 296–300

O
oat flour, about, 291–93
oatmeal. See also rolled oats
    apple pie overnight, 55
    homemade flour, 285
    overnight power bowl, 49
    sprouted, 37
    Tropical Overnight Oats, 57
oats, about, 293
Oh Em Gee Veggie Burgers, 159–60
oils
    avocado, 304
    coconut, 302
    olive, 304
    sesame, 304
ovens, xiii
Overnight Hot Oatmeal Power Bowl, 49

P
parsley
    crispy smashed potatoes, 123–24
    Hemp Heart and Sorghum Tabbouleh, 105
    Protein Power Rainbow Quinoa Salad, 99
pasta
    Fusilli Lentil-Mushroom Bolognese, 161–62
    Mac and Peas, 177
    sun-dried tomato, 185–86
pastry rollers, xvi
Peanut Better Balls, 231–32
peanut butter
    balls, 231–32
    and chocolate tart, 237–38
    cookies, flourless, 213–14
    and jam breakfast cookies, 41
Peanut Butter Lover's Chocolate Tart, 237–38
peanuts, about, 299
pear
    Reset Button Green Smoothie, 25, 27
    vanilla mint smoothie, 21
Pear Vanilla Mint Green Smoothie, 21
peas and macaroni, 177

sour cream, cashew, 261
soy milk: vegan mayonnaise, 269
soy products, about, 311
spelt
  flour, about, 293
  and molasses cookies, 219
  pumpkin cupcakes, 224–25
spelt berries
  cooking, 287
  Stuffed Avocado Salad, 109–10
spice mixes, 258
Spiced Buttercream Frosting, 227
spices and herbs, about, 308–20
spinach
  Green Tea Lime Pie Smoothie Bowl, 9
  Green-Orange Smoothie, 13
  Reset Button Green Smoothie, 25, 27
  Sun-Dried Tomato Pasta, 185–86
  sweet potato and chickpea coconut curry,
    179
Spiralized Courgette Summer Salad, 103
spring onions
  and marinated lentils, 129
  Protein Power Rainbow Quinoa Salad, 99
Sriracha, about, 316
strawberries
  Coconut Chia Seed Pudding, 67
  Glowing Rainbow Smoothie Bowl, 15
  oat crumble bars, 45–46
  and vanilla compote, 233–34
Strawberry Oat Crumble Bars, 45–46
Stuffed Avocado Salad, 109–10
sugar, about, 305–8
Sun-Dried Tomato and Garlic Super-Seed
    Crackers, 81–82
Sun-Dried Tomato Pasta, 185–86
sun-dried tomato(es)
  about, 316
  and garlic hummus, 85
  and garlic seed crackers, 81–82
  and marinated lentils, 129
  pasta, 185–86
  in quinoa salad, 99
  spiralized courgette salad, 103
sunflower seeds
  about, 299–300
  butter, 79–80

Endurance Crackers, 89
Strawberry Oat Crumble Bars, 45–46
Sun-Dried Tomato and Garlic Super-Seed
    Crackers, 81–82
Vanilla Super-Seed Granola with Coconut Chips, 33
Sweet Potato, Chickpea and Spinach Coconut
    Curry, 179
Sweet Potato Casserole, 133
sweet potatoes
  and carrot soup, 141
  casserole, 133
  chickpea and spinach coconut curry, 179
  loaded, 165
  Roasted Breakfast Hash, 53
  Secret Ingredient Chocolate Pudding, 229
  vegetable and 'cheese soup', 143
  veggie burger, 159–60
sweeteners, 305–7
Swiss chard: lentil stew, 145–46

T

tabbouleh
  bowl, 157
  hemp heart and sorghum, 105
tacos: green wraps, 191–92
tahini
  about, 299
  and lemon dressing, 265
tamari, about, 311
tart, peanut butter chocolate, 237–38
Thai Almond Butter Sauce, 249
Thai Crunch Salad, 101
toast, avocado hummus, 39
tofu
  about, 311
  cast-iron, 137
  marinated Italian, 135
  pressing, 271
tomato(es). *See also* cherry tomatoes; sun-dried
    tomatoes
  barbecue sauce, 255
  cabbage soup, spicy, 139
  Chilli Cheese Nachos, 169–70
  gazpacho, 147–48
  lentil stew, 145–46
  tomato sauce, 175

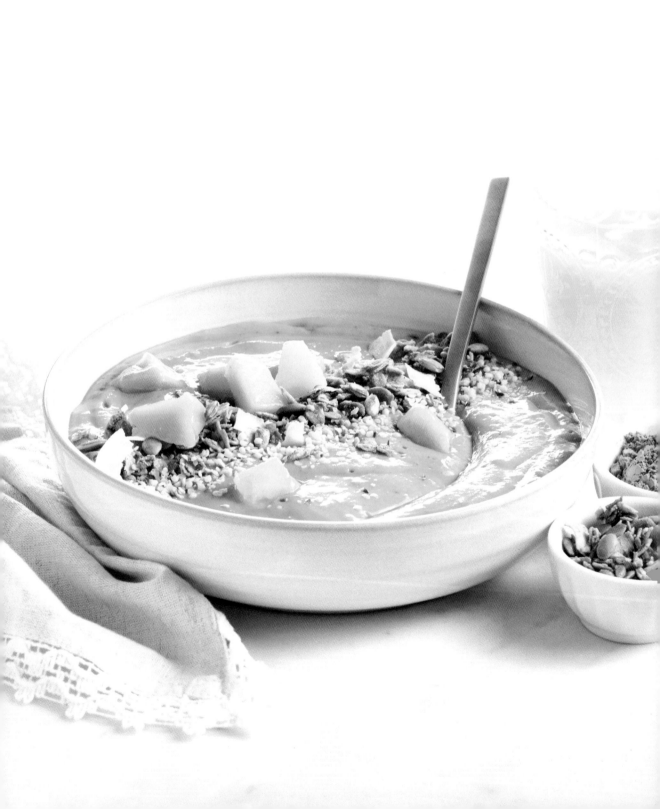

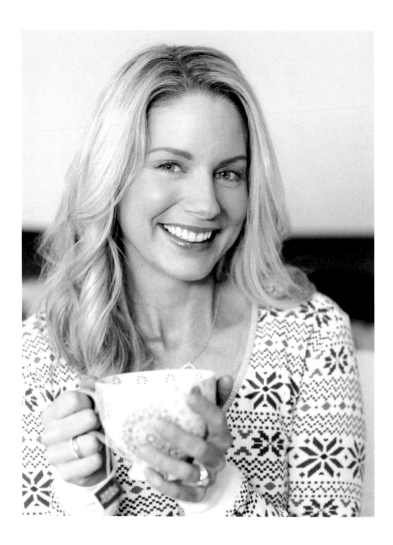

ABOUT THE AUTHOR

ANGELA LIDDON is the founder, recipe developer, photographer, and writer behind OhSheGlows.com—an award-winning destination for energizing, plant-based recipes, with millions of visitors each month. Her work has been featured in local and international publications such as *VegNews, O Magazine, Fitness, The Kitchn, Self, Shape, National Post, the Guardian, Glamour, the Telegraph, Barre3, T.O.F.U.,* and *Best Health*. She has also won several awards, including *VegNews*'s Best Vegan Blog 2012, 2014, and 2015, *Chatelaine*'s Hot 20 under-30 award, and Foodbuzz's Best Veg Blog and Best Overall Blog. Her first cookbook, *The Oh She Glows Cookbook*, is an international bestseller. It was selected as Indigo's Book of the Year for 2014, *VegNews*'s Favorite Cookbook of 2014, and appeared on the *New York Times* Best Seller list. Angela and her family live in Oakville, Ontario, Canada, and her blog can be found online at OhSheGlows.com.